Contents

List of Contributors

Jozé Braspenning PhD
Senior Researcher, Centre for Quality of Care Research (WOK), Radboud University Nijmegen Medical Centre, Nijmegen, The Netherlands

Jako Burgers PhD
Senior Researcher, CBO, Utrecht; Centre for Quality of Care Research (WOK), Radboud University Nijmegen Medical Centre, Nijmegen, The Netherlands

Marion Campbell BSc MSc PhD CStat FRSS
Professor, Deputy Director Health Care Research Unit and Director Health Care Assessment Programme, Health Services Research Unit, University of Aberdeen, Aberdeen, UK

Stephen Campbell BA MA PhD
Research Fellow, National Primary Care Research and Development Centre, University of Manchester, Manchester, UK

Martin Eccles MD FMedSci FRCP FRCGP
Professor, Centre for Health Services Research, School of Population and Health Sciences, University of Newcastle upon Tyne, Newcastle upon Tyne, UK

Glyn Elwyn BA MB BCh MSc FRCGP PhD
Professor, Department of Primary Care, Swansea Clinical School, Swansea, UK

Jeremy Grimshaw MBChB PhD FRCGP
Professor, Director Clinical Epidemiology Programme, Ottawa Health Research Institute, Ottawa, Canada

Richard Grol PhD
Professor, Director Centre for Quality of Care Research (WOK), Radboud University Nijmegen Medical Centre, Nijmegen, The Netherlands

Marlies Hulscher PhD
Senior Researcher, Centre for Quality of Care Research (WOK), Radboud University Nijmegen Medical Centre, Nijmegen, The Netherlands

Niek Klazinga PhD
Professor, Department of Social Medicine, Academic Medical Centre/University of Amsterdam, Amsterdam, The Netherlands

Miranda Laurant MSc
Senior Researcher, Centre for Quality of Care Research (WOK), Radboud University Nijmegen Medical Centre, Nijmegen, The Netherlands

Jody D Martens MSc
Research Worker, Integrated Care Unit, University Hospital Maastricht, Maastricht, The Netherlands

Craig Ramsay BSc PhD
Senior Statistician, Health Services Research Unit, University of Aberdeen, Aberdeen, UK

Johan L Severens PhD
Professor, Department of Health Organisation, Policy and Economics, and Department of Clinical Epidemiology and MTA, University Hospital Maastricht, Maastricht, The Netherlands

Trudy van der Weijden PhD
Senior Researcher, Centre for Quality of Care Research (WOK)/Department of General Practice, Maastricht University, the Netherlands

Michel Wensing PhD
Senior Lecturer, Centre for Quality of Care Research (WOK), Radboud University Nijmegen Medical Centre, Nijmegen, the Netherlands

Hub Wollersheim PhD MD
Senior Lecturer, Centre for Quality of Care Research (WOK), Radboud University Nijmegen Medical Centre, Nijmegen, the Netherlands

Improving Patient Care

The implementation of change in clinical practice

Richard Grol PhD

Professor and Director, Centre for Quality of Care Research (WOK),
Radboud University Nijmegen Medical Centre, Nijmegen, The Netherlands

Michel Wensing PhD

Senior Lecturer, Centre for Quality of Care Research (WOK),
Radboud University Nijmegen Medical Centre, Nijmegen, The Netherlands

Martin Eccles MD, FMedSci, FRCP, FRCGP

Professor, Centre for Health Services Research, School of Population and
Health Sciences, University of Newcastle upon Tyne,
Newcastle upon Tyne, UK

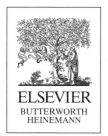

ELSEVIER
BUTTERWORTH
HEINEMANN

Edinburgh London New York Oxford Philadelphia St Louis Sydney Toronto 2005

ELSEVIER
BUTTERWORTH
HEINEMANN

An imprint of Elsevier Limited
© 2005, Elsevier Limited. All rights reserved.

ISBN 0 7506 8819 X
British Library Cataloguing in Publication Data
A catalogue record for this book is available from the British Library
Library of Congress Cataloging in Publication Data
A catalog record for this book is available from the Library of Congress

Note
Medical knowledge is constantly changing. Standard safety precautions must be followed, but as new research and clinical experience broaden our knowledge, changes in treatment and drug therapy may become necessary or appropriate. Readers are advised to check the most current product information provided by the manufacturer of each drug to be administered to verify the recommended dose, the method and duration of administration, and contraindications. It is the responsibility of the practitioner, relying on experience and knowledge of the patient, to determine dosages and the best treatment for each individual patient. Neither the Publisher nor the author assumes any liability for any injury and/or damage to persons or property arising from this publication.

For Butterworth Heinemann:
Commissioning Editor: Heidi Harrison
Development Editor: Catherine Jackson
Production Manager: Yolanta Motylinska
Project Manager: John Ormiston
Designer: Judith Campbell

The
Publisher's
policy is to use
**paper manufactured
from sustainable forests**

Printed in Spain by GraphyCems

Introduction

Richard Grol

Friesland is the homeland of the famous black-and-white Friesian cows, and the land of milk and cheese. For centuries these cows were milked by hand, which meant the farmer and his family awoke at 4 or 5 o'clock in the morning. Around 1890 reports of successful experiments with a milking machine appeared in the regional newspapers; according to the experts this machine had been shown to be both efficient and cost-effective. It milked cows with udders of different sorts very well. How quickly would this new technique spread among Friesian farmers?

The first machines were introduced in 1910, but it was not until the 1950s that they were adopted widely (Mak 1996). Why did farmers prefer to rise at the crack of dawn, even though everyone knew about the new machine? That it was the personal relationship they maintained with their cows is probably too romantic. The way to understand the causes of this, and what a successful implementation programme should have been directed towards, is to examine the farmers' motives and their living and working conditions at that time. One of the main reasons for non-adoption was that the milking machine cost money, whereas manpower provided by the family was free. At that time farmers were, for the most part, self-sufficient and their work involved little exchange of money. Perhaps more important was their system of standards and values: the most important aim of a farming enterprise was to guarantee the continuity of the family business, not to make a profit. Taking risks was therefore at odds with their mission; following a set routine developed by their forefathers was seen as a guarantee of success. According to Mak (1996), it was not until World War II, when these standards were subjected to enormous modification, that farming practices in Friesland changed. An earlier effective introduction of milking machines would have required changes at different levels: changes in standards and values, greater skill in dealing with money, increase in farm size and changes in milk and cheese production in the factories. In short, changes in the entire process from cow to consumer, a complete change in culture at all levels.

This example demonstrates, if one wants to introduce an innovation successfully, how crucial it is to have a clear understanding of, and insight into, the target group's living and working conditions and standards and values, as well as of the issues involved in the implementation of an innovation itself. Simply publishing (or otherwise distributing information on the innovation's usefulness) the effects or efficiency is usually not enough to guarantee a successful adoption. The real obstacles must be sought and tackled in a systematic way with a variety of appropriate methods and measures that have proved to be effective in practice. This is the message being delivered in this book.

In the field of healthcare an enormous number of valuable insights, procedures and technologies become available each year. They derive from well-planned scientific research or from careful experiments and evaluation in everyday practice. Only a (small) proportion of these methods and technologies are, in the short term, adopted into the daily practice of patient care. Thus patients, clients and care users are needlessly deprived of effective care or they receive unnecessary, outdated or, even worse, harmful care. Of course, not all innovations are improvements, but it is a general observation that in healthcare the situation is often one of 'underuse, overuse and misuse of care' (Bodenheimer 1999). Therefore, it is important that great care be taken when adopting valuable insights and procedures into daily practice; in so doing an important contribution can be made to the improvement of the quality of patient care.

Adopting valuable insights and procedures does not usually take place easily or completely. Implementation may be only partially successful and at times completely unsuccessful. There are many possible reasons for this, such as the nature of the proposed method of working or that it is new, or the target group or setting in which the intended change is to take place. However, there may also be structural, financial or organisational obstacles; equally, the way in which the change is implemented may be ineffective. Given that knowledge about effective implementation is growing, it is important to bring together this knowledge and to distil recommendations from it to aid implementation in routine patient care. This is the purpose of this book:

> This book is meant for care providers, staff involved in quality assessment, healthcare managers, policy makers and researchers who are concerned with the question of how to best design the implementation of valuable new and existing insights and procedures so that they contribute to optimal patient care.

WHICH CHANGES?

The book is directed at the implementation of various changes and improvements in patient care practices, including:

- Adoption of well-developed guidelines for use in practice, both those developed centrally and those developed within a local area or institution;
- Adoption of new, well-researched or tested procedures, technologies, care programmes and preventative programmes;
- Adoption of care protocols, care pathways or care processes that may lead to an improvement in patient care and that have been shown to work well ('best practices');
- Removal of undesirable (i.e. unnecessary, harmful or inefficient) routines and variations in the care provided.

In this book, the discussion moves between innovations, guidelines, new procedures and changes in care provision.

It is certainly not true to say that all new technologies, procedures, guidelines or recommendations from scientific research signify real improvements in patient care. Nor is it the case that the improvement of care provision can arise only from scientific information being made available.

In this book we concentrate on guidelines, insights and procedures based on scientific evidence, on careful evaluation or on good experience in practice – thus, on innovations that are firmly established as being able to contribute to better care for patients.

This does not mean that these innovations would be able to find their way into practice as they stand,

without further adaptation. In many cases active contributions from the target groups are necessary to adapt an innovation to their own setting and experiences. The importance of such 'two-way traffic between practice and science' is also discussed in this book.

GUIDELINES

As guidelines for practice are, currently, seen as one of the most important aids to introducing new insights into care and to achieving an optimal level of care for patients, they are considered separately in more depth. Guidelines are a way to translate research results and clinical experiences in practice into recommendations about care procedures. They work as an intermediary in the implementation process. They can be helpful to patients and care providers if they are of a high quality and are actually used in care practice. Guidelines do not have to apply only to new scientific insights; they can also focus on establishing good practice routines or on the improvement of existing practice methods.

THE BOOK'S MESSAGE

The messages delivered in this book can be summarised as:

- When formulating guidelines or developing a new working method, care protocol or programme to improve care provision, it is important, from the outset, to take into account how they are to be implemented.
- Know and understand as well as possible the target group and the setting in which implementation is to take place. Try to see the target group's perspective and involve them in both the development and implementation of the innovation.
- Usually many helpful and unhelpful factors play a role and determine whether an implementation is a success. Addressing these requires a well-planned intervention with a diversity of cost-effective strategies and measures.
- Thorough organisation of the implementation process and careful evaluation of the ensuing results are crucial to success.

THE BOOK'S BASIC PRINCIPLES

It is important for readers to keep in mind a number of principles that underpin this book.

- The book is about *optimising patient care*; thus, it is about the quality of care and quality improvement.

However, it is not a 'manual for quality improvement'. It concentrates on the implementation of insights and procedures with a 'proven' value.

■ The emphasis lies on the improvement of the *primary processes in care provision* by doctors, nurses and paramedics and the teams they work in. The patient is centre stage. Changes in the organisation of institutions or practices can be very important, but are discussed here predominantly in terms of whether they contribute to the improvement of direct patient care.

■ The immediate reasons for implementation may be the availability of new scientific insights and/or the availability of valuable procedures and experiences from daily practice. Changes may be initiated and realised both *top-down* and *bottom-up*.

■ The book takes the *perspective* of the *implementer* – the person who is, or who feels, responsible for the implementation of improvement in care provision. Through the book, however, processes and implementation are often also looked at through the eyes of the target group.

THE BOOK'S ORGANISATION

The book is organised into a number of parts, each of which contain several chapters:

■ Part I provides a general introduction, presents a series of theories on implementation and change in healthcare and finishes with a model for implementation that is used throughout the rest of the book.

■ Part II discusses the characteristics of new insights, guidelines and procedures that can contribute to their ultimate implementation. The characteristics and development of effective guidelines are examined in some detail and existing guideline programmes are compared.

■ Part III deals with the analysis of the target group and the setting, and discusses the range of factors that may play a role in implementation. Methods to carry out a 'diagnostic analysis' are also presented.

■ Part IV describes existing dissemination and implementation strategies and current scientific knowledge of their effectiveness.

■ Part V is about designing an effective implementation plan and organising its implementation in daily practice.

■ Part VI discusses how the implementations carried out and their effects could be evaluated, and makes a distinction between small-scale improvement projects, implementation studies and the evaluation of large-scale implementation programmes.

References

Bodenheimer T (1999). The American health care system. The movement for improved quality in health care. *N Engl J Med*. **340**:488–492.

Mak G (1996). *Toen God Verdween uit Jorwerd [When God Disappeared from Jorwerd]*. Amsterdam: Atlas.

Part I

Principles of implementation of change

Chapter 1

Implementation of changes in practice

Richard Grol

KEY MESSAGES

- Many patients do not receive optimal care – well-planned programmes are required to implement new or valuable scientific findings, guidelines, protocols, care processes or best practices.
- Different approaches to the implementation of change in patient care can be observed, each based on different assumptions and theories of human and organisational behaviour.
- A combination of rational, top-down and participative, bottom-up approaches is needed to improve practice successfully.

Box 1.1 AMC Guideline development

For years the Academic Medical Centre (AMC) in Amsterdam has been working on the systematic formulation and implementation of (evidence-based) guidelines and protocols for clinical practice. In keeping with this policy, the surgical department attempted to introduce guidelines on the use of antibiotics and thrombosis prevention and on the use of catheters and wound drains (Koelemay *et al.* 1996). Adherence to the guidelines was measured both before and after the period of adoption on the basis of a number of specific indicators. Before implementation, the adherence to the guidelines ranged from 49 to 94%. After drawing up guidelines within teams and receiving feedback on performance from the department, the only improvement was in the correct use of bladder catheters (from 49 to 74%). So, for departments to draw up guidelines and provide feedback to all members of staff does not appear to be sufficient to bring about change. The researchers gave different explanations according to the guideline involved:

- The guideline for thrombosis prevention was already well implemented and probably all that happened was that the standard working practice already in existence became formalised;
- The benefit of wound drains is unclear as evidence for promoting their use is not convincing, so this guideline should be discussed critically once again;
- Failing to adhere to the guideline for catheter use turned out to be based mainly on patients' wishes, as the catheter was left in place for too long.

This project clearly illustrates the complexity involved in the implementation of guidelines. Non-adoption may result from any or all of the quality of the guideline itself, the extent to which it fits in with existing care practice, the opinions of professionals and the wishes of patients, and the way in which the guideline is implemented and the conditions under which it is introduced.

INTRODUCTION

The number of new insights, procedures, programmes and techniques that have become available as a result of careful development and / or scientific research is enormous. It is estimated that around 2 million articles a year are published in medical journals (Mulrow 1994). The number of well-organised trials added to Medline, a large database of journals in the field of medicine, was 500 each year from 1975 to 1980, a figure that

reached almost 10,000 a year recently (Chassin 1998). In the same period the number of systematic literature analyses (meta-analyses) and the number of clinical guidelines also increased enormously (*Table 1.1*).

Knowledge about optimal patient care changes over time, influenced by both scientific developments and by social developments (*Box 1.2*). A great deal of knowledge that one absorbs over 5 years of training to be a doctor is obsolete by the time the course has been completed.

Table 1.1 Articles included in Medline between 1975 and 1997[a]

Article type	1975–1980	1993–1997
Randomised studies	500	8500
Meta-analyses	1	416
Clinical guidelines	1	454

[a]Average number of new articles a year (Chassin 1998; President's Advisory Commission 1998).

Box 1.2 Changing scientific arguments

In 1348, King Philip VI of France asked the medical faculty of the University of Paris for a scientific explanation of the plague epidemic, known as the Black Death, which killed about a third of the population of Europe. After extensive research, the Sorbonne came up with the cause – a threefold conjunction of Saturn, Jupiter and Mars in the fortieth grade of Aquarius. For a long time this was generally accepted as being the definitive explanation in both Europe and the Arab world.

What will we make of our explanations of the most important diseases of our time 100 years from now?

The production of new knowledge about patient care is progressing at an ever-increasing pace, but the percentage of valuable new insights subsequently introduced into routine patient care in the short term is considerably lower. In this respect healthcare does not differ from other areas of society. This was the case in the past and is still so today. 300 years ago a British naval captain called Lancaster, having carried out an experiment with four sheep, discovered that scurvy on long sea journeys could be prevented by drinking one teaspoon of lemon juice a day (Rogers 1983). Despite his discovery, it took another 200 years before his remedy became standard practice for the British Navy. Another example is that, even though Semmelweis had long before demonstrated the importance of antiseptics, many surgeons operating around 1900 still used their bare hands, with adverse consequences. Even today many institutions pay too little attention to washing and disinfecting hands before and after medical or nursing interventions (Teare et al. 2001).

The adoption of new ideas in this information age is probably taking place faster than it did in the past. Nevertheless, researchers and policy makers have noticed that it takes a variable and unpredictable amount of time before research results or insights related to effective and efficient care find their way to doctors, nurses and other care workers. In many cases healthcare professionals only find out gradually, which is understandable considering the overdose of information to which they are constantly exposed. The aver-

age doctor would have to read about 19 articles a day to keep pace with the literature. However, even enthusiastic academics spend only 2 hours per week, at the most, going through recent articles (Haines 1996). Even if one is informed about new insights on optimal patient care, no changes necessarily take place within daily routines. The scientific literature is full of examples from which it would appear that patients are not given the care that, according to recent scientific or professional insights, is desirable. Giving up smoking, taking aspirin and beta-blockers, receiving treatment for hypertension, lowering serum cholesterol and administering anti-coagulation drugs have all been proved valuable with specific (high-risk) groups of patients. Despite their proved effectiveness they are often not utilised adequately (Stalenhoef 1998). A European study of 4000 patients in 11 countries showed that, on average, only 46% of all patients were given the recommended beta-blockers after a heart attack (Woods et al. 1998), and women and older people were prescribed these medicines significantly less often. In primary care there are now reliable data on the implementation of guidelines, developed by the Dutch College of General Practitioners (NHG). On average, the guidelines were followed in 67% of the decisions made in practice (Spies and Mokkink 1999).

A literature review of 48 Medline articles on the quality of care provision in the USA showed that 50–70% of the patients in the USA were found to receive the recommended care, while 20–30% received unnecessary care (Schuster et al. 1998). Appropriate care is sometimes

Table 1.2 Action taken by urologists when presented with prostate complaints[a]

	Percentage of patients receiving treatment	
	Partnership with the highest percentage	Partnership with the lowest percentage
Ultrasound scan kidney	80	8
Ultrasound scan prostate	90	17
Surgery	48	20
Medication	36	0

[a]Differences between 12 partnerships (Casparie 1996).

not offered, but in many cases, contrary to recent insights, unnecessary care is. The consequences in terms of the personal and community costs of such inefficient practice are considerable. Studies sometimes show a large variation in practice – in some regions or hospitals the likelihood that one will be operated on for back problems, or that a hysterectomy or a trans-urethral resection of the prostrate will be carried out, are far greater than in others (*Table 1.2*). Baxter *et al.* (1998) found, in a comparison of 500 English general practitioners (GPs), that some GPs prescribed more than 50 times as much cholesterol-reducing medicines as others. Many clinical actions are, of course, in accordance with current thinking, but a substantial minority of patients do not receive the appropriate care, or receive unnecessary or (even worse) harmful care. Bodenheimer (1999) estimated that in the USA between 8 and 86% of operations are unnecessary. It has emerged that in about 20–30% of their decisions GPs in the Netherlands took unnecessary actions (Spies and Mokkink 1999). The types of action concerned were:

▪ Inappropriately prescribing antibiotics for acute ear infections (30%);

▪ Referral to a physiotherapist for acute back pain (20%);

▪ Not prescribing the first-choice medicine for stomach complaints (25%);

▪ Unnecessary prostate-specific antigen (PSA) testing for men suffering from micturition problems (71%).

Finally, patients may be unnecessarily harmed by poor practice and inefficient care processes, not to mention the frustrations or costs that are incurred. Figures from the USA reveal a high number of deaths as a result of poor practice. A US government report indicates about 44,000–95,000 deaths per year caused by medical (mis)management, of which about half are said to be preventable. Observations carried out on three wards of a top hospital in the USA showed that 480 of the 1047

patients observed had, more than once, been the victim of a complication as a result of inappropriate or wrong procedures. In 18% of cases there was, on at least one occasion, a serious failure in procedures with serious consequences (Andrews *et al.* 1997). Malpractice and inefficient working methods regularly led to complaints or disciplinary council hearings, particularly if they occurred in combination with poor communication and being impolite to the patient.

IMPLEMENTATION OF IMPROVEMENTS IN PATIENT CARE: VARIOUS APPROACHES

There is a high level of agreement between all parties involved in healthcare that the care given could be better (i.e. more effective, more efficient, safer and more patient-centred). However, when it comes to how this can be achieved, opinions differ. Various parties and disciplines propose a diversity of approaches (Grol 1997, 2001). Professionals are inclined to take improvements into their own hands and to promote good training and agreements among themselves. Epidemiologists believe more in cataloguing the scientific developments within a field and making this information available to professionals. Healthcare researchers, working on behalf of the government or formulating policy, usually feel the need to map out existing care and point out the variations between care providers, institutions and regions. Data corrected to accommodate population differences is then channelled back to care providers as feedback or 'mirrored information'. Experts from the management world focus less on the individual professional; instead, they look into how care processes can be optimised and how organisational conditions for optimal care can be created. Ethicists and lawyers place the patients centre stage and argue for more autonomy, better information provision and a more influential role for patients in decisions about their illnesses. Insurers and the government are responsible for controlling the cost of care and regularly apply instruments such as rule making and budgeting. Thus, in the daily practice of optimising patient care, different parties are inclined to opt for different strategies to improve care. The strategies chosen are an expression of the implicit assumptions that concern the effective implementation of improvements in care – assumptions concerning human behaviour and the functioning of groups or organisations.

Below (and *Table 1.3*) a number of approaches to the improvement of clinical practice are described, as well as the assumptions on which they are based (Grol 1997):

■ *The educational approach* is based on the assumption that change is mainly brought about through an internal motivation to achieve optimal competence and performance. Strategies to improve clinical practice therefore emphasise intrinsic motivation, for instance by basing them on experiences and problems that professionals are faced with in their daily work. 'Problem-based learning' and 'bottom-up' methods fit in well with this approach.

■ *The epidemiological approach* regards professionals as people who make decisions on the basis of weighing up rational arguments. If care providers do not adopt a particular working practice this is because they lack convincing information about its effectiveness. The most important strategy is therefore to provide them with this information in the form of summaries of scientific literature and (evidence-based) guidelines that can bear the scrutiny of criticism.

■ *The marketing approach* emphasises the importance of developing and disseminating an attractive proposal for change that accommodates the needs and wishes of the target group and helps them to achieve their personal goals. Such a proposal is adjusted to fit a local situation and disseminated along various channels, both through the mass media and through personal contacts.

Table 1.3 Approaches aimed at the implementation of improved care (Grol 1997)		
Approach	Focus	Selected strategies
Emphasis on internal processes		
Educational	Intrinsic motivation of professionals	Local consensus Interactive learning in groups Problem-based learning
Epidemiological	Rational decision making	Evidence-based medicine and guidelines
Marketing	Attractive product adjusted to needs of target group (segments)	Needs analysis Local adaptation Various distribution channels
Emphasis on external influences		
External influence	Conditioning	Feedback, reminders Economic incentives, sanctions
Social interaction	Influence by important others, role models	Peer review Outreach visits Opinion leaders Patient-directed methods
Managerial	Structural and organisational conditions	Redesign care processes Total quality management (TQM) and continuous quality improvement (CQI)
Control and compulsion	External motivation, avoiding negative consequences	Legislation and regulations Budgeting Disciplinary measures, complaints

■ *External influence approaches* are based on the principles of learning theory. In this approach human behaviour is seen as something that can be steered in a certain direction by outside influences, by information and by incentives before, during and after the performance of an action. Important strategies in this respect are feedback about performance (in comparison to others), reminders and material (or non-material) rewards and sanctions.

■ *Social interaction approaches* are based on the assumption that learning and change come about mainly by the example and influence of, and interaction with, other people considered to be important. Like most other people, care providers are constantly looking to colleagues and others for approval and support, and for exemplary behaviour that they can emulate. They have a need for information and feedback from others and are guided by them. Important strategies to improve practice include using opinion leaders, organising 'outreach visits' (visits by respected colleagues or experts), peer assessment and the influence patients have on professionals.

■ *The managerial approach* is directed less towards influencing individuals and more to creating the organisational conditions essential for change. The assumption is that poor quality care is a 'systems problem'. Changing the system, redesigning the care processes or changing roles and tasks, improving the internal culture and continuously monitoring and improving care are considered to form the set of methods required to optimise patient care.

■ *Control and compulsion* best sums up the final set of measures, which are based on the power of external control and compulsion to change people's performance. Many people do their utmost to avoid negative consequences of their actions and are sensitive to what happens to them in terms of earnings or privileges. Legislation and issuing rules, re-registration and accreditation, budgeting and contracts, and complaints procedures and disciplinary jurisdiction fit into this type of approach to the implementation of improved care.

Obviously, there are other approaches. It is important when reading this book to realise that the different approaches, and the strategies to improve practice

derived from them, are based on various theories about behavioural change. Some theories emphasise changing the behaviour of the individual professional, whereas others are more directed at organisational contexts and processes. Some assume that change must come about from the inside, from an inner need or motivation, whereas others assume just the opposite, that external influence or pressure from above produces the optimal result. Likewise, some theories put the emphasis on self-regulation and personal responsibility for those who have to change, whereas others take a critical stance and assume that this approach rarely leads to the desired result. In Chapter 2 we give an overview of theories in the field of change in healthcare. The problem is that, as far as optimising patient care is concerned, there is no convincing evidence that any one of the described approaches is more effective in a given situations than another (Grol and Grimshaw 2003). For this reason, the focus of this book is not on one specific approach, but on an integration of different approaches within a practically applicable implementation model or framework.

WHAT IS IMPLEMENTATION?

Implementation can be described as:

> a planned process and systematic introduction of innovations and/or changes of proven value; the aim being that these are given a structural place in professional practice, in the functioning of organisations or in the health care structure. (Zorg Onderzoek Nederland 1997)

Many terms for realising improvements in practice are in circulation, such as innovation, implementation, dissemination, diffusion, adoption, education, quality improvement and care modernisation. The diversity in terms reflects the variation in thinking in scientific circles and in the policies that cover this subject (*Box 1.3*). The term 'care modernisation' seems to be used mainly for organisational changes and changes such as those in home care or mental healthcare. Individual professional workers in the field are more inclined to speak about quality improvement, whereas clinical researchers, when they refer to implementation, think mainly in terms of the dissemination of their research results or knowledge uptake.

Box 1.3 Definitions related to 'implementation' (Davis and Tailor–Vaisey 1997)

Diffusion	Spreading information and natural adoption by the target group of guidelines and working methods.
Dissemination	Communication of information to care providers to increase their knowledge and skills; more active than diffusion; directed at a specific target group.
Adoption	Positive attitude and decision to change personal routine.
Implementation	Introduction of an innovation in the daily routine; this demands effective communication strategies and removal of hindrances to change by using techniques that are effective in practice.

In this book we adhere to the definition of implementation given at the beginning of this section, which recognises several important elements:

▓ *Planned process and systematic introduction.* The activities chosen and carried out are well thought through to achieve the adoption of a specific innovation or change. These types of strategies may be directed at care providers, at the patient–client or at organisational or structural aspects of care. Information or education on innovations may result in consciousness raising or attitude changes and is therefore a precondition for real adoption. However, on its own, it is not usual for this to lead to changes in behaviour in practice. Effective implementation therefore demands a planned process in which it is essential that effective dissemination, transfer of knowledge, attitude change and the like take place prior to the promotion of the actual implementation of the innovation.

▓ *Innovations and/or changes of proved value.* This concerns the introduction of procedures, techniques or processes that are new, better or different from those accepted in a specific setting. These may be new therapies or diagnostic procedures that have *proved* their worth in a well-designed study. This may also be a guideline based on a systematic review of the scientific literature, or a new form of organisation for a care process that has been found to work well and that leads to the desired end. This does not mean that the innovation always has to be developed fully and completely; the right time to adjust and tailor an innovation to suit the specific circumstances experienced in practice is during the implementation process.

▓ *Giving it a structural place.* Implementation should lead to sustainable change. However, in reality there is often a relapse, one reason being that support is withdrawn after a project has finished.

▓ *Professional practice, the functioning of organisations or the structure of healthcare.* Changes can take place at different levels. This book on implementation assumes that changes in the organisation or structure of the care provided are bound to have consequences for the patient and the primary care process. The changes are usually aimed at improved effectiveness or efficiency or at making the care more patient-centred, with direct effects for patients. This book considers organisational and structural changes from this perspective.

Two approaches to implementation

Broadly speaking, two contrasting approaches to implementation can be distinguished: the 'rational model' and the 'participation model' (Kitson *et al.* 1998; Van Woerkom and Adolfse 1998; *Table 1.4*). In implementation practice one usually recognises elements from

Table 1.4 Approaches to implementation (Van Woerkom and Adolfse 1998)

Rational approach	Participation approach
Linear implementation	Incremental implementation
Clear start to implementation	Unclear start
Steered from above	Steered from practice
Driven by supply of technology	Driven by need for technology
Often positive about innovation	Neutral about innovation
No attention paid to diversity of needs in practice	No attention paid to influences of macro-processes
	Chance that suboptimal technology is implemented

both models. When using the term *rational model*, one should think of the health technology cycle, which works as follows. After the primary research and synthesis of the research findings have taken place, dissemination and implementation follow. There is a clear point of departure, and steering takes place externally and mainly from above. The starting point is the availability of new insights or working methods that are considered to be worth introducing. Hopefully, through dissemination, increasing numbers of target group members become converted to adopting them. Criticism levelled at this model is that little attention is paid to the diversity of needs in the target group and it makes little use of the knowledge and experience present within that group.

The *participation model* uses the needs and experiences from practice as its departure point. The exact starting point for the change is often difficult to determine. It takes place step by step (incrementally); in some cases there may not be a strongly felt prior need to implement a concrete innovation or working method. Communication and feedback between people in daily practice determine whether the change will or will not be realised. The phases of development, testing, dissemination and introduction of an innovation intertwine. A criticism levelled at this model is that it does not always introduce the best patient care possible and that it does not pay enough attention to the structural factors that influence its introduction. The model actually describes how change is often brought about in practice, but offers few leads for a planned approach to implementation.

Important elements from both approaches are used in this book. Optimisation of patient care is seen as a two-way flow between practice and science. Inspiration for improvement of care comes both from practice (from the problems noted there and from developments experienced in the work place) and from research and projects on optimal care provision. The next section clarifies this two-way flow.

IMPLEMENTATION OF CHANGES IN CARE: TWO STARTING POINTS

The departure point for the implementation of change is that there is a range of desirable changes in patient care. These changes may involve evidence-based insights, procedures, techniques or guidelines for good care practice. Alternately, they may concern problems observed in routine practice that demand a solution, or (the opposite) good experiences using a certain working method that could be implemented on a wider scale.

Evidence–based medicine and guidelines

Many insights about optimal care derive from research carried out into the effectiveness and efficiency of certain routines in clinical, preventative or care practice. The evidence-based medicine movement is oriented towards helping care providers, patients and policy makers with decisions on how to act when faced with health problems by basing their decisions, wherever possible, on the best scientific evidence (Sackett *et al.* 1997). With this in mind, international work groups, within the framework of the Cochrane Collaboration, painstakingly summarise scientific insights within a specific area. Once located, the studies and the systematic analyses of the literature are added to a large database, the Cochrane Library, which already contains many hundreds of thousands of well-planned studies and a great number of reviews. In terms of ambitions, this world-wide activity has already been compared to the Humane Genome Project, in which all human genes are being mapped out. The idea is that clinicians consult these sorts of databases when they are at work and so develop a critical attitude towards using the scientific literature. Research has shown, however, that clinicians are eager to find support for their decisions, but find it difficult to consult databases such as these (Guyatt *et al.* 2000; Tomlin *et al.* 1999; McColl *et al.* 1998).

Studies looking into the effects of introducing such databases are still scarce (Wyatt *et al.* 1998). Methods are required to make access to literature easier. Compiling scientific evidence in the form of clinical practice guidelines is one such useful method. Guidelines are a potentially important resource for introducing insights into the best forms of patient care in an easily accessible form and for these being adopted. However, before this can be achieved they have to meet certain requirements. At the moment guidelines for care are being formulated all over the world by a wide range of parties, including governments, insurers, professionals and patients' organisations. These guidelines have different aims and development methods, and therefore their quality varies. In the past they were based mainly on the consensus views of experts; gradually, the procedures have become more systematic and attempts are being made to incorporate the most recent scientific insights into their development methods. Guidelines form an important resource with which to implement new, valuable insights and they are an important intermediate step in the process of implementation of scientific knowledge, and so Chapter 5 deals explicitly with guideline development. Nonetheless, they are also a new technology in itself and good implementation methods are needed to ensure that guidelines find their way into daily practice.

Care processes and total quality management

Many innovations in healthcare practice do not get into their stride as a result of the introduction of scientific findings or evidence-based guidelines. In many cases it is possible to conclude that the driving force behind the desired improvement in care (which may or may not be based on factual information about variations in care provision) is that existing practice is not leading to the intended result, that mistakes are being made, that patients are not satisfied or that working methods are inefficient. No matter how carefully the search for, and analysis of, scientific literature is carried out, there is good scientific evidence for only a proportion of current clinical actions and decisions (estimated to be less than 40–50%). There is a large grey area in which the experiences and preferences of those involved play a far more important role than any guidelines in determining what good care is (Naylor 1995). However, even if scientific research has been carried out, translating this into useful recommendations that link up with everyday practice can prove difficult. A great deal of research and a large number of guidelines are based around concrete actions carried out by individual professionals.

In daily practice, however, the reality is just as likely to involve longer running, complex care processes that include multiple care providers, doctors, paramedics and nurses, for which the approach consists of a logical series of linked interventions or actions (Van Weel and Knottnerus 1999). For example, a patient who suffers a stroke, should immediately be sent by their GP to a stroke unit, and after having received the proper treatment there, should rapidly be moved on to a rehabilitation centre. Good team work, clearly defined tasks, exchange of information and logistics, supported by so-called 'clinical pathways' or 'disease management systems' work better here than guidelines for separate procedures carried out by individuals on their own.

Regarding care provision as processes and chains of actions and the need to analyse and improve these processes and chains in their entirety takes pride of place

in the 'integrated care' or the 'total quality management' approach (Berwick 1998). Identified problems are tackled in concrete improvement projects, following a cyclical process of change (plan–do–study–act model) and are checked continuously to see if the desired result has been achieved. Use is made of good experiences and 'best practices' elsewhere. This approach has also been included in the model and the basic principles adhered to in this book.

CONCLUSIONS

We contend in this chapter that many patients do not receive optimal care and that specific, well-planned programmes are required to implement new or valuable scientific research, guidelines, protocols, care processes and procedures. Different approaches to implement improvement can be observed, each based on different assumptions and theories on human and organisational behaviour. Some focus on internal, others on external influences. Some believe in bottom-up processes of change, others in top-down approaches. Some see change as a rational process that can be planned well in advance, others as something that will happen incrementally without much planning.

Different views and theories, as well as their consequences for the practice of implementation, are presented in Chapter 2 and are used to formulate a model in Chapter 3.

Recommended literature

Grol R (1997). Beliefs and evidence in changing clinical practice. *BMJ* **315**:418–421.

Grol R and Grimshaw J (1999). Evidence-based implementation of evidence-based medicine. *Jt Comm J Qual Improv.* **25**:503–513.

References

Andrews L, Stocking C, Krizek T, *et al.* (1997). An alternative strategy for studying adverse events in medical care. *Lancet* **349**:309–313.

Baxter C, Jones R and Corr L (1998). Time trend analysis and variations in prescribing lipid lowering drugs in general practice. *BMJ* **317**:1134–1135.

Berwick D (1998). Developing and testing changes in delivery of care. *Ann Int Med.* **128**:651–656.

Bodenheimer T (1999). The American health care system. The movement for improved quality in health care. *N Engl J Med.* **340**:488–492.

Casparie AF (1996). The ambiguous relationship between practice variation and appropriateness of care: An agenda for further research. *Health Policy* **35**:247–265.

Chassin M (1998). Is health care ready for Six Sigma Quality? *Milbank Q*. **76**:565–591.

Davis D and Tailor-Vaisey A (1997). Translating guidelines into practice: A systematic review of theoretic concepts, practical experience and research evidence in the adoption of clinical practice guidelines. *Can Med Assoc J*. **157**:408–416.

Grol R (1997). Beliefs and evidence in changing clinical practice. *BMJ* **315**:418–421.

Grol R (2001). Improving the quality of medical care. *JAMA* **284**:2578–2585.

Grol R and Grimshaw J (2003). From best evidence to best practice: Effective implementation of change in patients' care. *Lancet* **362**:1225–1230.

Guyatt G, Meade M, Jaeschke R, *et al.* (2000). Practitioners of evidence based care. *BMJ* **320**:954–955.

Haines A (1996). The science of perpetual change. *Br J Gen Pract*. **46**:115–119.

Kitson A, Harvey G and McCormack B (1998). Enabling the implementation of evidence based practice: A conceptual framework. *Qual Health Care* **7**:149–158.

Koelemay M, Bossuyt P and Gouma D (1996). Implementatie van richtlijnen voor klinisch handelen op een afdeling chirurgie [Implementation of guidelines for clinical performance at a surgery department]. *Ned Tijdschr Geneeskd*. **140**(49):2454–2463.

McColl A, Smith H, White P, *et al.* (1998). General practitioners' perceptions of the route to evidence based medicine: A questionnaire survey. *BMJ* **316**:361–365.

Mulrow C (1994). Rationale for systematic reviews. *BMJ* **309**:597–599.

Naylor C (1995). Grey zones of clinical practice: Some limits to evidence-based medicine. *Lancet* **345**:840–842.

President's Advisory Commission (1998). *Quality First: Better Health Care for all Americans*. Final report to the President of the USA. Washington: President's Advisory Commission on Consumer Protection and Quality in the Health Care Industry.

Rogers E (1983). *Diffusion of Innovations*. New York: Free Press.

Sackett D, Richardson W, Rosenberg W and Haynes R (1997). *Evidence-based Medicine: How to Practice and Teach*. London: Churchill Livingstone.

Schuster M, McGlynn E and Brook R (1998). How good is the quality of health care in the United States? *Milbank Q*. **76**:517–563.

Spies TH and Mokkink HGA (1999). *Toetsen aan Standaarden. Het Medisch Handelen van Huisartsen in de Praktijk Getoetst. Eindrapport [Assessment of Guidelines. Medical Care of General Practitioners Assessed in Practice. Final Report]*. Nijmegen/Utrecht: Werkgroep Onderzoek Kwaliteit/Nederlands Huisartsen Genootschap [Centre for Quality of Care Research/Dutch College of General Practitioners].

Stalenhoef A (1998). *Cholesterol. Van Concept naar Consensus. Inaugurale Rede [Cholesterol. From Concepts to Consensus]*. Nijmegen: KUN.

Teare L, Cockson B and Stone S (2001). Hand hygiene. *BMJ* **323**:411–412.

Tomlin Z, Humphrey C and Rogers S (1999). General practitioners' perceptions of effective health care. *BMJ* **318**:1532–1535.

Weel C van and Knottnerus J (1999). Evidence-based intervention and comprehensive treatment. *Lancet* **353**:916–918.

Woerkom C van and Adolfse L (1998). Interactieve kennisontwikkeling en -benutting [Interactive knowledge developmental and use]. *SI* **1**:10–19.

Woods K, Ketley D, Lowy A, *et al.* (1998). Beta-blockers and antithrombotic treatment for secondary prevention after myocardial infarction. *Eur Heart J*. **19**:74–79.

Wyatt J, Paterson-Brown S, Johanson R, *et al.* (1998). Randomized trial of educational visits to enhance use of systematic reviews in 25 obstetric units. *BMJ* **317**:1041–1046.

Zorg Onderzoek Nederland (1997). *Met het oog op Toepassing [From the Perspective of Application]*. Beleidsnota Implementatie ZON 1997–1999. Den Haag: ZON.

Chapter 2

Theories on implementation of change in healthcare

Richard Grol, Michel Wensing, Marlies Hulscher and Martin Eccles

KEY MESSAGES

- Different disciplines propose different approaches to the implementation of innovations, based on different theories about changing professional and organisational performance.
- Some theories focus on change within the professionals, others on change within the social setting or within the organisational and economic context.
- A number of current, popular theories from different disciplines are presented in this chapter, ordered in three categories: theories that focus on individual factors, theories about social influence and theories about the influence of organisational and economic factors on changing healthcare.
- The conclusion of this chapter is that all the theories can potentially contribute to describing and explaining the effective implementation of changes in patient care. However, we need theories that predict change and an integrated model that offers direct support for designing and planning implementation activities in normal patient care.

Box 2.1 Reducing unnecessary antibiotic prescribing (Belongia and Schwartz 1998)

Unnecessary use of antibiotics in cases of viral infections can be seen widely and has led to an increased resistance to antibiotics. This may, in time, lead to reduced possibilities for the effective treatment of infections. Research has identified different causes of the unnecessary use of antibiotics. Some physicians are not informed about the optimal treatment or find it difficult to change their prescribing habits. Some do not know the natural course of viral infection, or they think that patients expect an antibiotic treatment and that to refuse such medication leads to dissatisfaction and problems with patients. Under time pressure, the physicians prefer to prescribe rather than inform patients about the best approach to their condition. Patients usually do not know the difference between a viral and a bacterial infection; they expect antibiotics to be effective for all infections and think that such medication is always required to treat certain symptoms. They believe that antibiotics can help them to recover quickly and return to work sooner. In many practices and hospitals control of the rational prescribing of antibiotics is limited – often repeat prescriptions are provided without proper evaluation by the physician. Also, pharmacies often lack a system that prevents the unnecessary use of antibiotics.

Evidently, different types of factors determine the rational or irrational prescribing of antibiotics: those related to the physician, those to patients and those to the social and organisational context. Different theories on the implementation of change can provide ideas to improve the prescribing routines in practice, based on assumptions about the factors that play a crucial role in current performance.

INTRODUCTION

The implementation of new scientific findings, new procedures or guidelines sometimes happens quickly and easily. An example is the finding from randomised controlled trials that myringotomy in cases of acute otitis media in children was no more effective than a conservative approach of waiting and giving medication. Publication of this finding was sufficient for almost all physicians to stop performing this procedure within a short time, perhaps because most children and parents disliked it so much. However, producing change is usually less easy, particularly if the innovation requires complex changes in clinical practice, better collaboration between disciplines, changes in patient behaviour or changes in the organisation of care.

New evidence, guidelines, best practices or procedures do not usually implement themselves. In most cases the interaction of a large number of factors determines whether or not implementation is successful. The following categories of factors can be identified in the literature (Davis and Taylor-Vaisey 1997; Grol 1992):

- Features of the innovation itself – some are more evidence based, better formulated, more credible and/or better adapted to the needs of clinical practice or fit better to the norms and values of the target group than do others;
- Features of the target group of professionals who should use the innovation – their knowledge, skills, opinions, attitudes, values, routines and/or personalities can facilitate or block implementation;
- Features of the patients – their attitude, knowledge, behaviour, capacities, coping skills, compliance, needs and preferences can also stimulate or hinder a successful implementation;
- Features of the social setting – the attitude of colleagues, the culture in the team or social network and the view of opinion leaders, as well as the style of leadership in the organisation, can be of influence;
- Features of the economic, administrative and organisational context can exert powerful influences on practice routines and on the successful implementation of innovations;
- Finally, features of the methods and strategies for dissemination and implementation used – these will have more or less effect dependent on the choice of the intervention methods, their intensity and duration, and the source and change agents involved.

Not all of these factors can be addressed within one theory or model of change. In addition, the complexity of implementing changes in patient care cannot be explained easily from a single perspective – different views on effective implementation need to be integrated as coherently as possible, if necessary tailored to the change at hand.

Theories on implementation of change explain under what circumstances the implementation will be successful. Such theories can be found in a large number of disciplines and scientific areas, for instance in the social sciences, the educational sciences, the health promotion field, the organisational, management, economic and engineering sciences, and the fields of marketing and political sciences. Many of the current popular theories used in healthcare have been derived from either the field of health promotion, where they were developed to explain life-style changes, or from organisational and management sciences that explain how organisations behave and change. Most of the theories are not directly applicable to changing patient care or implementing innovations, clinical guidelines or best practices in healthcare. New procedures, technologies or clinical guidelines can be seen as innovations with specific characteristics – our knowledge of the relative importance of these characteristics is as yet limited. In addition, many of the theories and views on changing clinical practice overlap to a greater or lesser extent; new ideas about implementation are usually built upon the views of other authors.

ABOUT THIS OVERVIEW OF THEORIES

We present in this chapter a set of current theories and views on the implementation of change in patient care. While some research findings are included, a systematic underpinning of the approaches with the relevant literature citations is not attempted here. Integration of the different theories is presented in Chapter 3. Some considerations need to be made when reading this overview of the theories:

- The overview is *not exhaustive*, as this is impossible within the context of a book chapter and other overviews can be consulted for further information (e.g. Ashford 2004). Rather, we have selected theories that may help to explain change in patient care.
- Also, as becomes clear from reading them, the theories are not distinct, but often overlap, sometimes to a large extent. Most of the theories and models presented here build on earlier theories or on more basic concepts.
- It is important to make a distinction here between *theories and models that describe or explain* how change takes place and which factors are crucial in such a process, on the one hand, and *theories and models that are used to plan* change, on the other. We introduce some models for planning change in Chapter 3 and restrict ourselves here to theories that predominantly focus on explaining factors, although it is sometimes difficult to categorise the theories (see, for instance, the PRECEDE/PROCEDE model of Green in Chapter 3).
- Another important distinction is between theories that are *related directly to improving patient care* and theories that discuss *how to improve conditions for good patient care* (e.g. by providing resources, by improving the general climate and working conditions in a hospital, by changing the management of a hospital or by cre-

ating an environment in which change of patient care can be facilitated). This chapter (and this book) does not focus on macro-organisational change, but on change in the primary (micro) processes of patient care. Macro-systems of reimbursement of healthcare are not addressed; reimbursement systems that directly influence the quality of patient care, however, might be. So, in this chapter we explore, first, factors in individuals, patients, teams and groups, organisations, and then the wider environment that may have a direct impact on changing primary processes of patient care.

To facilitate the consideration and discussion of these theories we need a taxonomy. Various proposals for ordering such factors can be found in the literature, such as the distinction between predisposing, enabling and reinforcing factors (Green *et al.* 1988). We take improvement and change of the direct provision of care to patients by professionals and teams as a starting point for our categorisation and make a distinction here between (*Table 2.1*):

▨ Theories on factors related to individual professionals (their cognitions, motivations, routines, styles of

Table 2.1 Theories on the implementation of change and relevant factors in the process of change

Theory	Factors
Individual professionals	
Cognitive theories	Mechanisms in the processes of thinking and deciding, and in balancing the advantages and disadvantages of specific performance
Educational theories	Individual learning needs, learning styles and motivation to learn and to change
Attitude theories: theory of planned behaviour	Attitude towards an innovation, perceived social norms, control and self-efficacy expectations, and intention to change
Motivation or stages of change theories	Different motivational stages with different factors that determine the motivation to change
Social interaction and context	
Social learning theory	Observed behaviour of role models, incentives, positive feedback, capacity to learn through experience and observation
Social network and influence theories	Network characteristics, such as weak ties and change agents, existing norms and values in social network, culture within network, expectation of peers and opinion leaders, opinions of key persons
Theories on patients, factors related to patients	(Perceived) patient expectations and needs, patient behaviour – patients can stimulate or trigger performance change when they are informed about optimal care or are involved in care decisions
Theories on professional development	Professions develop a body of knowledge and standards that guide individual professionals – the dynamics of professional development is influenced by specialisation, self-interest and multidisciplinary contacts
Theories on leadership	Leadership style, type of power, involvement and commitment of (top) management in innovation
Organisational and economic context	
Theories of innovative organisations	Extent of specialisation, decentralisation, professionalisation and functional differentiation; the type of organisation (large or small, profit or non-profit); internal or external communication
Theory of quality management	Culture in the organisation, leadership, team characteristics, organisation of care processes, customer focus
Process re-engineering theory	Optimally designed care processes, pathways and multidisciplinary collaboration
Complexity theory	Interactions between parts of a complex system, 'attractors' or behavioural patterns
Theory of organisational learning	Capacity of an organisation to stimulate continuous learning and information exchange at all levels of the organisation
Theories on organisational culture	To change clinical practice a change in culture is needed, particularly a flexible, externally oriented culture
Economic theories	Reimbursement systems, rewards and incentives

learning, etc.) that influence change in performance;
- Theories on the influence of the social context on the change process (social norms and values in the social network, influence of peers, opinion leaders and role models, and interaction within the system) – theories related to the social context can also concern theories on the influence of (the communication with) patients on professional performance and change;
- Theories of those factors related to the organisational, administrative or economic context (culture within the organisation, resources, systems of reimbursement, organisation of processes, etc.).

Some of the theories include factors related to more than one of these categories; these are grouped under one of the headings. To set the stage we start with an example of an evidence-based routine that has not yet found its way into daily practice (*Box 2.2*).

We address this clinical problem of poor hand hygiene throughout this chapter using the different theoretical perspectives presented here and then offer an implementation plan based on these perspectives.

THEORIES ON FACTORS RELATED TO INDIVIDUAL PROFESSIONALS

Factors related to the change of individual professionals focus on the way professionals make choices or decisions, on their (lack of) knowledge or skills, their attitudes and motivation, or on their routines and habits in daily professional life. Social or structural conditions may be important in these theories, but only in the way that these are perceived by the individuals. We discuss the following theories:

- Cognitive theories;
- Educational theories;
- Attitude theories – theory of planned behaviour;
- Motivation or stages of change theories.

Cognitive theories

Cognitive theories of change management focus on the (rational) processes of thinking and deciding by individual professionals and offer links to changing these processes. Rational decision-making theories assume that professionals consider and balance the advantages and disadvantages of different alternatives to provide optimal care. If, for instance, decision analyses show that a specific operation (trans-urethral resection of the prostate) for benign prostatic hyperplasia can improve symptoms in about 75% of the patients, but that the risk of complications lies between 3 and 35%, the physician and patient can, on the basis of balancing the benefits and risks, decide on the best management (AHCPR 1994). Within such a theory, the provision of convincing information on risks and benefits and pros and cons is seen as crucial to performance change. In our example of hand hygiene, this theory views the lack of compliance with existing guidelines primarily as a knowledge problem: the professionals are considered to be not well informed about or not convinced about the scientific evidence on the consequences of inappropriate hand hygiene. As one doctor wrote in the *British Medical Journal* (1999): 'If there is such compelling evidence for the need to wash hands between each patient contact, then why do I and the vast majority of my colleagues not do it? Firstly, I have never seen any convincing evidence that

---

Box 2.2 The complexity of changing practice: the case of hand hygiene

In many countries the priorities for healthcare include the reduction of hospital-acquired infections. Such infections are estimated to affect about one in 11 patients, with a 13% mortality and an increased length of stay in the hospital by a factor of 2.5. The extra cost per patient with an infection in the UK is about £3000 (Stone 2001). Between 15 and 30% of the infections are considered to be preventable. One of the main possible improvements is better handwashing and disinfection by professionals between contacts with patients. We have been aware of the importance of hand hygiene since the mid-1800s, starting with Ignaz Semmelweis who found that hand disinfection reduced maternal morbidity in obstetric departments. Since then we are regularly confronted with evidence of the importance of good hand hygiene, as in a recent review of nine randomised trials (Pratt *et al.* 2001, Stone 2001). The treatment effect is so great that "if hand hygiene were a new drug it would be used by all". Nevertheless, compliance by health workers in general and physicians in particular is known to be poor (Teare *et al.* 2001). Many hospitals have guidelines on the prevention of infections, but these are often not followed. Physicians largely overestimate their own routines in hand hygiene (Handwashing Liaison Group 1999).

Thus, a well-established evidence base is available, summarised in disseminated clinical guidelines on the prevention of hospital infections. Most clinical professionals have been educated, at least by formal methods, on its importance. Yet performance is poor.

What is the problem and what can be done about it?

handwashing between each patient reduces infection rates …'. The perceived benefits of regular washing do not weigh up against the disadvantages of the extra work involved for this physician. Providing relevant information is the preferred strategy in this theory.

Other cognitive theories are more descriptive and show how decisions are actually made. A cognitive–psychological approach, developed in education, states that clinicians do not act rationally, but decide on the basis of previous experiences and contextual information (Schmidt 1984). When they diagnose a health problem they use so-called 'illness-scripts', cognitive structures in which they have organised the knowledge about a specific health problem and in which previous experiences with specific patients are seen as crucial to further decisions. Put simply, when a patient presents with a problem, the physician opens some mental drawers that contain the details of previous patients and compares the current case to some similar cases. This then determines the physician's further thoughts and actions. Experienced doctors diagnose patients more quickly because they have more cases available and better use the contextual information of such cases (Hobus 1994). However, professionals can also use obsolete information or inadequate experiences as the basis of their performance.

Other theories also describe cognitive mechanisms that may prevent rational decision making. For instance, people prefer consistency in thought and action, and so make choices that may not be rational, but fit well within existing opinions, needs and behaviours (Festinger 1954). When they do not like handwashing or doubt the effect of it, they interpret or seek information that confirms their beliefs. People may also seek external explanations for specific events or behaviours, instead of internal ones, to make the outcome more acceptable to themselves or make more in line with existing perceptions.

To develop a successful implementation strategy it is important, according to the cognitive theories, to discover cognitive mechanisms that play a role in inappropriate performance. Using cognitive theories, a lack of hand hygiene by physicians can be explained by a lack of relevant (scientific) information, by incorrect expectations about the consequences of their behaviour or by attributing infections to causes outside their control, etc. Therefore, it may be important, in changing performance, to focus on the way professionals think and make decisions about their daily work and to support more effective ways of decision making.

Educational theories

Cognitive theory of learning and education was developed simultaneously with general cognitive theory. The fundamental idea of the theory is that learning is an active, constructive cognitive process, which must be studied to optimise it. Learning can only happen if learners actively use the new knowledge and link it to pre-existing knowledge.

Other educational theories focus less on cognitions and more on the motivation to learn. For instance, *adult learning theories* state that people learn better and are more motivated to change when they start from problems that they have experienced in practice, rather than when they are confronted with abstract information (Merriam 1996; Mann 1994; Norman and Schmidt 1992). Principles in adult learning are:

- Effective change in healthcare is achieved better by focussing on concrete problems in practice than by focussing on abstract issues such as diseases, a guideline or a specific action (e.g. a test, a prescription, an operation technique; Holm 1998);
- Professionals have a large reservoir of experiences that can be used as a source for learning and changing (Smith *et al.* 1998) – particularly professionals who are older, have acquired more experience, have more individual learning needs and have increased competence in self-directed learning;
- Professionals are more motivated to change by internal motivation than by external pressure or stimuli.

Such principles of problem-based and self-directed learning can be used effectively in the implementation of change or innovations in healthcare, although the fundamental assumptions behind the theory remain largely speculative (Norman 2002). Applied to our example, to improve hand hygiene in a hospital the care providers involved first need to experience a problem, such that their behaviour leads to infections in patients, and they need to develop a motivation to do something about it. However, the theory can also be used to discuss with them how, based on their experience, this complicated problem can be solved within their own work setting.

'Problem-based learning' and 'self-directed learning' are increasingly popular in healthcare, in the undergraduate training of physicians, nurses and paramedics and in postgraduate training and continuous medical education. In some countries (e.g. UK and Canada) projects are conducted in which physicians plan, perform, monitor and evaluate their own learning and change process, so-called portfolio learning (Holm 1998). For successful implementation a change strategy needs to be tailored to the individual who directs – under supervision – his or her own change process. Not all care providers have the competence to do this. According to Merriam (1996), they need to be methodical, logical, reflective, analytical, flexible, responsible, creative, independent, open and motivated – not a simple set of requirements for a successful implementation process. Evidence suggest that at least one critical component of adult learning, self-assessment, is not easy (Norman 2002).

Also to be taken into account is that professionals may have different motives in relation to (self-directed) learning and changing (Stanley *et al.* 1993). Tassone and Heck (1997) identified a number of motives:

- Social interaction – participation in education and learning to facilitate interaction with others and become part of a group;
- External expectations – participation as a reaction to the expectations or demands of others or leaders in the work setting;
- Social well-being – participation to be able to serve others or society better;
- Professional competence – participation to increase personal skills, acquire a better professional status or obtain a certificate;
- Escape – participation to prevent boring routines or frustration in the job;
- Cognition – participation to improve knowledge.

Tassone and Heck (1997) showed that the most important reason among nurses and physiotherapists for taking part in education was the wish to improve professional competence. If this was a legal requirement there would be more involvement, but voluntary participation resulted in more change than compulsory participation. Other authors (Fox and Bennett 1998; Holm 1998) also emphasise the wish to be competent as the most important driver. It is potentially important to understand such motives when planning change in professional performance. Fox and Bennett (1998) distinguished between the role of different factors in the change processes of physicians, for instance curiosity, personal and financial well-being, career planning, wish to improve competence, pressure from patients and pressure from colleagues. Personal factors seem to be related to large and complex changes, while professional and social factors are related to smaller, simpler changes.

Another factor seen as important in educational theories is that the change process is linked to the *personal learning style* of the professionals. Different learning styles have been distinguished (Lewis and Bolden 1989):

- Activist style – people who like new experiences and therefore accept, but also abandon, innovations quickly (attention to the maintenance of a change is important in this group);
- Reflective style – people who want to consider all the options very carefully before changing (data are collected methodically before they decide, but they may wait too long before acting);
- Theoretical style – people who prefer a rigorous analysis and logical arguments to explain why a change is needed;
- Pragmatic style – people who prefer to act on the basis of practical experience with an innovation.

Practising physicians and trainees proved to prefer a pragmatic learning style, while trainers scored higher on a theoretical style (Lewis and Bolden 1989; Owen *et al.* 1989; Nylenna *et al.* 1996).

In conclusion, according to educational theories, implementation of innovation and change in patient care should account for the individual learning needs and personal motives of professionals as well as for their personal learning styles. This implies that these needs and motives need to be understood, and that strategies for change need to be tailored to the identified needs of defined subgroups of learners. Therefore, in developing a programme to improve hand hygiene it may become clear, for example, that physicians have different motives for change and different learning styles compared to those of nurses, so change strategies should address those differences.

Attitude theories – theory of planned behaviour

Some theories focus strongly on the role of attitudes, perceptions and intentions towards the desired performance. For instance, the theory of planned behaviour states that any given behaviour of professionals is influenced by their individual intentions to perform that specific behaviour, and these intentions are determined largely by attitudes concerning the behaviour, by perceived social norms and by perceived control related to the behaviour (*Figure 2.1*; Ajzen 1991). All these factors can be addressed in implementation. The attitude concerning a specific behaviour, such as handwashing before and/or after each contact with a patient, is determined by the expected outcomes of this behaviour (opinion that it leads to fewer infections in the hospital) and the positive or negative appraisal of these

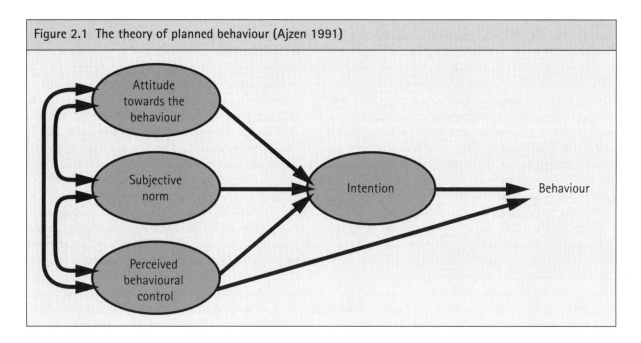

Figure 2.1 The theory of planned behaviour (Ajzen 1991)

outcomes (this is worth the extra effort or not). The perceived social norms are influenced by the norms seen in others (whether others wash or disinfect their hands regularly and, particularly, whether physicians do it or not) and the importance attached to these norms. The perceived or experienced control, or self-efficacy expectation (Maibach and Murphy 1995; Bandura 1986), represents the belief that one can really achieve the desired change in the specific setting (regular handwashing under time pressure, for example). Self-efficacy expectations can be related to the behaviour itself ('Am I able to perform this?'), to the social context ('Can I resist social pressure?') and to the pressure related to the behaviour ('Can I perform the behaviour under pressure?'). Extensions of the theory include, for instance, the 'experienced personal moral obligation or accountability' as a predictor of change ('it is unacceptable when patients acquire an infection in our hospital') and the distinction between concrete plans for change (implementation intention) and the new behaviour (goal intention). To achieve better hand hygiene, concrete plans that relate to 'when', 'what', 'where' and 'how' the change will be performed need to be made (Gollwitzer and Oettingen 1998; Orbell et al. 1997).

The theory of planned behaviour has, so far, mostly been used within the field of health promotion. Research on its use within the field of implementation of change is yet limited. Mann (1994) found that the self-efficacy expectations of physicians about the prevention of cardiovascular disease influenced their

efforts in this area. Walker et al. (2001) used the theory of planned behaviour in a study to examine family physicians' intentions to prescribe antibiotics to patients who presented with an uncomplicated sore throat. The multiple correlation coefficient between the intention to prescribe and the beliefs and perceptions of the physicians was high (0.69).

The attitude theories offer a useful model for diagnosing implementation problems that relate to professional attitudes, opinions and personal experiences, and for developing concrete programmes for change on the basis of this diagnosis.

Motivation or stages of change theories

Motivation theories focus not so much on the determinants of change, but on differences in the motivation or intention to change between professionals, or on the process of change and the motivational steps that individuals need to take to accomplish real change. Many such models are available, and an overview of models of step-wise change processes is provided in Chapter 3. These theories suggest that professionals need to go through specific phases in their motivation before they can start subsequent phases. Each phase requires different strategies for change. Such theories lead to the characterisation of different subgroups or segments in a target group (care providers who work in a hospital or nursing home), with different motivations to change their handwashing and disinfection routine and each subgroup needing different approaches. For instance, the innovation–diffusion theory of Rogers (discussed in more detail in Chapter 3), makes a distinction between *innovators, early adopters, early majority, late majority* and *laggards.* These groups differ with respect to searching for information on innovations and the extent to which they are motivated to try and adopt new guidelines, techniques and procedures (Rogers 1983). 'Innovators' represent a small segment of the target group who are strongly focussed on new ideas and information. They try to influence the 'early adopters', an active group with high status within the target group and a reference group for the innovators. The 'early majority' is composed of people who are not the leaders in the field, but who have close contact with and are influenced by the early adopters. The 'late majority' is composed of people who have a more sceptical attitude towards change and new ideas; they are not particularly sensitive to information sources and put more confidence in the opinion of colleagues or public opinion. Finally, the 'laggards' are a group who resist change. In improving hand hygiene it is important to find the early adopters and involve them in influencing the rest of the target group.

One of the stages of change theories, widely used in health promotion and stop-smoking programmes, is the *trans-theoretical model* or the 'stage of readiness to change model' of Prochaska (Prochaska and Velicer 1997). It distinguishes six phases in the motivation to change:

- *Pre-contemplation* – the individual is not motivated or has no plans to change hand-hygiene routines in the near future. Reading, talking or thinking about the proposed new performance is avoided. Implementation activities in this phase have to focus on creating awareness (e.g. by presenting infection rates), increasing emotional commitment and stimulating thinking about the consequences of the poor hand hygiene for others (particularly for patients).
- *Contemplation* – the individual considers that he or she will change in the near future. Pros and cons of different hand-hygiene routines are considered, but the individual is not ready for concrete action. In this phase implementation can be supported by activities that focus on creating positive attitudes, for instance by discussing evidence and barriers to change concerning hand hygiene.
- *Preparation* – the individual intends to change routines in the immediate future and is sensitive to interventions that support a trial of the change. Implementation can be stimulated particularly by strengthening the self-efficacy expectations ('it is possible') and the commitment to the change.
- *Action* – the individual has actually tried the new hand-hygiene routines. Further implementation can be facilitated by incentives, social support and providing new skills or resources (e.g. new equipment or alcohol rub).
- *Maintenance* – the individual tries to consolidate the change and prevent relapse into previous habits or routines, which may take quite a while and may be stimulated by regular feedback.
- *Completion* – the change is now part of a new normality and falling back into old routines is impossible.

So, when applying such segmentation theories to our case of hand hygiene a crucial step is to determine the motivation and change intentions with respect to hand-hygiene routines within the target group and to find segments that have to be treated differently within the implementation programme (*Box 2.3*).

Box 2.3 Proposal for interventions linked to Prochaska's 'stage of readiness to change model' (after NHMRC 2000; Moulding *et al*. 1999)

Stage	Focus on individuals	Focus on populations
Pre-contemplation and contemplation	Local opinion leaders Individual instruction Workshops or conferences Small discussion groups Local consensus Involve users in change proposal	Dissemination through internet, post, newspapers, journals Adoption by official organisations National opinion leaders Media campaigns Public information through local education
Preparation and action	Personal audit and feedback Administrative interventions Computerised systems to support behaviour Reminder systems	Feedback on care processes and outcomes General reminders to physicians and patients by mail Media campaigns

Some authors propose that this model be applied to performance change in healthcare (Moulding *et al*. 1999; Cohen *et al*. 1994); others criticise the lack of empirical support for it (Weinstein and Rothman 1998; Bandura 1997). A review of the use of the stage model in stop-smoking interventions showed that it was not effective in most of the studies (Riemsma *et al*. 2003).

THEORIES ON FACTORS RELATED TO SOCIAL INTERACTION AND CONTEXT

Theories that focus on the influence on change processes of others within the environment usually discuss determinants of change in the interaction between an individual professional and others, such as the influence of key individuals and opinion leaders, participation in social networks, the influence of patients, leadership, cultural factors and mutual influence by peers. The (partly related) theories presented here are:
- Social learning theory;
- Social network and influence theories;
- Theories on factors related to patients;
- Theories on professional development;
- Theories on leadership.

Social learning theory

The social cognitive or social learning theory of Bandura (1986) is an extension of classic behavioural theories and of the theory of planned behaviour, and explains the behaviour of individuals in terms of personal factors, behavioural factors and context-related factors. *Personal factors* are those concerned with the skill of the individual to learn by experience, by doing and by observation of the behaviour of others. It encompasses, for instance, the capacity to:
- Store knowledge (symbolic capacity);
- Develop a mental representation of future events (forethought capacity);
- Learn through observation of the actions of others (vicarious capacity);
- Reflect on and analyse actions (self-reflective capacity);
- Develop guidelines for future behaviour and focus energy on achieving this behaviour (self-regulatory capacity).

Behavioural factors are concerned with the possibilities of actually showing the desired performance, while *contextual factors* are concerned with factors in the setting that reinforce this performance. Important contextual factors are material or non-material rewards of others (e.g. positive comments by peers or opinion leaders), as well as modelling of the behaviour by others. Such modelling means that one can observe in others that it is possible to demonstrate the behaviour, and that this leads to the expected results.

Within this social learning theory the basic assumption is that there is a continuous interaction between a professional, his or her performance and the social environment. They need each other and reinforce each other in changing performance. Relating this to our example of inadequate hand hygiene, this theory particularly addresses the issue of care providers observing each other and observing the performance of 'leaders' in the setting, as well as the importance of (positive) reinforcement of the desired performance by peers and important others in the work setting.

Social network and influence theories

Theories on the diffusion of innovations state that the adoption of new ideas and technologies is influenced largely by the structure of social networks and of specific individuals in or at the margins of these networks (Rogers 1995). The theories are based on a social network approach, which suggests that the behaviour of individuals cannot be seen in isolation from the behaviour of others in the networks in which they operate. Work on networks has explored the influences of the strengths of the links between individuals within a network and the threshold effects of adoption of innovations (Gladwell 2000; Valente 1996). Relevant network characteristics that may influence an effective transfer of information and support may include:
- The strength of the ties between members of the network. 'Weak ties' between individuals may increase the transfer of information in ways not usually available within networks of individuals bonded by 'strong ties'.
- Heterophily, or the difference between interacting individuals in certain attributes. Some degree of heterophily is necessary within networks for diffusion to occur. In networks of individuals who are alike (homophilous), innovations are less likely to be adopted. However, once adopted by one participant, there is a higher probability that the innovation will be adopted in such networks.
- The proportion of the population that has already adopted an innovation (Valente 1996). Threshold models of diffusion propose that an individual

engages in a behaviour based upon the proportion of people already engaged in that behaviour. Individuals with a low threshold engage in collective behaviour before others do, and those with higher thresholds only after a large proportion of the population has adopted it. Therefore, the rate of adoption depends *both* upon individual thresholds and the proportion of individuals who have adopted an innovation.

To improve hand-hygiene routines, it may be very important to enhance interaction and exchange information (or staff) between departments that have changed their performance and those that have not yet achieved this.

Related to social network theories are *social influence theories*. These are theories that focus on existing norms and values in the social network of professionals. They assume that performance in daily practice is not usually based on a conscious consideration of (dis)advantages of specific behaviour, but on the routines that are observed in others and on the social norms in the network that define appropriate performance (Mittman *et al*. 1992). Professional cultures in a specific work setting often develop collective solutions for collective problems in the network (Greer 1988). Daily work in healthcare brings about many uncertainties as to the best management. In solving these uncertainties, most care providers are not influenced primarily by the scientific literature, but more by an exchange of opinions with peers and important others in the network, for instance during formal meetings or informal contacts. Change often takes place only after the achievement of local consensus. Local communication, interactions within the social network, the views of opinion leaders, the expectations of significant peers and the availability of local education are all important factors in an effective implementation of innovations or changes. For our example of hand hygiene, this means that we need to study interactions within the teams, opinions of the leaders within the teams and the way people influence each other. So, barriers to better hand hygiene may be the lack of mutual control and accountability or the lack of leaders with a positive attitude towards regularly washing and disinfecting their hands. Implementation strategies need to be adapted to the specific characteristics of the social setting and to the patterns of interaction and influence in that setting.

The role of *local opinion leaders* is seen as particularly important in these social network and social influence theories. They are considered, within their setting,

as respected persons with great influence in a specific field. They are not the innovators, but can be regarded as role models for the network, and they act as facilitator, supporter and problem solver in the change process. Through their place in the network or their informal contacts they can easily facilitate the diffusion of information. Opinion leaders represent the social norms within the network and therefore others trust them to appraise innovations against existing social norms and the specific demands of the local situation. The presence of such important key persons within social networks in healthcare has been confirmed in a number of studies (Stross 1996). Paulussen (1994; Paulussen *et al*. 1995), for instance, studied the dissemination of information about acquired immune deficiency syndrome (AIDS) in high schools. He showed that contact between colleagues and social norms within the group were the best predictors of the awareness and use of the information in the classroom. Interestingly, while Grimshaw *et al*. (2000) were able to identify opinion leaders in a number of secondary care settings within the UK health service, they were unable to identify such individuals within primary care.

A programme to improve hand hygiene in hospitals using social influence theories needs to focus on ensuring that the key persons in the network are on board and to give them a modelling role. It also needs to focus on changing the social norms with respect to hand hygiene within the teams, as well as mutual control and accountability with respect to the desired behaviour.

Theories on factors related to patients

Patient expectations and behaviours, or the perception of care providers of these expectations and behaviours, can have a strong influence on the care provided and therefore on achieving changes in patient care. Patients influence the care delivered by their decisions to seek healthcare by expressing, explicitly or implicitly, their expectations, preferences or demands for specific diagnostic or therapeutic actions, by their adherence to treatment and advice, and by the way they manage and cope with their illness. Patients can be seen as co-producers of the outcomes of care, as well as co-producers of the type of care provided. So, patients can also influence change in clinical practice, particularly when they are informed about the desired performance, adhere to it and demand it from their care providers. In the case of poor hand hygiene, patients could remind or even demand that nurses and doctors wash or disinfect their hands before touching them.

Currently, no theories are available that directly focus on changing clinical practice and implementing innovations through the patient as the mediator (patient-mediated interventions). Theories that indirectly relate to this type of change interventions are, for instance, theories on healthcare seeking, the 'Health Belief Model', theories on self-management and coping with illness, or theories on patient empowerment and shared decision making. For instance, patients may be motivated directly by change agents to seek or demand specific treatment or advice from their care providers.

The Health Belief Model suggests that individuals consider the advantages and disadvantages of specific actions and then take a rational decision (Janz and Becker 1984). Change is often the result of a trigger, a 'cue to action', which may be derived from the mass media or a social network. The change agent may make use of such triggers to influence the health beliefs of the community. In a study by Domenighetti et al. (1988) in Switzerland, an attempt was made to reduce the number of hysterectomies, first by feedback on variations in operations done to the gynaecologists involved. This was not successful. Next, a campaign through the mass media (journal, radio, television) was used to inform the public in one county about unnecessary hysterectomies. This patient-mediated action reduced the number of hysterectomies in subsequent years by 26%, while it stayed at the same level in the rest of the country. The hypothesis was that the mass media campaign influenced both patients and doctors, the latter because they anticipated new knowledge and expectations from their patients. Mass media campaigns have proved to be influential, particularly on patient participation in achieving high vaccination and screening rates (Grilli et al. 1998).

One hypothesis, often found in the literature, is that to provide information to the public on the quality and outcomes of hospitals or practices influences patient behaviour and will also influence improvements in healthcare through changes in patient demands – so-called public reporting (Marshall et al. 2000a,b). For instance, public reporting about infection rates and hygiene in different hospitals may influence patient decisions as to the hospital in which they want to be treated or operated on. However, research shows that people seldom behave as rational decision makers (Lupton et al. 1991; Salisbury 1989; Hibbard 1988). A review on the effect of public reporting showed that lay people often

do not understand the information and do not use it in their decisions to seek healthcare (Marshall et al. 2000a).

Theories on increased autonomy and empowering of patients emphasise the positive effects of increasing the role and involvement of patients in their care. By giving them a larger role, they influence the performance of professionals as well. The preferences of patients can be included in or be decisive in decisions as to what type of care is provided. Care providers may give extensive information on alternative treatments and share the final decision with the patient (Elwyn et al. 1999; Charles et al. 1997; Coulter 1997). Specific 'decision aids' can be used to provide information on the effects and risks of treatments. However, the effects of empowering patients and shared decision making are, as yet, largely unclear (Wensing and Grol 2000). This approach probably only works with well-informed and well-educated patients who are not seriously ill. Factors important in the effective involvement of patients in healthcare probably have to do with both the skills of the care providers and the age, skills, knowledge and attitude of the patients, but these factors need to be further investigated. For our case of hand hygiene, this suggests that patients could be actively involved and might be given a role in checking and improving handwashing and disinfection routines.

Theories on professional development

Professionals (such as physicians and nurses) have a body of knowledge that is not easily accessible to non-professionals and that is highly valued by society because of its practical relevance to citizens. Theory on professional development specifies the development of professions and professionals, which comprises a number of factors that may influence changes in professional behaviour (Freidson 1970). This theory has its background in sociology, but more recently it has been elaborated in other disciplines such as management science (Mintzberg 1996). Professions have usually succeeded in obtaining a monopoly of practice in their field of work and a certain degree of autonomy in their decisions. Access to the professions is based on training and examination, which are controlled by members of the profession.

Professional development can influence behaviour change in different ways. Firstly, professional standards influence the behaviour of individual professionals, so innovations consistent with these standards are easier to implement. That professions have a strong internal orientation means that members' main loyalty often tends to be given to their profession rather than to the healthcare organisations in which they practice (Blane 1982). Standards on hand hygiene set by surgeons or by nurses and controlled by surgeon leaders or by nurse leaders are very important in a change of handwashing and disinfection routines. Professions also produce, assess and transfer new knowledge in their field by being involved in research, theory and knowledge transfer. Innovations consistent with the developing body of knowledge in a profession are more likely to be implemented than are other innovations.

The degree of professional development (weaker or stronger) can be characterised in terms of a number of factors, which can be seen as indicators of more or less influence over individual professionals, such as:

- Obligatory training programmes with examinations for individuals who want to become professionals;
- Protection of the area of practice from non-professionals through laws and regulations;
- Established systems for dealing with medical errors and patient complaints;
- Explicit professional standards, such as clinical guidelines and protocols;
- Obligatory continuing education, quality improvement, accreditation and recertification schemes.

The dynamics of professional development are influenced by different factors (Raad voor de Volksgezondheid en Zorg 2000), such as the extent of specialisation of knowledge [the expanding knowledge base stimulates further (super)professionalisation],of self-interest (avoiding changes that threaten their professional autonomy and status, particularly in competition with other professions regarding specific areas of work) or of the extent of contact with other professions (professional development is influenced by interdisciplinary contacts).

For our example on hand hygiene, this theory particularly emphasises the importance of using professional pride, professional standards and professional loyalties and self-interest to transfer the idea that something needs to be done about poor hand hygiene. National guidelines should be 'reinvented' by a profession and adopted as the professional standard. Perhaps, even, use could be made of competition between professions in meeting the standards.

Theories on leadership

Formal or informal leaders can be very influential in changing clinical practice or the implementation of new procedures or processes. Effective leadership is assumed to promote, guarantee or (in some circumstances) block an innovation. Such power or influence can be based on different sources (Donaldson 1995):

- Formal authority;
- Control over scarce resources;
- Possession of information, expertise or skills needed to achieve specific, valued aims;
- Being part of a strong social network;
- Belonging to a dominant culture.

It is probable that specific types of leadership are effective for specific innovations in specific settings. For instance, to change the culture and mission of a hospital on the prevention of infections a different leader may be required to that needed to implement a new operation technique or a new antibiotics protocol.

Ross and Offerman (1997) make a distinction between two types of leadership – transactional and transformational leadership. The first type of leader provides support in achieving concrete targets, while the second type is particularly effective in changing the culture in the organisation and the ambitions of the people who work there.

Surveys, case studies and general management literature all underline the importance of the involvement and commitment of leaders (the top management) of a healthcare organisation in the implementation of valuable changes in patient care (Weiner *et al*. 1997; Rodgers *et al*. 1993). A systematic review of 39 studies showed that, when the leaders of an organisation became involved in management by objectives, the productivity increased by a factor of five (Rodgers *et al*. 1993). Satisfaction of the staff was also influenced by the extent of active involvement of the top managers.

So, effective implementation of guidelines on infection prevention or hand hygiene requires a good understanding of who the formal and informal leaders in an organisation or team are, how they use their power or influence and how this can be used optimally within a plan aimed at specific changes in patient care. The following factors represent an elementary summary of the main characteristics of leaders within leadership theories:

- Leader traits (e.g. their intelligence, initiative and self-confidence);
- Leader behaviours (e.g. the degree of orientation towards tasks, and the relationships with others);
- Power-sharing styles [e.g. autocratic (or structuring) or democratic (participative)];
- Contingencies (e.g. how much the organisation or group likes and trusts the leader, or how powerful the

leader is with respect to the group or organisation);
- Perceptions of and attributions made to leaders by others;
- Transformational leader behaviours (e.g. intellectual stimulation or inspirational motivation).

Inadequate hand hygiene could, at least in part, be traced back to a lack of interest and commitment in this area by the managers and leaders in the teams and hospitals (*Box 2.4*). They need to make the active prevention of infections part of the mission and culture of the hospital, and they need to support it intellectually as well as by providing resources for it and by setting up registration systems on infections (Teare *et al.* 2001).

Box 2.4 The case of hand hygiene

The first step in introducing a national, evidence-based guideline to control hospital infections in the Netherlands was to select six key recommendations concerning washing and disinfecting hands, for which it was assumed there were considerable implementation problems. These were described in concrete terms and subsequently presented in a written questionnaire to 120 doctors, nurses and paramedics from hospitals and nursing homes. The aim was to identify the most important problems impeding optimal use of the guidelines in daily care. The problems were within the care providers themselves, their social context and the organisational context (table below). A variety of problems were relevant in the implementation of this complex issue, which needed a variety of strategies and measures to be effective in changing performance. The problems can be explained within the context of various theories presented in this chapter.

Interventions aimed at improving hand hygiene
On the basis of the analysis of implementation problems and the theories presented in this chapter a well-balanced plan to improve hand hygiene could be drawn up, and include activities like:
- Folder with an attractive layout that contains the concrete guidelines and relevant scientific evidence, as well as the concrete benefits of the new actions;
- Team meetings to discuss the guidelines, to translate these into concrete targets for improvement, to find out where the problems in using the guidelines lie and to draw up a plan together to ensure that guidelines are better implemented;
- Formal protocol for the hospital, prepared by the teams themselves, but endorsed by management and spread throughout the entire institution;
- New soap and towels to reduce skin irritation of the hands, with disinfectant next to each patient's bed;
- Continuous monitoring and registration of infections, with regular feedback at team and hospital level, and comparison between teams;
- (Opinion) leaders and team managers to observe the hand-hygiene routines regularly and give feedback;
- Reminders for physicians, nurses and paramedics at specific moments and locations;
- External support to help the team to achieve its targets.

Consideration has to be given to the adequate mix of strategies and measures that would prove feasible, affordable and lead to the best results, and careful thought should be given to the order in which these are used and how progress is determined.

Problems experienced in following hand–hygiene guidelines (*N* = 120; Grol and Grimshaw 2003)			
Level	Relevant factors	Problems/barriers to change	Percentage considering an item as a real problem or barrier to implementation
Individual professional	Cognitions	I seldom see any complications	61
		Hard evidence for guideline is lacking	43
	Attitudes and motivation	Repeated washing harms and irritates hands	81
		Takes more time, which we do not have	50
	Routines	I forget to do it because of pressure of work	65
		I quickly revert to old routines	49
Team/unit	Social influence and leadership	Nobody pays attention or checks up on it	50
		Management is not interested in the subject	45
Hospital	Organisational and systems factors	There is no time for it during normal work	61
		No guidelines on this area in hospital	49
	Economic factors	Limited sanitary facilities in hospital	42

THEORIES ON FACTORS RELATED TO THE ORGANISATIONAL AND ECONOMICAL CONTEXT

Theories on factors related to the organisational and economical context are particularly relevant to change in patient care in structural, administrative, economic or organisational conditions and reforms (e.g. a better organisation of the care processes, a different division of tasks and roles, a change in the culture in the work setting or the collaboration between professionals) and in economic factors (e.g. the available resources, equipment or reimbursement system). The following (largely related and overlapping) theoretical approaches are explained in this section:
▪ Theories of innovative organisations;
▪ Theory of quality management;
▪ Process re-engineering theory;
▪ Complexity theory;
▪ Theory of organisational learning;
▪ Theories of organisational culture;
▪ Economic theories.

Theories of innovative organisations

Theories of innovative organisations focus on the characteristics of organisations that determine whether and to what extent they are able to implement innovations (Wolfe 1994). Some organisations adopt innovations quicker and more easily than other organisations do. A considerable number of studies have been conducted in this area; for instance, a systematic review of 23 studies on the influence of different features of organisations on the innovativeness of organisations was conducted by Damanpour (1991). The results of that review are summarised in *Table 2.2*. Innovativeness seems to be predicted by, for instance, a high level of specialisation, by functional differentiation and a high level of professionalism, by decentralised decision

Table 2.2 Expected relationships between characteristics of organisations and innovativeness (Damanpour 1991)		
Characteristic	Expected relation	Explanation
Specialisation	Positive	A diversity of specialists leads to more knowledge and exchange of ideas
Functional differentiation	Positive	Growth of coalitions between professionals working in different units who collaborate on improving the systems
Professionalism	Positive	More professionalism increases self-confidence and willingness to change existing situations
Formalisation	Negative (not confirmed)	Flexibility and less emphasis on regulations promote innovation, partly by a greater openness
Centralisation	Negative	Concentration of power blocks innovation, while involvement of shop-floor workers increases commitment to change
Attitude of management towards change	Positive	Positive attitude in management leads to a culture that stimulates innovation
Available technical competence	Positive	More technical knowledge and skills lead to better understanding of new technical concepts and to easier implementation
Management intensity for innovation	Positive	More managers provide the leadership, co-ordination and support required
Budget, reserves	Positive	More budget and reserves make it possible to finance innovations and the costs of their implementation, to overcome problems and to explore new ideas
External communication	Positive	Good communication with other organisations stimulates exchange of innovations
Internal communication	Positive	Good internal communication stimulates diffusion and acceptance of new ideas
Vertical differentiation	Negative (not confirmed)	Hierarchy and different levels in organisation hamper communication as well as dissemination of innovations

making, by better technical knowledge, by good internal and external communication, and by a positive attitude to change among the leaders and managers. Such characteristics of innovative organisations differed, however, between commercial and not-for-profit organisations, between industry and service organisations and between single and multifaceted innovations.

Scott (1990) applied organisational models to healthcare organisations. He underlined the importance of a distinction between different types of innovation (e.g. medical, technical or administrative change) and different types of healthcare organisations that need to implement changes. Improvement of hand hygiene demands both technical (e.g. new equipment or materials) and administrative innovations (monitoring systems for infections, new guideline arrangements at the team level). The size of a hospital proved to be related to successful implementation of both technical and administrative innovations. Most healthcare institutions are professional bureaucracies in which professionals have considerable autonomy and authority. Specific individuals, more than the organisation as a whole, were shown to be responsible for and influential in achieving specific changes. Decision making about innovations often takes place in specific units, for example technological innovations, such as introducing new imaging equipment, are dominated by specific professionals (e.g. radiologists). To change hygiene routines it is important to determine the people in the hospital who are likely to be most influential in the process of change (e.g. microbiologist, infection-control managers, nurse leaders). Centralisation and strict hierarchical relations proved to block change. More innovations were found in specialised hospitals and in larger hospitals. In hospitals with larger budgets more technological innovations were observed, while in hospitals with smaller budgets more administrative innovations were seen. Contacts between institutions also influence the extent to which innovations spread.

Theory of quality management

Total quality management (TQM), sometimes presented under the title of continuous quality improvement (CQI), is a theory on the continuous improvement of (multidisciplinary) processes in healthcare with the aim to better meet the needs of the customers (Blumenthal and Kilo 1998; Shortell *et al*. 1998). TQM emphasises the understanding and improvement of work processes and systems aimed at changing the organisation as

a whole. Inadequate performance is not seen as an individual problem, but as a system failure; real change can only be achieved by changing the system (Berwick 1989). Changing the organisational culture, a clear leadership and team building are important components of this approach. It was introduced into healthcare around the 1990s, after successful use in other industries (Batalden and Stoltz 1993; Berwick *et al*. 1990; Berwick 1989; Laffel and Blumenthal 1989). Basic principles of TQM are (Plsek *et al*. 2003):

- *Comprehensive, organisation-wide effort to improve quality.* Systematic activities at all levels of the organisation; everybody is involved.
- *Understanding processes and systems.* All work in healthcare involves the execution of processes. Processes need to be defined continuously and redesigned to improve patient care. Processes are embedded within one another and linked in complex ways.
- *Patient- (or customer-) centred focus.* Processes and systems exist to produce outputs that provide a benefit for or meet the needs of patients, families and society. Customers can be internal (e.g. a laboratory technician) or external (a patient, a pharmacist who must provide a medication). TQM encourages such customer thinking throughout the organisation.
- *Understanding variation.* The outcomes of processes and systems are variable (e.g. patients will not always take medication or physicians do not always provide the required care). Some of the variation results from intended and some from unintended causes; some is desirable and some is not, and some may even be harmful. TQM focuses on understanding the causes of variation.
- *Pursuit of continuous improvement.* An effective TQM system should facilitate continuous improvements and redesigns of care processes by encouraging alternating cycles of change, followed by relative stability, followed by more change and so on (Berwick 1998).
- *Management by facts and continuous learning.* Fundamental to TQM is the commitment to using data and a logical process to build knowledge and promote ongoing learning in the organisation. The concept of systematically building knowledge through disciplined data collection, evidence-based practice and experimentation lies at the foundation of all effective TQM.
- *Positive view of people.* While some see individual professionals as the cause of all problems and inefficiencies, TQM sees them as the ultimate source of knowledge on how to improve work. TQM seeks to

engage the people who actually do the work in efforts designed to improve the work. This requires ongoing training for all staff, an understanding of processes and systems and multidisciplinary teamwork.

- *Key role of leadership*. The need for an effective and visionary leadership is a central theme in TQM. Without strong leadership and an organisational infrastructure to support quality management, improvement may not happen or may quickly dissipate. Leaders must be actively involved in the initiation and support for all improvement activities (Berwick and Nolan 1998).

To succeed in making TQM into a success the care providers involved need knowledge about the desired improvement, about the care processes and about variation in performance (content knowledge), as well as technical knowledge on improvement methods and techniques (Batalden and Stoltz 1995).

Berwick and Nolan (1998) and Batalden and Stoltz (1995) strongly emphasise the use of Plan–Do–Study–Act cycles (PDSA cycles) to improve processes in care provision. Such cycles use continuous learning about change, by introducing a change and next reflecting on it. Improvements in a system usually demand various cycles of change, instead of achieving the implementation of change by one great design. Before starting a PDSA cycle, three crucial questions need to be asked (Langley *et al.* 1996):

- What do we want to achieve – the formulation of specific, ambitious targets for change, in the definitions of which leaders play an active role;
- How do we know that the change is an improvement – by measuring or monitoring performance, particularly to support change;
- Which changes lead to improvement – selection of optimal strategies for change.

Relating the theory to our example of improving hand hygiene, we do not need to focus so much on professional behaviour, but on understanding the processes in the organisation related to hand hygiene and infection control, setting ambitious targets for change and applying PDSA cycles while continuously monitoring the progress made. Leaders in the organisation need to support these activities and create a culture in which such change in hand-hygiene routines is possible.

Shortell *et al.* (1995) examined the relationships between organisational culture, quality-improvement processes and selected outcomes in hospitals. They found that what really matters is whether or not a hospital has a culture that supports quality-improvement work. A participative, flexible, risk-taking organisational culture significantly relates to quality-improvement implementation. Quality-improvement implementation, in turn, is positively associated with greater perceived patient outcomes and human resource development.

Gustafson and Hundt (1995) analysed a series of studies and showed that successful innovation in an organisation is related to a customer focus (particularly understanding their needs), to support of the innovation by the top leaders, to keeping to the mission of the organisation and to gaining information about best practices in other organisations.

Despite the high expectations, quality-management initiatives have not been very successful so far, according to Blumenthal and Kilo (1998) who interviewed many experts in this field. One of the reasons is that, while most managers were very positive about the approach, it proved crucial to involve physicians and to focus the change efforts on clinical, patient-oriented improvements instead of on reduction of costs or changes in the organisation of care.

Process re-engineering theory

Theories on process re-engineering, such as business process redesign (BPR) and disease management, focus on better organising and managing the care processes for specific patient categories in such a way that optimal care is provided, patients needs are better met and costs are reduced when possible. Effective change is often better achieved by redesigning or better organising multidisciplinary care processes than by influencing professional decision making, according to these theories. It usually includes top-down, management driven approaches, in which current practices and processes are analysed, reconsidered and basically redesigned (Rogers 2003). Most of the time these approaches include the organisation of new collaborations between care providers, a different allocation of tasks, the efficient transfer of information, the efficient scheduling of appointments and contacts, and the use of new types of health professionals. The patient and his or her disease is put at the centre and not the interests of different, involved care providers and professionals (Hunter 2000). Often one person (the case manager) coordinates the process. The approach is mostly applied to change and improve the care for chronically ill patients (Wagner *et al.* 1996). The theory behind disease management is that resources can be used more effectively if the patient becomes the pivot around which healthcare is organised

(Hunter 2000; Hunter and Fairfield 1997). Specific guidelines and care pathways are used to determine exactly what care should be provided by whom at what time, and in what setting, for each part of the care process. Traditional boundaries between disciplines are thus less relevant, and multidisciplinary collaboration is crucial. Wagner (2000) studied the influence of care teams in chronic disease management and found that effective chronic care generally relies strongly on multidisciplinary teams. By the delegation of responsibilities from physicians to other team members, critical elements of care that doctors may not have the training or the time for are performed competently.

Successful intervention programmes for patients with chronic diseases shared specific characteristics (Casalino *et al*. 2003; Wagner *et al*. 1996), such as case management, performance feedback to individual care providers, use of clinical practice guidelines and explicit protocols and pathways, use of disease registries, electronic or chart-based reminder systems, and reorganisation of the practice to better meet the needs of patients. In current clinical practice, however, non-physician personnel, who need to perform many new tasks, do not have the time to do so and have not acquired enough skills and knowledge for the new jobs. Usually, incentives to improve care processes are missing and many doctors are reluctant to share care with others (Wagner *et al*. 1996).

To improve hand hygiene, the consequence of these theories is that infection control and hand hygiene are seen as processes that encompass a series of related actions and that these processes need to be analysed, reconsidered and redesigned. Handwashing and disinfection need to be organised in a way that they fit more logically into the normal care-provision activities. Many professionals complain about the lack of time and the lack of practical tools for hand hygiene. Redesigning the care processes must lead to more efficient use of time.

Complexity theory

Complexity theory, a recent approach, is a theory of systems behaviour and systems change, which starts from the assumption that the world of healthcare has become increasingly complex and that it is important to observe and improve systems as a whole instead of focussing on separate parts or components. The theory sees most systems in healthcare, whether it be a hospital, a primary care team or the care organised around a specific disease (stroke, diabetes), as 'complex adaptive systems'. These are defined "as a collection of individual agents (components, elements) with the freedom to act in ways that are not always totally predictable, and whose actions are interconnected, so that one agent's actions changes the context for the other agents" (Plsek and Greenhalgh 2001). Other examples of such systems are a flock of birds, a colony of termites, a family, the financial market or the immune system.

Complex systems have a large number of components that continuously interact, and these interactions are more important than the discrete actions of the individual agents or components (Sweeny and Griffiths 2002). Therefore, such systems cannot be understood adequately by analysis of their constituent parts. In addition, the boundaries of such systems are fuzzy; they are embedded in other systems and members of one system can simultaneously be members of other systems. Therefore it is difficult to understand a system without reference to the other systems.

One of the conclusions of the theory is that, to improve patient care in such complex systems, comprehensive plans with detailed targets for parts of the systems are seldom very effective. The focus should be the system as a whole with simple goals or minimum specifications (Plsek and Wilson 2001). This is because the behaviour of a complex system is usually very unpredictable over time. Small influences in one part of the system often have a large impact on other parts of the system and outside the system in other systems. In the UK, one scandal in healthcare (the Bristol case) and the subsequent analysis of this case (the Bristol Inquiry) had a nationwide effect on quality-improvement policies. A single report linking the mumps–measles–rubella (MMR) vaccine with the subsequent development of autism had a large impact on the national MMR vaccination rate in the UK (Sweeny and Griffiths 2002). Particularly when there is disequilibrium, new behaviour is often produced in an unpredictable way, without a coordinated plan. In countries such as the UK and the Netherlands, geographically centralised offices for out of hours and emergency care have emerged spontaneously, without central planning, as a reaction to workload and a shortage of primary care doctors.

This does not mean that such systems are completely unsuitable for analysis and improvement – observation of complex systems (such as a flock of birds, a family or a team in a hospital) shows a large amount of self-organisation. The agents within the system seem to follow a few, simple, shared rules of behaviour. Overall patterns of behaviour can be seen – a set of internalised rules that seem to guide the system in a certain direction. Everyone in the system seems to know how to behave adaptively to fulfil the aim of the system. These patterns may be studied and used in setting up change within the system, because they relate to the intrinsic motivation of the system. They are called 'attractors': good practice spreads more quickly when leaders and change agents acknowledge and respect these patterns or attractors. Change is adopted more easily when compatible with the attractors of a team, a practice or an organisation.

Infection control in a hospital, including hand-hygiene routines, may be seen as a complex system in which many components and agents influence each other, a system embedded in other wider systems, such as the hospital as a whole. According to complexity theory it is important not to focus on single parts of this system, such as the handwashing routines of nurses. Rather, it is important to set broad targets for change, observe the system as a whole, find the attractors and link actions to these.

We were involved in a hospital where, on the basis of the publication of a new national infection guideline, the staff were not motivated to spend much time on hand hygiene. This changed after the occurrence of an uncontrollable infection on one of the wards. This small event, which linked well with the intrinsic motivation about the kind of care provided at the hospital, resulted in new, hospital-wide policies on hand hygiene, a plan for improvement with the commitment of all the staff, and large improvements in handwashing and disinfection.

Theory of organisational learning

A 'learning organisation' has been defined as 'an organisation skilled at creating, acquiring and transferring knowledge, and at modifying its behaviour to reflect new knowledge and insights' (Ashford 2004). Most authors who have written about organisational learning seem to agree that both the individuals and the organisation learn. Individuals learn as agents for the organisation and the knowledge acquired is stored in the memory of the organisation (e.g. embedded in routines; Örtenblad 2002). Learning is seen as a characteristic of the organisation because knowledge and expertise is kept, even though individuals leave the organisation (DiBella *et al.* 1996; Nevis *et al.* 1995). Effective organisations continuously aim to improve knowledge within the organisation (Garside 1998).

The boundaries between the concepts of *organisational learning* and *knowledge management* are unclear. A review of the organisational literature on both concepts shows that learning organisations are associated mostly with training, organisational development and human resources development, while knowledge management is associated mostly with information technology, intellectual capital and the use of information systems (Scarbrough and Swan 2001). So, in knowledge management there is a stronger emphasis on information and communication technology that can support knowledge transfer within organisations (Garavelli *et al.* 2002). The key of both theories is that it is only through the learning of individuals that organisational routines are changed. Therefore, improving organisational learning ability should first include the creation of favourable conditions for learning by individuals (Lähteenmäki *et al.* 2001; Senge 1990). The literature appears, however, to be richer on descriptions of types of learning organisations than on factors associated with increased learning ability and on how to apply the theory within healthcare organisations. Ashford (2004) mentions the following barriers to effective organisational learning:

- Fragmentation: the traditional analytical approach to problem solving in which the idea is to break problems down into manageable pieces and analyse them independently of interactions – redesign of delivery processes has little effect if the underlying 'mental models' adopted in the organisation are not changed;
- Reactiviness: the tendency to change only in reaction to outside forces, rather than try to strive for continuous improvement of products and services;
- Competition: a focus on competition rather than cooperation leads to emphasis on looking good rather than being good, and to short-term measurable results over addressing underlying problems.

Organisations usually have formal and informal structures for the acquisition, dissemination and integration of knowledge in the organisation (DiBella *et al.* 1996; Nevis *et al.* 1995). Whether these structures are effective depends on the culture in the organisation (see below). Learning organisations can be distinguished from non-learning organisations by, for instance:

- External orientation, awareness of conditions and practices outside the organisation;
- Shared perception of the gap between actual and desired performance;
- Striving for specific, quantifiable measures, using measurement as a source of learning;
- Experimental mind-set, curiosity about trying new things, 'failures' are not punished;

- Climate of openness, accessibility of information, sharing errors and problems, debate and conflict are acceptable;
- Continuous education, ongoing commitment to education, growth and development at all levels of the organisation;
- Variety of methods, procedures and systems used;
- New ideas and methods supported by many employees at all levels;
- Involved leadership, frequent interactions with members of organisation, actively involved in education.

According to Weggeman (1997) the most important task of the leaders of a 'knowledge intensive organisation', such as healthcare institutes and practices, is concerned with facilitating collective learning experiences of individuals in the organisation. Success factors that achieve this include involving professionals in defining the collective ambitions of the organisation, a structure with teams and groups that are largely self-responsible for their work, investment in information exchange (using many media) and continuous feedback.

We may hypothesise on the basis of these theories that improving hand-hygiene routines will be more successful in a learning organisation, where effective infection control belongs to the collective expertise of the hospital, where people at different levels are eager to acquire the knowledge about best practices in infection control and how to solve the problem of poor hand hygiene, and where experiences and information about better hand hygiene are shared and exchanged between different units and teams.

Theories on organisational culture

Theories on organisational culture are based on the assumption that culture is related to performance and that a culture can or should be altered to change that performance (Scott *et al.* 2003a). As a consequence, there is increasing interest in managing organisational culture as a lever for healthcare improvement (Scott *et al.* 2003b). However, there is little consensus among scholars over the precise meaning of 'organisational culture'. Among the many overlapping and competing definitions, two broad streams can be distinguished. The first sees culture as 'something an organisation possesses' – an 'attribute' of organisations – while the second stream tends to regard 'culture' as defining the whole character and experience of organisational life (basically, an organisation 'is' a culture; Scott *et al.* 2003b; Cameron and Quinn

1999). Scott *et al.* (2003a) reviewed the evidence for a relationship between organisational culture and healthcare performance. They found that four of ten studies provided supportive evidence that culture and performance are linked. For example, cultures in healthcare that emphasise group affiliation, teamwork and coordination have been associated with better implementation of CQI practices and higher functional health status in coronary artery bypass graft patients. By contrast, organisational cultures that emphasise formal structures and regulations appear to be associated negatively with quality improvement activity.

Scott *et al.* (2003b) identified a number of possible facilitators that could stimulate planned change in the culture of an organisation, such as a critical mass of employees in favour of the programme aimed at changing the culture, realistic time frames to implement the types of complex and multi-level changes and consideration of the impact of change on the different subgroups that exist within a culture, and the design of appropriate policies to accommodate this.

A conceptual model to describe different types of organisational culture is *the competing values framework* (Quinn and Rohrbaugh 1981), characterised by a two-dimensional space that reflects different value orientations. The first dimension is the flexibility–control axis, which shows the degree to which the organisation emphasises change or stability. The second is the internal–external axis, which addresses the organisation's choice between focusing on activities that occur within the organisation or outside in the external environment. This typology leads to four ideal cultural orientations that correspond to four major models in organisational theory (*Figure 2.2*; Stock and McDermott 2001):

- Group or clan culture emphasises flexibility and change and is further characterised by strong human relations, affiliation and a focus on the internal organisation;
- Developmental culture also emphasises flexibility, but is externally oriented – the focus is primarily on growth, creativity and adaptation to the external environment;
- Rational culture is also externally focused, but is control oriented – the emphasis is on productivity and achievement, with objectives typically well-defined and external competition a primary motivating factor;
- Hierarchical culture emphasises stability with the focus on the internal organisation – this orientation is characterised by uniformity, coordination, internal efficiency and a close adherence to rules and regulations.

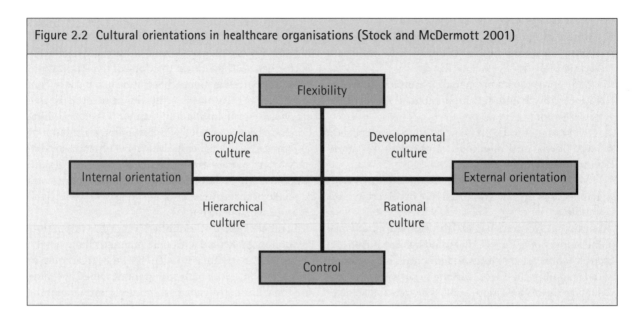

Figure 2.2 Cultural orientations in healthcare organisations (Stock and McDermott 2001)

Stock and McDermott (2001) found that higher levels of internal orientation, whether reflecting flexibility (group culture) or control (hierarchical culture), were negatively related to operational success and competitive outcomes in technology implementation. Higher levels of external orientation were positively related to competitive success. Marshall *et al.* (2003) asked managers in Primary Care Trusts in the UK about their perception of the culture of primary care practices and concluded that the culture is aimed mostly at internal stability and loyalty to the 'clan'.

To improve hand-hygiene routines, this theory emphasises the importance of creating an organisational culture that stimulates improvement of this aspect of healthcare delivery. Specific activities may be undertaken to make infection control a priority of the whole organisation, something that people in the organisation experience as part of their culture.

Economic theories

Economic theories have as their basis the assumption that individuals aim for optimisation of their goals; they make choices on the basis of shortage. People are sensitive to prices if a product concerns a large part of their income. Reimbursement can be used, therefore, to influence professional or organisational performance, and also healthcare. The type of reimbursement may determine whether innovations are implemented and changes achieved or not. Different reimbursement systems exist

(Barnum *et al.* 1995) and other systems have been proposed (Sonnad and Foreman 1997; Shaughnessy and Kurowski 1982). Reimbursement systems may be prospective (capitation, salary or budgets) or retrospective (fee-for-service or case-based payment). These may include some level of cost-sharing by patients (co-insurance rates, deductibles or prescription charges). Economic theory suggests that retrospective reimbursement systems provide incentives for an increased provision of services, development towards a more expensive mix of services and reluctance to use other services or providers. Prospective reimbursement systems provide incentives for decreased provision of services and avoidance of high-risk patients. Cost-sharing by patients provide incentives for reduced demand for healthcare, which leads to a reduced volume of services provided.

A review (Rice and Morrison 1994) showed that when patients have to pay extra out-of-pocket fees for their medical care, the consumption of care decreases, particularly for people with a low income. Physicians, however, may try to compensate a decreased consumption by patients through offering extra services, since they too strive to optimise their goals.

The type of reimbursement or reward can stimulate the implementation of changes and innovation in healthcare (Barnum *et al.* 1995). A distinction can be made between a fixed budget per period or per patient (salary, budget, capitation or subscription) and a fee-for-service system. Each has advantages and disadvantages. Fee for service stimulates additional actions and may lead to more contacts, prescriptions and referrals, and therefore to higher costs. Fixed budgets, however, have been shown to reduce the volume of care (prescriptions, admissions to hospital, etc.; Chaix-Couturier *et al*. 2000), but they may lead to reduced attention to patients, waiting lists, selection of low-risk patients or use of cheaper, less effective treatments (Barnum *et al*. 1995; Shimmura 1988). Fundholding for general practitioners has led, in the UK, to fewer prescriptions, although an effect on referral could not be demonstrated (Dixon and Glennerster 1995). The expectation is that financial incentives can improve the quality and volume of preventive care (Hughes and Yule 1992; Shimmura 1988). Besides reward, financial risks can also influence performance, because most care providers try to limit such risks (Kirkman-Liff *et al*. 1997).

In improving hygiene routines, the financial cost of hospital infections may be used as a motivator to induce change. However, rewards and incentives (both material and non-material) may be given to teams that succeed in improving their hygiene routines and in reducing the number of infections.

In summary, rewards, incentives and financial systems and measures can all influence both performance and the implementation of innovations, but their mechanism and predictable effect is not yet clear.

CONCLUSIONS

A number of theories on the implementation of innovations and change in practice are presented in this chapter along with some evidence for their value (*Box 2.5*). Although this overview is not exhaustive, it is clear that many of the theories described are not totally distinct, but overlap and build on previous theories or on basic concepts of change. However, this overview offers a broad description of the factors that

---

Box 2.5 Interventions aimed at improving hand hygiene: the evidence

What interventions to improve hand-hygiene practices might be effective? We found one specific systematic review of 22 studies that evaluated interventions to improve hand hygiene (Naikoba and Hayward 2001; see below). Most (15/22) took place on intensive care units and only three were randomised controlled trials. The main findings were:

- Educational interventions (training sessions, newsletters, classes and videos) were used in 11 studies and appeared to have only a short-term effect on handwashing practice;
- Reminders (posters, coloured signs, labels with messages, patients reminding staff) were evaluated in seven studies and shown to have a modest, but sustained, effect;
- Performance feedback (both personal and non-personal, both oral and written) was used in nine studies – the results suggest that this intervention can improve practice, but the effect stops if feedback is not continued;
- Introduction of new soap or hand rub and the adjustment of sinks had small or unclear effects only;
- Multifaceted interventions were applied in 11 studies, with programmes that combined, for instance, education, written materials, feedback and reminders. Some were hospital wide (Pittet *et al*. 2000; Larsson *et al*. 1997). Most of these programmes had a marked and sustained effect on both hand-hygiene practices and hospital-acquired infections.

Although some caution is needed when interpreting the evidence, the results show that a comprehensive plan, which targets different problems and barriers to change, with strategies at different levels (professional, team, patient and organisation), is probably required to achieve lasting changes in hand-hygiene routines.

Interventions	Number of studies	Conclusions
Education and/or information	11	Only short-term effects
Reminders	7	Modest, but sustained effects
Performance feedback	9	Effective, but effect stops if feedback is not continued
New soap and/or hand rub	3	Small effect for hand rub
Adjusted sinks	3	Unclear effect
Multifaceted interventions	11	Marked effects on practice and outcomes

may influence the success of change implementation. The different theories are based on different assumptions about human behaviour and behavioural or organisational change. The empirical evidence behind these assumptions is, for most of the approaches, limited, particularly in as far as their effectiveness and feasibility in healthcare is concerned. Nevertheless, it is possible to draw useful lessons from each of the theories and approaches. These are summarised in *Table 2.3*, along with specific lessons for improving hand hygiene, the illustrative condition used throughout this chapter.

However, as identified above, the different theories and models overlap, sometimes to a considerable extent. Some are eclectic and make use of several theories from social sciences, economics and organisational or management sciences (e.g. TQM). This is very logical – processes of change in healthcare are often very complex, too complex to be covered by a single model or theory. Therefore, in Chapter 3 we use elements from a number of different approaches to develop and underpin a comprehensive, step-wise approach to the implementation of innovations, guidelines, procedures and new practices in patient care.

Table 2.3 Lessons about implementation of change (derived from different theories) and to improve hand hygiene

Theory	Lessons for change implementation	Lessons for improving hand hygiene
Individual professionals		
Cognitive theory	Implementation needs to take into account the decision processes of professionals; they need good information and methods to support their decisions in practice	Provide convincing information to professionals and support their decision making on hand-hygiene routines
Educational theories	Implementation should be linked to the needs and motivation of professionals; intrinsic motivation is crucial; people change on the basis of experienced problems in practice	Involve professionals in finding solutions to the infection problem; define personal targets for improvement as well as individual 'learning plans'
Attitude theories – theory of planned behaviour	Implementation needs to focus on attitudes, perceived social norms and experienced control related to desired performance	Convince professionals about the importance of handwashing and show that they can do it and others feel it important that they do it
Motivation and stages of change theories	Implementation takes place in different (motivational) steps; analyse segments in target groups	Determine segments in the target groups who have different motivations to changing hygiene routines and tailor interventions to these motivations
Social interaction and context		
Social learning theory	Changing performance takes place through demonstration and modelling, and through reinforcement by others	Modelling of hand hygiene by 'leaders' and positive feedback of desired routines
Social network and influence theories	Local adaptation of innovations and use of local networks and opinion leaders in dissemination; identify innovators and key persons in the social network	Study the interaction in the team, determine the opinion leaders and use these to improve hygiene routines
Theories on patient influence	Implementation needs to focus on informing patients about optimal care and on involving them in the design of and in deciding on care	Patients are actively involved in reminding care providers about hygiene and in the redesign of routines
Theories on professional development	Importance of professional loyalty, pride, consensus; 'reinvention' of change proposal by professional body	Use of professional pride, standards and consensus; defining hand-hygiene targets and control by profession
Theories on leadership	Importance of involvement and commitment of leaders and (top) management in change process	Top management actively initiates and supports activities aimed at changing hygiene routines (*cont.*)

Table 2.3 (*cont.*) Lessons about implementation of change (derived from different theories) and to improve hand hygiene

Theory	Lessons for change implementation	Lessons for improving hand hygiene
Organisational and economic context		
Theory on innovative organisations	Implementation should take into account the type of organisation; decentralised decision making (teams) about innovation is crucial	Involve the most influential people in changing hygiene; teams develop their own plans for change
Theory of quality management	Improvement is a continuous cyclical process; plans for change are adapted continuously on the basis of previous experience; organisation-wide measures aimed at improving culture, collaboration, customer focus and processes	Reorganise work processes around hygiene and infection control; develop hospital-wide system to prevent infections; monitor progress and adapt plans for change continuously on the basis of new data
Process re-engineering theory	Change multidisciplinary care processes and collaboration, instead of individual decision making	Analyse and redesign the work processes related to hand hygiene, make these more efficient and practical
Complexity theory	Focus on the system as a whole, find patterns in behaviour (attractors) and link change plan to these	See infection control in hospital as a system with many agents; find patterns or attractors, define minimum specifications for change
Organisational learning theory	Create conditions within the organisation for continuous learning at all levels	Continuous learning and exchange of information about infections and better hygiene at all levels of the organisation
Theories on organisational culture	Changes in the culture can stimulate changes in performance: more teamwork, flexibility and external orientation	Work on improving the general culture in the hospital, in which infection control is seen as a priority
Economic theories	Importance of attractive rewards and (financial) incentives for effective implementation	Reward the decrease of infections with non-material or material and/or financial incentives (extra budget, staff, sabbatical leaves)

References

AHCPR (1994). *Benign Prostatic Hyperplasia: Diagnosis and Treatment*. AHCPR Publication 94-0583. Lockville: US Department of Health and Human Services.

Ajzen I (1991). The theory of planned behaviour. *Organ Behav Hum Dec*. **50**:179–211.

Ashford AJ (2004). *Behavioural Change in Professional Practice. Supporting the Development of Effective Implementation Strategies*. Newcastle upon Tyne: Centre for Health Services Research.

Bandura A (1986). *Social Foundation of Thought and Action: A Social Cognitive Theory*. New York: Prentice-Hall.

Bandura A (1997). The anatomy of stages of change. *Am J Health Promot*. **12**:8–10.

Barnum H, Kutzin J and Saxenian H (1995). Incentives and provider payment methods. *Int J Health Plan M*. **16**:23–45.

Batalden PB and Stoltz PK (1993). A framework for the continual improvement of health care. *J Qual Imp*. **19**:424–452.

Batalden PB and Stoltz PK (1995). Quality management and continual improvement of health care: a framework. *J Cont Educ Health Prof*. **15**:146–164.

Belongia EA and Schwartz B (1998). Strategies for promoting judicious use of antibiotics by doctors and patients. *BMJ* **317**:668–671.

Berwick DM (1989). Continuous improvement as an ideal in health care. *New Engl J Med*. **320**(1):53–56.

Berwick DM (1998). Developing and testing changes in delivery of care. *Ann Intern Med*. **128**:651–656.

Berwick DM and Nolan TW (1998). Physicians as leaders in improving health care. *Ann Intern Med*. **128**:289–292.

Berwick DM, Godfrey AB and Roessner J (1990). *Curing Health Care*. San Francisco: Jossey-Bass.

Blane D (1982). Health professions. In: Patrick DL and Scambler G (Eds). *Sociology as Applied to Medicine*. London: Bailliére Tindall.

Blumenthal D and Kilo CM (1998). A report card on Continuous Quality Improvement. *Milbank Q*. **76**:625–648.

Cameron KS and Quinn RE (1999). *Diagnosing and Changing Organizational Culture. Based on the Competing Values Framework*. Reading: Addison-Wesley.

Casalino MD, Gillies RR, Shortell, *et al*. (2003). External incentives, information technology, and organized processes to improve health care quality for patients with chronic diseases. *JAMA* **289**:434–441.

Chaix-Couturier C, Durand-Zaleski I, Jolly D, *et al*. (2000). Effects of financial incentives on medical practice: Results from a systematic review of the literature and methodological costs? *Int J Qual Health Care* **12**:133–142.

Charles C, Gafni A and Whelan T (1997). Shared decision making in the medical encounter: What does it mean? (Or it takes at least two to tango). *Soc Sci Med*. **44**:681–692.

Cohen SJ, Halvorsson HW and Gosselink CA (1994). Changing physician behavior to improve disease prevention. *Prev Med*. **23**:284–291.

Coulter A (1997). Partnerships with patients: The pros and cons of shared clinical decision-making. *J Health Serv Res Policy* **2**:112–121.

Damanpour F (1991). Organizational innovation: A meta-analysis of effects of determinants and moderators. *Acad Manage J*. **34**:555–590.

Davis DA and Taylor-Vaisey A (1997). Translating guidelines into practice: A systematic review of theoretic concepts, practical experience and research evidence in the adoption of clinical practice guidelines. *Can Med Assoc J*. **157**:408–416.

DiBella AJ, Nevis EC and Gould JM (1996). Understanding organizational learning capability. *J Manage Stud*. **33**:361–379.

Dixon J and Glennerster H (1988). What do we know about fundholding in general practice. *BMJ* **311**:727–730.

Domenighetti G, Luraschi P, Casabianca A, *et al.* (1988). Effect of information campaign by the mass media on hysterectomy rates. *Lancet* **ii**:1470–1473.

Donaldson L (1995). Conflict, power, negotiation. *BMJ* **310**:104–107.

Elwyn G, Edwards A and Kinnersley P (1999). Shared decision-making in primary care: The neglected second half of the consultation. *Br J Gen Pract*. **49**:477–482.

Festinger 1954 (1954). A theory of social comparison processes. *Hum Relat*. **7**:117–140.

Fox RD and Bennett NL (1998). Learning and change: Implications for continuing medical education. *BMJ* **316**:466–468.

Freidson E (1970). *Profession of Medicine*. New York: Dodds, Mead.

Garavelli AC, Gorgoglione M and Scozzi B (2002). Managing knowledge transfer by knowledge technologies. *Technovation* **22**:269–279.

Garside P (1998). Organisational context for quality: Lessons from the fields of organisational development and change management. *Qual Health Care* **7**(Suppl):S8–S15.

Gladwell M (2000). *The Tipping Point*. New York: Little Brown.

Gollwitzer PM and Oettingen G (1998). The emergence and implementation of health goals. *Psychol Health* **13**:687–715.

Green LW, Eriksen MP and Schor EL (1988). Preventive practices by physicians: Behaviorial determinants and potential interventions. *Am J Prev Med* **4**(Suppl):101–107.

Greer AL (1988). The state of the art versus the state of the science. The diffusion of new medical technologies into practice. *Int J Technol Assess Health Care* **4**:5–26.

Grilli R, Freemantle N, Minozzi S, *et al.* (1998). Impact of mass media on health services utilisation. The Cochrane Library, Issue 3. Oxford: Update Software.

Grimshaw JM, Greener J, Ibbotson T, *et al.* (2000). *Is the Involvement of Opinion Leaders in the Implementation of Research Findings a Feasible Strategy?* Mimeo. Aberdeen: Health Services Research Unit.

Grol R (1992). Implementing guidelines in general practice care. *Qual Health Care* **1**:184–191.

Grol R and Grimshaw J (2003). From best evidence to best practice: Effective implementation of change in patients' care. *Lancet* **362**:1225–1230.

Gustafson DH and Hundt AS (1995). Findings of innovation research applied to quality management principles for health care. *Health Care Manage Rev*. **20**:16–33.

Handwashing Liaison Group (1999). Handwashing: A modern measure with big effects. *BMJ* **318**:686.

Hibbard JH (1988). Consumers in a competition-based cost containment environment. *J Public Health* **16**:233–249.

Hobus P (1994). *Expertise van Huisartsen [Expertise of General Practitioners]*. Thesis. Maastricht: Universiteit Maastricht.

Holm HA (1998). Quality issues in continuing medical education. *BMJ* **316**:621–624.

Hughes D and Yule B (1992). The effect of per-item fees on the behaviour of general practitioners. *J Health Econ*. **11**:413–437.

Hunter DJ (2000). Disease management: Has it a future? It has a compelling logic, but it needs to be tested in practice. *BMJ* **320**:530.

Hunter DJ and Fairfield G (1997). Managed care: Disease management. *BMJ* **315**:50–53.

Janz NK and Becker MH (1984). The health belief model: A decade later. *Health Educ Q*. **11**:1–57.

Kirkman-Liff BL, Huijsman R, Grinten T van der and Brink G (1997). Hospital adaptation to risk-bearing: Managerial implications of changes in purchaser–provider contracting. *Health Policy* **39**:207–223.

Laffel G and Blumenthal D (1989). The case for using industrial quality management science in health care organization. *JAMA* **262**:2869–2873.

Lähteenmäki S, Toivonen J and Mattila M (2001). Critical aspects of organizational learning research and proposals for its measurement. *Br J Manage*. **12**:113–129.

Langley G, Nolan K, Nolan T, *et al.* (1996). *The Improvement Guide*. San Francisco: Jossey Bass.

Larsson E, Bryan J, Adler L, *et al.* (1997). A multi-faceted approach to changing hand-washing behavior. *Am J Infect Control* **25**:3–10.

Lewis AP and Bolden KJ (1989). General practitioners and their learning styles. *J Roy Coll Gen Pract*. **39**:187–189.

Lupton D, Donaldson C and Lloyd P (1991). Caveat emptor or blissful ignorance? Patients and the consumerist ethos. *Soc Sci Med*. **33**:559–568.

Maibach E and Murphy DA (1995). Self-efficacy in health promotion research and practice: Conceptualization and measurement. *Health Educ Res*. **10**:37–50.

Mann KV (1994). Educating medical students: Lessons from research in continuing education. *Acad Med*. **69**:41–47.

Marshall M, Shekelle P, Leatherman S, *et al.* (2000a). The public release of performance data. *JAMA* **283**:1866–1874.

Marshall M, Shekelle P, Leatherman S, *et al.* (2000b). Public disclosure of performance data: Learning from the US experience. *Qual Health Care* **9**:53–57.

Marshall M, Marrion R, Nelson E and Davies H (2003). Managing change in the culture of general practice. Qualitative case studies in primary care trusts. *BMJ* **327**:599–602.

Merriam SB (1996). Updating our knowledge of adult learning. *J Cont Educ Health Prof*. **16**:136–143.

Mintzberg H (1996). *Organisational Structures*. New York: Prentice Hall.

Mittman BS, Tonesk X and Jacobson PD (1992). Implementing clinical practice guidelines: Social influence strategies and practitioner behaviour change. *Qual Rev Bull*. **18**:413–422.

Moulding NT, Silagy CA and Weller DP (1999). A framework for effective management of change in clinical practice: Dissemination and implementation of clinical practice guidelines. *Qual Health Care* **8**:177–183.

Naikoba S and Hayward A (2001). The effectiveness of interventions aimed at increasing handwashing in healthcare works – a systematic review. *J Hosp Infect*. **47**:173–180.

Nevis EC, DiBella AJ and Gould JM (1995). Understanding organizations as learning systems. *Sloan Manage Rev*. **36**:73–85.

NHMRC (2000). *How to Put the Evidence into Practice: Implementation and Dissemination Strategies*. Canberra: NHMRC.

Norman G (2002). Research in medical education: Three decades of progress. *BMJ* **324**:1560–1562.

Norman GR and Schmidt HG (1992). The psychological basis of problem-based learning: A review of the evidence. *Acad Med*. **67**:557–565.

Nylenna M, Aasland OG and Falkum E (1996). Keeping professionally updated: Perceived coping and CME profiles among physicians. *J Cont Educ Health Prof*. **16**:241–249.

Orbell S, Hodgkins S and Sheeran P (1997). Implementation intentions and the theory of planned behavior. *Pers Soc Psychol Bull*. **23**:945–954.

Örtenblad A (2002). A typology of the idea of learning organization. *Manage Learn*. **33**(2):213–230.

Owen PA, Allerly LA, Harding KG, *et al*. (1989). General practitioners' continuing medical education within and outside their practice. *BMJ* **299**:238–240.

Paulussen TGW (1994). *Adoption and Implementation of AIDS Education in Dutch Secondary Schools*. Proefschrift. Maastricht: Universiteit Maastricht.

Paulussen T, Kok G, Schaalma H, *et al*. (1995). Diffusion of AIDS curricula among Dutch school teachers. *Health Educ Q*. **22**:227–243.

Pittet D, Hugonnet S, Harbarth S, *et al*. (2000). Effectiveness of a hospital-wide programme to improve compliance with hand hygiene. *Lancet* **356**:1307–1312.

Plsek PE and Greenhalgh T (2001). Complexity science: The challenge of complexity in health care. *BMJ* **323**:625–628.

Plsek PE and Wilson T (2001). Complexity, leadership, and management in healthcare organisations. *BMJ* **323**:746–749.

Plsek P, Solberg L and Grol R (2003). Total quality management and continuous quality improvement. In: Jones R, *et al*. (Eds). *Oxford Textbook of Primary Medical Care*. Oxford: Oxford University Press.

Pratt RJ, Pellowe C, Loveday HP, *et al*. (2001). The EPIC project: developing national evidence-based guidelines for preventing healthcare associated infections. Phase I: Guidelines for preventing hospital-acquired infections. Department of Health (England). *J Hosp Infect*. **47**(Suppl):S3–S82.

Prochaska JO and Velicer WF (1997). The transtheoretical model of health behavior change. *Am J Health Promot*. **12**:38–48.

Quinn R and Rohrbaugh I (1981). A competing values approach to organizational effectiveness. *Public Prod Rev*. **5**:122–140.

Raad voor de Volksgezondheid en Zorg (2000). *Professionals in de Gezondheidszorg [Professionals in Health Care]*. Zoetermeer: RVZ.

Rice T and Morrison KR (1994). Patient cost sharing for medical services: A review of the literature and implications for health care reform. *Med Care Rev*. **51**:235–287.

Riemsma RP, Pattenden J, Bridle C, *et al*. (2003). Systematic review of the effectiveness of stage based interventions to promote smoking cessation. *BMJ* **326**:1175–1177.

Rodgers R, Hunter JE and Rogers DL (1993). Influence of top management commitment on management program success. *J Appl Psychol*. **78**:151–155.

Rogers EM (1983). *Diffusion of Innovations*. New York: The Free Press.

Rogers EM (1995). *Diffusion of Innovations*, Fourth Edition. New York: The Free Press.

Rogers S (2003). Continuous quality improvement: Effects on professional patient outcomes (Protocol for a Cochrane review). The Cochrane Library, Issue 2. Oxford: Update Software.

Ross SM and Offerman LR (1997). Transformational leaders: Measurement of personality attributes and work group performance. *Pers Soc Psychol Bull*. **23**:1078–1086.

Salisbury CJ (1989). How do people choose their doctor? *BMJ* **299**:608–610.

Scarbrough H and Swan J (2001). Explaining the diffusion of knowledge management: The role of fashion. *Br J Manage*. **12**:3–12.

Schmidt H, Ed (1984). *Tutorials in Problem-Based Learning*. Assen/Maastricht: Van Gorcum.

Scott WR (1990). Innovation in medical care organizations. A synthetic review. *Med Care Rev*. **47**:165–192.

Scott T, Mannion R, Marshall M and Davies H (2003a). Does organisational culture influence health care performance? A review of the evidence. *J Health Serv Res Policy* **8**:105–117.

Scott T, Mannion R, Davies H and Marshall MN (2003b). Implementing culture change in health care: Theory and practice. *Int J Qual Health Care* **15**(2):111–118.

Senge PM (1990). *The Fifth Discipline. The Art and Practice of the Learning Organization*. London: Random House.

Shaughnessy PW and Kurowski B (1982). Quality assurance through reimbursement. *Health Serv Res*. **17**:157–183.

Shimmura K (1988). Effects of different remuneration methods on general medical practice: A comparison of capitation and fee-for-service payment. *Int J Health Plan Manage*. **3**:245–258.

Shortell SM, O'Brien JL, Carman JM, *et al*. (1995). Assessing the impact of continuous quality improvement/total quality management: Concept versus implementation. *Health Serv Res*. **30**(2):377–401.

Shortell SM, Bennett CL and Byck GR (1998). Assessing the impact of continuous quality improvement on clinical practice: What it will take to accelerate progress. *Milbank Q*. **76**:593–624.

Smith F, Singleton A and Hilton S (1998). General practitioners' continuing education: A review of policies, strategies, and effectiveness, and their implications for the future. *Br J Gen Pract*. **48**:1689–1695.

Sonnad SS and Foreman SE (1997). An incentive approach to physician implementation of medical practice guidelines. *Health Econ*. **6**:467–477.

Stanley I, Al-Shehri A and Thomas P (1993). Continuing education for general practice. 1. Experience, competence, and the media of self-directed learning for established general practitioners. *Br J Gen Pract*. **43**:210–214.

Stock GN and McDermott CM (2001). Organizational and strategic predictors of manufacturing technology implementation success: An exploratory study. *Technovation* **21**:625–636.

Stone S (2001). Hand hygiene – the case for evidence based education. *J Roy Soc Med*. **94**:278–281.

Stross JK (1996). The educationally influential physician. *J Cont Educ Health Prof*. **16**:167–172.

Sweeny K and Griffiths F, Eds (2002). *Complexity and Health Care: An Introduction*. Abingdon: Radcliffe.

Tassone MR and Heck CS (1997). Motivational orientations of allied health care professionals participating in continuing education. *J Cont Educ Health Prof*. **17**:97–105.

Teare L, Cookson B and Stone S (2001). Hand hygiene. *BMJ* **323**:411–412.

Valente TW (1996). Social network thresholds in the diffusion of innovations. *Soc Networks* **18**:69–89.

Wagner EH (2000). The role of patient care teams in chronic disease management. *BMJ* **320**:569–572.

Wagner EH, Austin BT and Van Korff M (1996). Organizing care for patients with chronic illness. *Milbank Q*. **74**(4):511–544.

Walker AE, Grimshaw JM and Armstrong EM (2001). Salient beliefs and intentions to prescribe antibiotics for patients with a sore throat. *Br J Health Psychol*. **6**:347–360.

Weggeman MCDP (1997). *Kennismanagement. Inrichting en Besturing van Kennisintensieve Organisaties [Knowledge Management. The Management of Knowledge Intensive Organisation]*. Schiedam: Scriptum.

Weiner B, Shortell S and Alexander J (1997). Promoting clinical involvement in hospital quality improvement efforts: The effects of top management, board and physician leadership. *Health Serv Res*. **32**(4):491–510.

Weinstein ND and Rothman AJ (1998). Stage theories of health behavior: Conceptual and methodological issues. *Health Psychol*. **17**:290–299.

Wensing M and Grol R (2000). Patients' views on health care: A driving force for improvement in disease management. *Dis Manage Outcomes* **7**:117–125.

Wolfe RA (1994). Organizational innovation: Review, critique and suggested research directions. *J Manage Stud*. **31**:405–431.

Chapter 3

Effective implementation: a model

Richard Grol and Michel Wensing

KEY MESSAGES

- The effective implementation of guidelines, valuable procedures or other innovations, be they new or old, requires a systematic approach with good preparation and planning.
- The following steps are important in a systematic approach to implementation:
  - Formulation of a concrete, well-developed and attainable proposal for change in practice, with clear targets.
  - Analysis of the target group and the setting: what are the problems in care provision, and what factors are stimulating or hampering the process of change?
  - Development or selection of a set of strategies for change: strategies for both the effective dissemination and the effective implementation and maintenance of change.
  - Developing and executing an implementation plan that contains activities, tasks and a timetable.
  - Evaluation and, if necessary, revision of the plan: continuous monitoring on the basis of indicators.
- These are brought together in a model. Various theories and approaches related to the effective implementation of change are integrated into this model.

Box 3.1 Introduction of a guideline for the management of depression (Baker *et al.* 2001)

Depression is a common disorder among patients who attend primary care. However, although generally effective treatment is available, patients do not always receive adequate care. Some patients are not diagnosed correctly, some do not receive a therapeutic dose of antidepressant and some do not receive treatment for a sufficient length of time. Baker and colleagues conducted a study to determine whether an intervention tailored to overcome obstacles to change and based on psychological theories was more effective than dissemination alone in the implementation of guidelines for the management of patients with depression in primary care.

In a randomised controlled trial design, 34 physicians were allocated to the intervention and 30 to the control group. Each practitioner in the intervention group had an in-depth interview 6 weeks after dissemination of the guidelines to identify their obstacles to implementing them. The content of the interviews was reviewed to identify comments that indicated particular obstacles to change. For each such comment, a psychological theory to explain aspects of the individual behaviour change was suggested. If a practitioner faced several obstacles, they received several implementation

methods. Thus, if a physician reported anxiety about assessing suicide risk and uncertainty about the form of questions to use, the theory identified would be self-efficacy theory and the implementation method might include the provision of scripts of questions used to assess suicide risk for the physician to use in consultations. The implementation methods were delivered to each practitioner 4–6 weeks after their interview. Practitioners identified patients who presented with depression before and after the intervention. The main outcome measures were the record of adherence to guideline recommendations in clinical records and the proportion of patients with Beck Depression Inventory (BDI) score less than 11 at 16 weeks after diagnosis.

In the group of practitioners who received the tailored intervention, there were significant increases in the proportion of patients assessed for suicide risk and the proportion of patients with BDI scores of less than 11 at 16 weeks. The authors concluded that this tailored approach was effective, but required further evaluation, particularly in terms of its cost-effectiveness.

INTRODUCTION

The interaction of many different factors determines whether or not implementation of an innovation succeeds or fails. We mention the following categories of factors in Chapter 2:

- Features of the innovation itself;
- Features of the target group of professionals who should use the innovation;
- Features of patients who have to accept or contribute to using the innovation;
- Features of the social setting and social network;
- Features of the economic, administrative and organisational context;
- Features of the methods and strategies for dissemination and implementation of the innovation used.

In Chapter 2 we present a series of theories that describe or explain how change takes place and which factors are crucial in such a process. In this chapter we present some theories and models that can be used to *plan and manage change (Box 3.2).*

ELEMENTS OF EFFECTIVE IMPLEMENTATION

Examination of the models and theories used in the field of planning the implementation of innovations shows that some crucial elements or principles for successful implementation recur through most publications (e.g. Grol and Grimshaw 2003; Ferlie 2001 and Shortell; Feder *et al.* 1999; Moulding *et al.* 1999; NHS 1999; Ovretveit 1999; Cretin 1998; Davis and Taylor-Vaisey 1997; Langley *et al.* 1996; Robertson *et al.* 1996; Grol 1992, 1997; Mittman *et al.* 1992; Green and Kreuter 1991; Kotler and Roberto 1989; Lomas and Haynes 1988). The scientific basis of these principles is still sketchy, but they provide a framework for setting up an implementation plan. These elements (summarised in *Box 3.3,* with an example model in *Box 3.4*) are:

- When changing routines in practice and implementing (new) procedures and processes of care it is important to take into account the complex reality of the practice. Usually, a large number of different factors play a role that may stimulate or hamper change. To steer the implementation process in the right direction,

---

Box 3.2   Some models for planning or managing change

- PRECEED/PROCEED model (Green and Kreuter 1991);
- Marketing theory (Kotler and Roberto 1989);
- Continuous improvement, PDSA cycles (Ovretveit 1999; Langley *et al.* 1996);
- Stages of change theories (Prochaska and Velicer 1997; Grol 1992; Rogers 1983);
- Persuasion–communication models (Kok 1987; Rogers 1983; McGuire 1981);
- Intervention mapping (Bokhoven *et al.* 2003; Bartholomew *et al.* 2001);
- Organisational development (Garside 1998).

Box 3.3   Elements of effective implementation described in the literature

- A systematic approach to and good planning of implementation activities is needed most of the time.
- Focus on the innovation – is it a 'good product'?
- Subgroups within the target group may be at different stages of the change process and have different needs – segmentation within the target group should be allowed for.
- Diagnostic analysis of the target group and setting should take place before the start of the implementation.
- The target group should be involved in the development and adaptation of the innovation, as well as in planning the implementation.
- The choice of implementation activities should link with the results of the diagnostic analysis.
- Usually, a single method or measure is insufficient – search for a cost-effective mix of methods tailored to the identified obstacles and incentives to change.
- Make a distinction between the phases of implementation (dissemination, implementation and integration) – different measures and strategies are effective at different stages.
- Take the appropriate measures for each of the various levels – national, local, team, practice and professional.
- Continuous evaluation of both the implementation process and its results required.
- Make implementation an integral part of the existing structures.

Box 3.4 The PRECEDE/PROCEDE model (Green and Kreuter 1991; Green *et al.* 1988)

The PRECEDE/PROCEED model, developed by Green and colleagues (Green and Kreuter 1991; Green *et al.* 1988) is a theory on behavioural change that can be used both to plan and to explain change in patient care. As far as planning is concerned, the model distinguishes nine steps to be taken in a process of change. The first three steps are 'social diagnosis', 'epidemiological diagnosis' and 'behavioural and environmental diagnosis', all aimed at determining important factors that influence behaviour. A distinction is made between *predisposing factors* for a specific behaviour (e.g. the knowledge, attitudes and values held in the target group), *enabling factors* (such as capacity, availability and accessibility of services) and *reinforcing factors* (opinions and behaviours of others). In the fourth and fifth steps of the model, the best approach to influence performance is explored; step six is the actual implementation, while steps seven to nine are the evaluation of process, impact and effect.

Green considers a series of important principles that underlie the effective change of behaviour. Firstly, strategies for the implementation of change should be based on an analysis of crucial determinants of behaviour (diagnostic principle). A 'hierarchical principle' is important here as well – there is a natural order in the factors that influence change (first predisposing, then enabling and finally reinforcing factors). Implementation strategies should be structured in that order. A third principle is that of 'cumulative learning' – to influence the performance of professionals a series of learning experiences need to be planned in a way that earlier experiences are used optimally in later experiences. A fourth principle is called 'participation' – a target group that defines both its own need for change and the preferred method for change increases the chance of success. The principle of 'situational specificity' comprises the idea that no strategy is uniformly superior or inferior for achieving change. The ultimate impact always depends on specific circumstances, characteristics of the target group, the timing, the commitment of opinion leaders and the change agents in the setting, and so on. The sixth principle is that of 'multiple methods' – as existing performance is determined by a variety of factors, a suitable strategy for each of these factors needs to be selected. The principle of 'individualisation' emphasises the importance of tailoring the implementation of change to the needs and experiences of individuals in the target group. And, finally, the 'feedback principle' identifies the necessity of direct feedback to individuals on the progress of the desired change.

This model is frequently used in health care, particularly in the field of health promotion. In a study on effective prevention, Green *et al.* (1988) found motivation and self-confidence in care providers, opinions about patient autonomy and self-efficacy expectations to be important predisposing factors. Important enabling factors were the resources available for prevention, reimbursement for preventive contacts and the availability of staff, time and administrative services. As far as reinforcing factors were concerned, positive feedback by patients, the support of colleagues and visible results were important. Two systematic reviews on the implementation of guidelines and change showed combined interventions that focus on all three types of factors to be more effective than interventions that focus on only one type of factor (Davis *et al.* 1992, 1999; Solomon *et al.* 1998).

The model of Green offers a comprehensive view on understanding and planning the implementation of change. Elements of it are used in this chapter, as well as in the framework used to structure this book.

---

implementation activities require *a systematic approach and good planning* most of the time. A one-off activity is sometimes effective, but often not. A well-planned process is nearly always required, in which all the relevant factors are considered, and in which there is regular monitoring to see what progress is being made in achieving the goals set out.

- It is important that specific attention be given to the *innovation* that is to be implemented. This means the process of development (who is involved, what is the status of the body developing it?), its scientific basis and the ultimate form in which the innovation is to be presented.

- For the target group, care providers and teams, implementation usually means following a *step-by-step process*. The factors that one must tackle successively to move forward in that process follow a natural order of progression. Different problems have to be surmounted in each step, for which different measures are required. Individuals or groups within the implementation's target group may be in different *phases* of a process of change. The needs and willingness to change may vary, as well as the problems people experience with change. For this reason, it is important when introducing change to differentiate between subgroups, and so-called *segmentation* may be practised. Different groups may different approaches.

- Before embarking upon implementation it is essential to know about the various target groups. It is advisable to start implementation with a *diagnostic or problem analysis*. This should provide insights into the:

- – Characteristics of the target group and, if applicable, subgroups within it;
- – Setting in which the implementation is to take place;
- – Most important departures from the desired performance;
- – Most important factors that could hamper or stimulate the change in performance;
- – Wider (social and/or organisational) context;
- – Important parties involved in the process of implementing the innovation.

■ *Commitment from the target group* to the entire process ultimately contributes to successful implementation. Planning of the implementation requires an understanding of the perceptions, needs, worries and realities of the working situation of those people or groups who must ultimately carry it out. The target group should ideally be involved in the development of a proposal for change. If national guidelines are involved, it is possible to adjust them locally to suit the situation and the specific needs experienced there. Ideally, the target group is also involved in mounting the implementation plan, and in developing and testing the measures and strategies to be used in that plan before applying them on a large scale.

■ *The choice of measures and strategies* to bring about change is linked, as far as possible, to the results of the diagnostic or problem analysis and to the stimulating and hampering factors that have been identified. On the basis of this, an efficient mix can be devised, such as education, rewards, feedback and organisational or practical measures. The approach has to be optimised to the needs and situation of the various subgroups within the target group.

■ Usually, a single method is not sufficient because subgroups within the target group are at various stages in terms of their willingness to change, and experience different problems in realising change in practice. Therefore, successful strategies often need to be *multifaceted*. However, this comes at a price. The necessary resources must be available if the plan is to go ahead. Just as in clinical practice, a balance must be sought between effectiveness and costs incurred in implementation activities. More interventions do not automatically lead to more success. A complete programme with scores of activities is not always the most efficient approach, and may even be frowned upon by the financiers or target group, who may feel that too much resource is being spent on an implementation.

■ When selecting suitable measures and strategies to support the implementation it is useful to *distinguish* between effective *dissemination* (spreading the information, keeping people informed and obtaining acceptance of the innovation) and effective *implementation* (actual adoption and integration into normal routines or care processes). For both steps different methods and measures are suitable and effective. In addition, the *level* at which the measures can best be deployed must be considered. Some changes can best be tackled at the national or regional level (for instance, financial compensation for extra work), while others are best done at a professional, practice or team level (for instance, feedback on current performance).

■ Each systematic attempt to change clinical practice should be accompanied by a plan to monitor progress and to *evaluate* to what extent the intended changes are being achieved. In doing so, it is important to use appropriate indicators and easily accessible data sources. On the basis of this information, the plan can be adjusted or, if it fails to succeed, the problems involved in its introduction can be re-analysed.

■ Finally, it is crucial that programmes to introduce innovations *become an integral part of existing structures* for professional development, quality control and quality improvement. It is important to be constantly aware of the change to avoid regression or diversification. The ultimate success criterion for an implementation is its sustainability in the long term.

PLANNING AND EXECUTING AN IMPLEMENTATION PROCESS: A MODEL

An implementation process is usually initiated for one of two reasons:

■ Firstly, new scientific information that indicates patient care can be provided more effectively or efficiently may become available. This information may come from a single well-designed study, or from a systematic review of the literature (for instance, undertaken within the framework of the Cochrane Collaboration). Sometimes care or prevention programmes have been tested out and evaluated, or sufficient experience has been gained on a wide scale. Such new information may be incorporated into guidelines for practice, care protocols or pathways in which the desired care is described for a department, team or practice.

■ Secondly, the starting point for the implementation may also be 'bottom-up', from dissatisfaction with the current routines within a work setting. Examples of this are the occurrence of critical or undesired incidents in an institution, or data from 'audits' or patient questionnaires that express the view that care could be improved. This may mean that there are also ideas or experiences from the work setting on how patient care could be better organised or made more efficient ('best practices') and from this, proposals are developed to improve the care processes. These proposals may be integrated with the available evidence or guidelines into a multidisciplinary care protocol.

Both situations, the one more 'top-down', the other more 'bottom-up', can start a process of change that subsequently should be tackled *systematically,* in as far as this is possible. The process of implementation of desired changes in patient care can be approached from two perspectives:

■ That of the 'implementer', the person, group or organisation that wants to plan and conduct the change and needs to follow specific consecutive steps to be successful;

■ That of the professional, team or target group that needs to go through a process of change and needs to take different (consecutive) steps to arrive at integrating new performance within fixed routines.

Both perspectives can be used to plan the implementation of change in patient care. The literature offers a variety of models for planning change, taking either the perspective of the 'implementer' or the perspective of the target group as a starting point. We discuss both perspectives and integrate these within the context of the model or framework presented below (Grol and Wensing 2004).

The model is given in a diagrammatic form in *Figure 3.1* and the various steps are discussed in detail next.

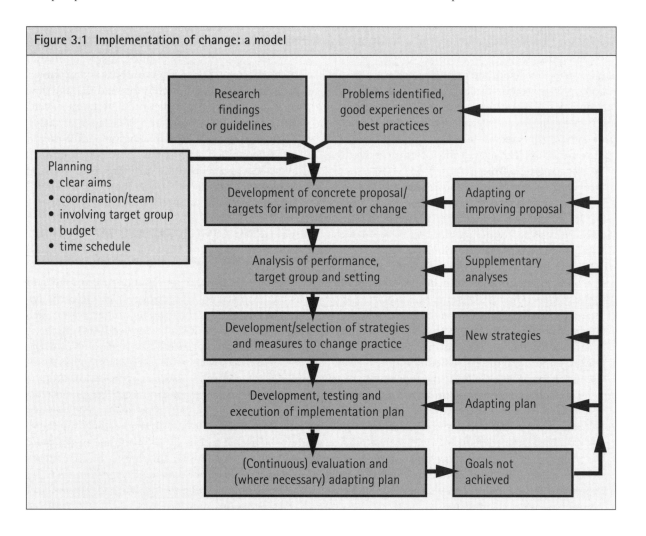

Figure 3.1 Implementation of change: a model

It is important to be aware that this is a model – the reality may demand a different sequence of events and supplementary steps! The various steps in this model are explained below and subsequently developed in the rest of the book.

PLANNING OF THE IMPLEMENTATION PROCESS

Planning is important to the whole process of implementation. Successful implementation of innovations or changes requires good preparation and planning of all of the steps in the implementation process, represented in the cyclical model shown in *Figure 3.1*. This is as true for introducing an evidence-based guideline, new procedure or best practice into clinical practice as for remedying indicated shortcomings in patient care. What this planning should look like, of course, varies according to whether the implementation programme is large scale, national or regional, or a smaller scale project aimed at improving care in a single ward or practice. There are also differences between a (controlled) implementation study, on the one hand, and an improvement or 'breakthrough' project with simple monitoring of its success, on the other. Nevertheless, on the basis of experiences from a wide range of implementation projects, a number of common points require attention:

- Ensure that a clear, overall aim is formulated for the project or programme:
  - What is the purpose of the activity;
  - What does one want to achieve;
  - When is the implementation a success?
  This aim acts as a continuous touchstone for all those involved in the implementation.
- Put together a team that has both sufficient expertise and motivation to co-ordinate and stimulate the project. Depending on the scale and the budget, they may have to have expertise in the fields of:
  - Leadership (someone who plays a central role in communicating the aim and involving the target group in the implementation);
  - Co-ordination (the daily organisation of activities);
  - Technical expertise (specific knowledge and skills in the areas of, for instance, literature analysis, data gathering or computer use);
  - Administrative support to organise meetings, plan social activities or develop products).
  The team should make a plan in which different tasks and responsibilities are worked out, and this should be committed to paper.

- Ensure that the target group is identified clearly and that, in all stages of the project or programme, the target group is involved in the implementation process. The group of people who experience the consequences of an implementation is often far larger than one imagines beforehand (Lomas 1997). It is worth compiling a list of people and organisations whose opinions are important and whose co-operation is desirable. This could be done by forming one or more brainstorming groups made up of a variety of people involved, who can look at it from their viewpoint and thus provide useful input. These may be different people at different stages in the process. The phase in which a proposal for improvement in care practice is being developed requires different inputs from those at the stage of analysis of the target group and setting, which are different again from those at the stage of planning and introduction of an implementation strategy (Hall and Eccles 2000).
- Finally, a realistic timetable must be drawn up: when is what happening? Take into consideration that most implementation paths and change processes require a certain amount of time, and that the time required is often underestimated beforehand (Evans and Haines 2000; Wye and McClenahan 2000). Change takes place slowly; nevertheless, the project must be tackled with some speed and vigour to avoid loss of momentum. Most target groups want to see quick results, otherwise they may lose motivation and return to the old practice.

DEVELOPING A PROPOSAL AND TARGETS FOR CHANGE

The development and determination of a concrete and feasible proposal and targets for the desired change in existing practice is the first step in the model. Such a proposal may include (or be derived from) guideline recommendations for effective or efficient care, the introduction of new valuable techniques or procedures into existing clinical work or insights concerning the organisation of patient-care processes (*Box 3.5*). Just like other innovations, they must be developed carefully, be of good quality, fit in with the needs of the target group, be usable and easily available and be designed attractively. A good understanding of the characteristics of an innovation, or plan for change, that are likely to affect its ultimate adoption is required. The range of characteristics includes the:

- Way in which the development has taken place – the quality and credibility of the process;
- Developers – the amount of support for the innovation;
- Design – its accessibility and attractiveness;
- Scope for adapting it to suit the local situation.

Most of the literature in this area is reflective and based on research undertaken outside the field of healthcare.

Specific theories do, however, provide useful insights. For instance, communication theory identifies the importance of the message being of understandable, well phrased and easy to remember. Marketing theories highlight the importance of a good 'product', developed and adapted on the basis of the needs and circumstances of the target group (*Box 3.6*; Kotler and Roberto 1989).

Box 3.5 Improving the quality of care for acute myocardial infarction (Mehta *et al.* 2002)

Management of acute myocardial infarction in hospitals was observed to be inadequate for items such as early aspirin use, discharge aspirin use, prescribing beta-blockers and angiotensin-converting enzyme inhibitors at discharge from the hospital and smoking counselling. Analyses showed that the responsible physicians and nurses lacked practical tools to support their performance. Therefore, a toolkit was developed, based on the guidelines of the American Medical Association, that contained standard orders, clinical pathways, pocket guides, patient information materials, discharge forms and chart stickers. For each hospital included in the intervention arm of the project, local physicians and nurse opinion leaders were recruited to help adapt the toolkit to local settings, to develop an implementation plan and to support actual implementation. The toolkit was introduced during the 'grand rounds' by personal site visits, by providing feedback on actual performance and by a meeting at which use of the tools was discussed. This intervention programme was effective, particularly when the tools were actually used in practice (difference in adherence to guidelines with a control group was 11–42% for different indicators). Key elements of success were, according to the authors, the systematic approach, use of national evidence-based guidelines as a basis for the practical tools, flexibility to adapt the tools, active involvement and local ownership, the tools as reminders and implementation built into the normal work of busy practitioners.

Box 3.6 Social marketing theory (Kotler and Roberto 1989)

Within social marketing theory, to relate to and satisfy the needs and culture of a target group is crucial to induce change. Good 'marketing' (implementation of an innovation), therefore, does not start with a ready 'product' (a guideline, a new procedure or best practice). First, data on the improvement of patient care need to be collected systematically, and knowledge about optimal patient care must be translated into the practices of the target group. A change agent has different tasks to perform as part of the implementation efforts (Dickinson 1995; Kotler and Roberto 1989):

- Exploring the setting – what are the problems, the strengths and weaknesses? Who is influential in the process of change and can be involved in that process?
- Diagnosing the target group – exploring their needs and identifying 'segments' in the target population with different needs and different routes for change.
- Identifying competitive messages or performances and the satisfaction linked to these.
- Developing a change strategy optimally suited to the target group and setting. Part of the plan are the seven Ps that need to be taken care of – product (quality, name, style, format, etc.), price (necessary investments), place (dissemination channels, service and help desk, etc.), promotion (public relations, advertising, special events), personnel (who is to disseminate, and the source

of information), presentation (how and where is the innovation to be introduced) and process (phases that a target group needs to complete to adopt the innovation).
- Planning – preparation of the implementation plan.
- Actual implementation – organising, controlling and evaluating the activities.

Dickinson (1995) applied the framework of social marketing theory to the implementation of guidelines in health care. The approach of 'moving knowledge to practice' should, in his view, be replaced by an approach in which professionals are central to implementing the change. They should be involved in developing the new practice routines as well as in developing the plans for change, instead of being the target of information or warnings when they deviate from guidelines.

The theory provides a useful framework for setting up implementation plans, and particularly emphasises the importance of an attractive proposal for change that meets the needs of the target group and can compete with existing routines. In the example of improving hand hygiene, presented in Chapter 2, the challenge is to translate evidence-based recommendations for practice into attractive and feasible proposals for new performance routines and new procedures that can improve upon the existing routines (for instance, providing alcohol disinfectant next to each bed instead of hands being washed at a sink) and that meet the needs of the target group in an optimal way.

Various authors have identified characteristics or qualities of innovations that stimulate or hamper their use in practice. Rogers (1995) suggests the following crucial characteristics of a successful innovation:

- It has more advantages than existing routines;
- It is consistent with existing standards and values that define good care;
- It is easy to understand, and its introduction is considered feasible and not too difficult;
- It is possible to experiment with it on a small scale before actually introducing it;
- The results of the new procedure are easily visible, to the user as well as to others.

These types of characteristics are considered in more detail in Chapters 4 and 5.

ANALYSIS OF PERFORMANCE, TARGET GROUP AND SETTING

The second step in the model is an analysis of the context within which changes in the routines are to take place, the characteristics of the target group, the factors that stimulate and hamper change and the aspects of performance that show the greatest deviation from the proposed behaviour (*Box 3.7*). The factors that determine whether the implementation of an innovation is successful or not are many and varied. Factors may be connected to the setting in which the innovation is to be implemented, the relationship between individuals within the setting, the goals of the implementation, the actual care provision proposed, the professionals who have to carry out the innovation, the patients who have to co-operate with the implementation, the resources available and the organisational or structural conditions for its effective introduction. Each target group or setting is, in some sense, unique. Not everyone in the target group can be placed in the same category. Some members or subgroups will be further advanced in the process of acceptance and adoption of an innovation than others. Effective implementation, therefore, cannot take place without an analysis of the setting and the target group in which the implementation is to take place. One must, as it were, according to Greer (Kaegi 1997), get inside the heads of the people and the institution that must change. This type of *diagnostic or problem analysis* may relate to the:

- Aims and settings of the implementation – who wants what change, where and for what reasons?
- (Variation in) existing care provision – to what extent does this deviate from the recommended care, what is most divergent and where is change most needed?
- Segments within the target group – what phase of change are they now in?
- Stimulating and hampering factors that affect the change.

Aims and settings of the implementation

Firstly, it is important to consider the aims of the implementation, the people involved and the roles played by those involved in the process. It makes a considerable difference whether a regional health insurer plans on introducing a guideline to reduce the costs of antibiotic use, whether a national commission on antibiotic use, which consists of doctors and pharmacists, is

---

Box 3.7 Continuous quality improvement in teams (Ovretveit 1999)

Ovretveit (1999) proposes a model for quality improvement to be carried out in teams, in which a clear distinction is made between a diagnostic phase and a solution or therapeutic stage. The model has nine steps:

Investigation:
1 Choosing the problem or improvement.
2 Formulating the problem and forming the team.
3 Guessing the causes of the problem.
4 Gathering data to find the cause.
5 Deciding on the real cause.

Solution:
6 Planning the solution.
7 Implementing the change.
8 Evaluating the results.
9 Finishing or continuing.

People are often inclined to skip over the problem and its causes and move on to plans for solutions far too quickly.

going to launch guidelines to combat antibiotic resistance in institutions, or whether a local hospital committee wants to improve antibiotic prescribing because of increasing resistance. The players are different and the goals vary. This influences the level of acceptance that might be anticipated when the innovation is introduced. This information is important when formulating an implementation plan, particularly with regard to making decisions about the tasks of those involved. It is important to have an overview, a 'social map' of the people and organisations that play a role or have an interest in the implementation. This information is also required to develop a successful, feasible plan.

(Variation in) existing healthcare

Secondly, it is important to gather knowledge about current practice – what pattern of care is provided now, to what extent is this in accordance with the proposed care, where are the important deviations to be found, what are the most important items that have to be tackled and which aspects of the care routines have already been implemented acceptably? Most proposals for change contain a number of concrete recommendations for optimal patient care. An efficient way to approach improving matters is to concentrate mainly, or solely, on the (main) deviations from the recommended care – those that can reasonably be expected to alter and produce a change for the better for patients. Various theories point out the importance of gaining insight into the discrepancies between actual and optimal care and then using this as a motivator for a change in practice. Most people overestimate their performance quality and are surprised when confronted with the reality.

Segments within the target group and stages of change

Thirdly, in various theories on change (see Chapter 2) attempts have been made to identify specifically recognisable subgroups within a target group that are different in character and therefore require a different approach. The most familiar classification is that provided by Rogers (1983), which divides people into:

- 'Innovators' – a small group that is very keen on new ideas;
- 'Early adopters' – an active group that often carries a good deal of status within the target group and that functions as a point of reference for most innovators;

- 'Early majority' – a group that does not consist of leaders, but that has close contact with 'early adopters' and allows them to lead the way;
- 'Late majority' – a group that is sceptical about change and not susceptible to information sources, and has more faith in public opinion or is more influenced by pressure from colleagues;
- 'Laggards' – a conservative group that puts up a great deal of resistance to change.

Rogers (1983) also describes that change takes place through social networks within the target group, which is the means whereby various subgroups influence one another. Within this social network, the availability of real 'innovators' and 'change agents' is of great importance for effective implementation within the total group.

Subgroups or individuals in the target group may be at different stages of a process leading to change. A number of theories in the field of implementation of innovations take the perspective of the target group as a starting point, see change or implementation as a stepwise *process* that individuals, groups (teams) or organisations (institutions, practices) must go through ultimately to arrive at the desired practice (see Chapter 2). Even though they originate from differing disciplines or subject areas (organisation studies, marketing, communication sciences, health information services, management sciences and psychology), the similarity in steps that evidently play a role in these sorts of processes is striking. Although the emphasis may vary and different terms be used, nonetheless a number of steps emerge that should be kept in mind when introducing guidelines and changes in clinical practice. Within each of these steps important problems or bottlenecks can arise that must be solved before the subsequent step can be taken. In this sense they follow a set sequence. We summarise a number of models in *Table 3.1*.

Examples of steps in the change process are to be found in the Rogers' innovation diffusion theory and in Prochaska's trans-theoretical model (see Chapter 2). Rogers' model distinguishes the following phases:

- 'Knowledge' – one reads and hears about the innovation;
- 'Persuasion' – one adopts a positive or negative attitude to it;
- 'Decision' – one carries out a trial of the innovation;
- 'Implementation' – one adopts or rejects it;
- 'Confirmation' – one has positive experiences when working with the innovation; one decides to continue along the same lines.

Table 3.1 Steps in a process of change

Author	1	2	3	4	5	6	7	8	9
Zaltman and Duncan (1977)	Knowledge/ awareness	Knowledge/ awareness		Attitude formation	Decision	Initial imple- mentation		Sustained im- plementation	
McGuire (1981)	Exposure/ interest	Comprehen- sion	Skills	Attitude change/ agreement	Decision	Behaviour change	Reinforce- ment	Consolidation	
Rogers (1983)		Knowledge		Persuasion	Decision	Implementation		Confirmation	
Kok (1987)	Attention	Under- standing		Attitude change	Intention to change	Behaviour change		Sustained change	
Orlandi (1987)		Seeking information		Persuasion about relevance	Decision to adopt	Change of practice		Sustained change	
Cooper and Zinud (1990)		Initiation			Adoption	Acceptance/ use		Incorporation	Infusion (wide use)
Grol (1992)	Awareness/ interest	Knowledge	Insight in- to own per- formance	Positive attitude	Intention to change	Implementation (trial)		Maintenance of change	
Spence (1994)	Awareness/ interest			Evaluation		Trial		Adoption	
Pathman et al. (1996)	Awareness			Agreement		Adoption		Routine adherence	
Prochaska and Velicer (1997)	Pre- contemplation			Contempla- tion	Prepara- tion	Action		Maintenance	

Prochaska's *Stage of readiness to change model* (Prochaska and Velicer 1997) focuses mainly on the motivation of those who have to adopt the innovation. Within health education, this model is used to influence smoking behaviour, safe sex and other risky behaviour. A distinction is made between the phases of:

■ 'Pre-contemplation' (the person is not planning to adopt new behaviour for lack of the basic knowledge and attitude);

■ 'Contemplation' (in the near distant future, such as within 6 months, the person is considering adopting the innovation and is mainly in need of emotional support);

■ 'Preparation' (in the short term, such as within 1 month, the person is considering adopting the innovation and is mainly concerned with how potential problems can be dealt with);

■ 'Action' and 'maintenance' (because of positive experiences the new behaviour is to be continued).

If we summarise the different step-by-step models described in the literature, the phases described next can be distinguished in the process of change that most individuals, groups or institutions probably go through if an innovation, clinical guideline or desired change in behaviour is to be integrated into practice routines (Grol and Wensing 2004). It is this planning model that has been developed by us for this book (*Box 3.8*). Not all the steps are always taken or taken in the order presented, but the model can help to differentiate between groups with different 'preparedness to change'.

Orientation

■ *Promote awareness of the innovation* – first and foremost, care providers, teams or institutions must be aware that there is an innovation, even if they do not know the details. It should be publicised in such a way that as many people from the target group as possible (professionals, patients, managers, policy makers, etc.) are aware that this is going on and are conscious of the existence of the innovation.

■ *Stimulate interest and involvement* – curiosity about the innovation is aroused. New working methods

---

Box 3.8 Phases in the process of change for care providers and teams (Grol and Wensing 2004)

Orientation	Promote awareness of the innovation Stimulate interest and involvement
Insight	Create understanding Develop insight into own routines
Acceptance	Develop a positive attitude, a motivation to change Create positive intentions or decisions to change
Change	Promote actual adoption in practice Confirm the benefit, value of change
Maintenance	Integrate new practice into routines Embed new practice within the organisation

---

and techniques are presented in such a way that relevant people think 'this is interesting, I would like to find out more about this'. They should also have the feeling that it is important for their own work.

Insight

▨ *Create understanding* – subsequently, the target group, particularly the clinical professionals, must know exactly what the recommended care involves and what is expected in terms of new behaviour. The transfer of information in this phase must be such that people have a clear understanding of what the innovation entails.

▨ *Develop insight into own routines* – equally, the target group should develop clear insight into their own performance and know which features differ from the new proposals.

Acceptance

▨ *Develop a positive attitude, a motivation to change* – the target care providers, the team or the institution, including all those involved, must weigh up the advantages and disadvantages of the new working method and be convinced that it is valuable, effective or useful, or that it leads to savings in time or money.

▨ *Create positive intentions or decisions to change* – the target group resolves to work differently in the short term. If they are to live up to this decision, they have to have a good idea of how the innovation can be applied to their own work-setting, what problems may arise in so doing and how these can be solved. The feeling must grow that they are able to carry through the change and that applying it to their own work setting is feasible.

Change

▨ *Promote adoption in practice* – an opportunity to try out the new working method on a small scale is provided to allow the target group to gain experience in using it, to learn the skills involved and to carry out practical and organisational adaptations.

▨ *Confirm benefit, value of change* – having implemented the new routines, the care provider or team conclude whether it works, whether it is satisfactory and whether it can be implemented without major problems, costs or damage.

Maintenance

▨ *Integrate new practice into routines* – subsequently, the performance has to be integrated with existing care protocols or care plans. Reverting to old routines or forgetting the guideline or innovation must be avoided.

▨ *Embed practice in the organisation* – finally, the new routines must be embedded and supported by the care organisation to such an extent that continuous implementation is possible. Organisational, financial and structural conditions to maintain implementation are fulfilled.

Barriers and facilitators to changing practice

Fourthly, different factors may be important at each phase or step in the process. Both stimulating and hampering factors may play a role in determining the success of the implementation. Insight into these factors is of great importance to inform how implementation strategies should be designed and to understand what kind of activities should be developed (*Box 3.9*). Factors may be related to the:

> ## Box 3.9 Implementing changes in the management of urinary tract infections and sore throat (Flottorp *et al*. 2003)
>
> In a study in 142 primary care practices in Norway, 72 were given interventions to implement recommendations for urinary tract infections (UTIs) and 70 were given interventions to implement recommendations for sore throat, serving as controls for each other. The outcomes were measured in about 25,000 consultations. The project aimed to reduce unnecessary antibiotic use for sore throats, reduce unnecessary laboratory tests for UTIs and increase the management of UTI by telephone. An intensive study was undertaken among physicians, assistants and patients to identify barriers to change (see Chapter 8). The interventions were tailored to those barriers and included a combination of strategies:
>
> - Summary of recommendations in electronic and poster format;
> - Patient-education materials;
> - Computer-assisted decision support and reminders;
> - Increase in the fee for telephone consultations;
> - Interactive course for doctors and practice assistants;
> - Credit points for CME.
>
> The changes were, however, small (1–5%) and not significant. The reasons for this lack of effect are not clear – perhaps more active support by, for example, outreach visitors may be needed for greater success. Further analysis of the barriers to change and the feasibility of the recommendations for practice change may also be needed.

- Individual care providers – their knowledge, skills, attitudes, values, self-confidence, habits and personalities;
- Social context – patients (their knowledge, attitude, behaviour, expectations, needs, experiences and priorities), attitude and behaviour of colleagues, culture in the social networks, opinion of leaders and key figures and the presence of innovators.
- Economic, administrative and organisational context – financial resources, equipment, qualified personnel, policies, task divisions and logistic processes.

The theories outlined in Chapter 2 provide insight into all sorts of potentially important factors in the implementation process. A systematic inventory (using quantitative and/or qualitative methods) is usually required to find out exactly which activities should be given priority in the implementation plan. Methods for doing this are described in Chapter 7.

Various sorts of barriers and facilitators may play a role in the different phases of a process of change (see Chapter 6) and may thereby activate the need for diverse strategies and interventions (see Chapters 9–14). Indicators to evaluate the success of the implementation activity can also be derived from this process (see Chapter 16). In this way, we can link the perspective of the 'implementer' to the perspective of the target group.

DEVELOPMENT OR SELECTION OF STRATEGIES

Linking up the factors identified in the previous stages and any other relevant information, a cost-effective mix of measures, methods and strategies for implementation is developed or selected, and possibly tested out on (part of) the target group. Different phases of implementation usually require different strategies:

- Dissemination – increasing interest in and understanding of the innovation, and encouraging a positive attitude and willingness to adapt existing routines;
- Implementation – encouraging its actual adoption and making sure that the recommended performance becomes a set part of daily routines.

The literature gives a great number of different strategies that can be used when introducing innovations and changes. Examples include the development of local protocols, audit and feedback, reminders, computer-supported decision making, educating patients, financial incentives or sanctions, organisational measures, redesigning care processes and disease management systems. The Cochrane Effective Practice and Organisation of Care Group (EPOC) has categorised these strategies into:

- Interventions directed at individual professionals (for instance, continuous medical education, practice visits, audit and feedback, or reminders);
- Financial interventions, directed at care providers and/or patients;
- Organisational interventions (structural measures and interventions directed at organisational changes);
- Issuing of laws and formal regulations.

This type of classification, which is dealt with in more detail in Chapter 8, does little justice to the reality of introducing changes into practice, nor to all manner of new developments in this area. In practise, there are normally a number of influential factors and, therefore, if success is to be achieved, what is usually required is a set of methods and measures that link well to these factors. A mix of activities is usually selected, in line with the results of the diagnostic analysis (see previous section); possibly, new measures and strategies are thought up and tested on a small scale (*Box 3.10*). In practice, a balance must be reached between the possibility of achieving the desired effects and the amount of money, time, effort and personal commitment invested and the commotion they may cause.

DEVELOPMENT, TESTING AND EXECUTION OF AN IMPLEMENTATION PLAN

When making an implementation plan, attention has to be paid to effective dissemination (to arouse interest in it and to guarantee sufficient knowledge about the guideline), both to encourage its acceptance (to foster a positive attitude and willingness to bring about real behavioural change) and to promote the actual implementation and integration into normal working routines and care processes.

In planning implementation activities (when, where and how does what happen and who does what?) it is helpful to consider the following points:
■ Begin on a small scale with a limited number of motivated people, teams or institutions. The implementation plan and the various interventions should be tested with these for suitability and feasibility, and then be adjusted in the light of this experience.
■ Plan according to the different phases of the change process – what must still be done to inform and interest specific subgroups, what must be done to overcome resistance and what is needed to incorporate a change into existing care processes?
■ There is a need to establish at what level interventions and measures can best be planned. This is different for national programmes, institution-directed programmes, ward or team projects and projects aimed at local groups or practices.

■ Involving the target group – it is not only important to involve the target group in the development of an innovation or protocol or in analysing problems in implementation. Representatives of the target group can play an important part in designing and testing the implementation plan. They may often know best what is possible and can think creatively about suitable interventions.
■ Planning of activities over time – a timetable is set out and a logical sequence devised for the different activities.
■ Distributing tasks, procedures and responsibilities – who does what, where and who checks it has been done, must be established clearly.
■ The implementation plan is built into the existing structures and channels for contacting or training the target group.
■ The plan's long-term aims are identified and used to guide the ongoing evaluation.
■ Structures, resources and personnel – whether it is a small-scale ward or practice implementation project, or alternatively a large-scale implementation project, adequate resources and ample expertise are needed.
■ Finally, the organisational culture in the setting in which the implementation is to take place may require attention. Clear leadership, good collaboration between professionals and a culture in which continuous learning and improvement of care can occur are all desirable and often a pre-requisite to achieving change.
We discuss these aspects in more detail in Chapter 15.

EVALUATION AND (POSSIBLE) ADAPTATIONS TO THE PLAN

A final step in the implementation of innovations in care is to evaluate the results – have the goals been

---

Box 3.10 Improving the quality of care for patients with acute myocardial infarction (Qasim *et al.* 2002)

An audit in one hospital showed that most patients with acute myocardial infarction (AMI) did not receive thrombolysis within 30 minutes of arrival in the hospital, although this was the official guideline set by the NHS in the UK (average 'door-to-needle' time was 45 minutes). An analysis of the process of care for these patients showed many inefficiencies. Therefore, a new pathway and new responsibilities were designed: when a patient with AMI arrived at the hospital a first assessment was performed by a specially trained thrombolysis nurse. In cases of AMI, the nurse started the thrombolysis treatment. In cases of uncertain problems, a specialist could arrive within a very short time. The new protocol was first tested and proved to be safe. After implementation, the average 'door-to-needle' time was reduced to 15 minutes (100% within 30 minutes).

achieved? This is a crucial step that often does not receive the attention it deserves. The results of this sort of evaluation are needed to determine whether the energy that has been invested has led to the desired degree of change and, where this is not the case, to consider what can be done to ensure better success. The evaluation may result in (*Figure 3.1*):

- Adaptation of the proposal for change, for instance by revising the goals if these prove to be unrealistic;
- Supplementary analyses of stimulating and hampering factors;
- Further strategies and measures to bring about change – more potentially effective strategies to be developed;
- Revise the plan and conduct the implementation – the way in which it has been introduced or the way

in which the process of change has been organised is revised.

Evaluation is not the final step in an implementation project. Ideally, one is continuously assessing whether care is improving and revising procedures on the basis of these findings (*Figure 3.2*). How the evaluation is tackled depends on whether it is a small-scale practice improvement or ward-improvement project, whether it is an implementation study in which the effectiveness of a specific intervention is determined or whether it is a large-scale implementation project. The aims of these different projects vary, as do the populations and the evaluation designs. In all cases, one really wants to know if the goals formulated beforehand have been attained in the project or programme:

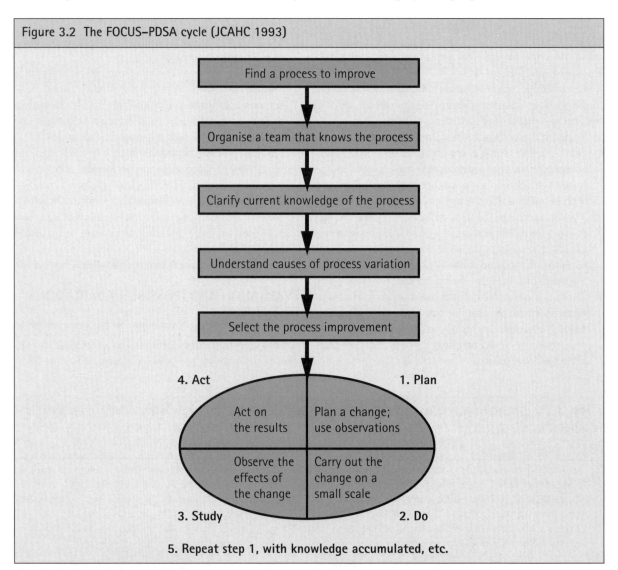

Figure 3.2 The FOCUS–PDSA cycle (JCAHC 1993)

Find a process to improve

Organise a team that knows the process

Clarify current knowledge of the process

Understand causes of process variation

Select the process improvement

4. Act

1. Plan

Act on the results

Plan a change; use observations

Observe the effects of the change

Carry out the change on a small scale

3. Study

2. Do

5. Repeat step 1, with knowledge accumulated, etc.

- Short-term aims – have the conditions for implementation been met, does the target group know about the change and has it been accepted?
- Intermediate aims – is the proposed change in performance actually being applied?
- Long-term goals – what is the effect in terms of health benefits, greater well-being and patient-satisfaction or cost-reduction?

To find out whether the goals have been reached they must be made measurable. For this purpose 'indicators' and criteria for goal attainment need to be formulated and selected – how this is done is described in Chapter 16. A second question is how the evaluation of 'effects' can best be set up and which methods and instruments might be useful for this, as explained in Chapters 17 and 18. To interpret whether the goals have or have not been attained, it is important to examine, by means of a so-called 'process evaluation', whether the implementation plan has been carried out as intended and which factors influenced its success or failure (Chapter 19). Finally, the cost or the level of investment needed to change care processes effectively must be examined (see Chapter 20).

An example of an overall process is shown in *Box 3.11*.

Box 3.11 A step–by–step approach to implementation of improvement in blood transfusion policy in Royal Melbourne Hospital (NHMRC 2000; Tuckfield *et al*. 1997; Metz *et al*. 1995)

A step-by-step process of proceeding is described on the basis of a number of questions.

	Question	Solution
1	What is the aim? What do you want to achieve?	Reduction in the use of incorrect blood products
2	Who can help to do this?	Team was formed with head of Haematology as co-ordinator and doctors from the Transfusion Committee
3	What is the existing care practice, and does it differ from elsewhere or from guidelines?	Use of blood products was incorrect for 16% of red cell transfusions, 13% of platelet transfusions and 31% of the 'fresh frozen plasma' transfusions
4	Who should be involved in the improvement?	Haematology ward, medical staff and hospital managers
5	What are key messages and recommendations?	Follow the blood transfusion protocol to the letter
6	Which concrete goals are being aimed at?	Reduction of the number of incorrect blood transfusions to an acceptable level (<5%)
7	Is the information about the improvement suitable for the target group(s)?	Draft protocol was produced based on the literature and presented to the Transfusion Committee for comments; the subsequent draft was distributed throughout entire hospital for comment, and final recommendations were printed on the application form
8	What are the bottlenecks in terms of its introduction?	Doctors are not used to having to make decisions according to protocols, nor to being required to check them – it takes extra time
9	What are the possible suitable interventions and measures?	Audit and feedback, using opinion leader, educational materials, reminders, administrative measures (application form) and feedback if guideline not adhered to
10	Is there sufficient support for the change?	The Transfusion Committee with all members involved continuously supporting the process
11	What does the change cost and is it worth it?	(Not calculated)
12	Did it work?	Incorrect red-cell transfusion rates fell from 16% to 3%; incorrect platelet transfusion rates fell from 13% to 2.5%; for fresh frozen plasma, incorrect transfusion rates fell from 34% to 15%, but this was still thought not acceptable.

CONCLUSIONS

In Chapters 1–3 of this book a description is given of what 'implementation' involves in practice, the theoretical points of view regarding changes in care practice and how – in general terms – a programme or project aimed at the introduction of new working methods or changes in practice could be set up. We have seen that – regardless of whether it is a large-scale or small-scale project and no matter whether it involves the introduction of guidelines, protocols, new care procedures, best practices or aims to solve problems in care practice – good preparation and planning are always important. All the steps in the implementation process must be given the required amount of attention. Precisely what this may mean and what science and experiences in practice can teach us is discussed in the rest of the book.

Recommended literature

Dunning M, Abi-Aad G, Gilbert D, *et al.* (1999). *Experience, Evidence and Everyday Practice*. London: King's Fund.

Grol R (1997). Beliefs and evidence in changing clinical practice. *BMJ* **315**:418–421.

Grol R and Grimshaw J (2003). From best evidence to best practice: Effective implementation of change in patients' care. *Lancet* **362**:1225–1230.

Rogers E (1996). *Diffusion of Innovations*. New York: Free Press.

References

Baker R, Reddish S, Robertson N, Hearnshaw H and Jones B (2001). Randomised controlled trial of tailored strategies to implement guidelines for the management of patients with depression in general practice. *Br J Gen Pract.* **51**:737–741.

Bartholomew L, Parcel G, Kok G and Gottlieb N (2001). *Intervention Mapping. Designing Theory and Evidence Based Health Promotion Programmes*. Mountain View: Mayfield.

Bokhoven M, Kok G and van der Weijden T (2003). Designing a quality improvement intervention: A systematic approach. In Grol R, Moss F and Baker R (Eds). *Quality Improvement Research*. London: BMJ Books.

Cooper R and Zinud R (1990). Information technology implementation research: A technological diffusion approach. *Manage Sci.* **36**:123–129.

Cretin S (1998). *Implementing Guidelines: An Overview*. Report. Santa Monica: RAND.

Davis DA and Taylor-Vaisey A (1997). Translating guidelines into practice: A systematic review of theoretic concepts, practical experience and research evidence in the adoption of clinical practice guidelines. *Can Med Assoc J.* **157**:408–416.

Davis DA, Thomson MA, Oxman AD, *et al.* (1992). Evidence for the effectiveness of CME: A review of 50 randomized controlled trials. *JAMA* **268**:1111–1117.

Davis DA, O'Brien MA, Freemantle N, *et al.* (1999). Impact of formal continuing medical education: Do conferences, workshops, rounds, and other traditional continuing education activities change physician behaviour or health care outcomes? *JAMA* **282**:867–874.

Dickinson E (1995). Using marketing principles for health care development. *Qual Health Care* **4**:40–44.

Evans D and Haines A (2000). *Implementing Evidence-Based Changes in Health Care*. Abingdon: Radcliffe Medical Press.

Feder G, Eccles M, Grol R, *et al.* (1999). Using clinical guidelines. *BMJ* **318**:728–730.

Ferlie E and Shortell S (2001). Improving the quality of health care in the United Kingdom and the United States: A framework for change. *Milbank Q.* **79**:281–315.

Flottorp S, Havelsrud K and Oxman A (2003). Process evaluation of a cluster randomised trial of tailored interventions to implement guidelines in primary care. Why is it so hard to change practice. *Fam Pract.* **20**:333–339.

Garside P (1998). Organisational context for quality: Lessons from the fields of organisational development and change management. *Qual Health Care* **7**(Suppl):S8–S15.

Green LW and Kreuter MW (1991). *Health Promotion Planning: An Educational and Environmental Approach*. Palo Alto: Mayfield Publishing.

Green LW, Eriksen MP and Schor EL (1988). Preventive practices by physicians: Behaviorial determinants and potential interventions. *Am J Prev Med.* **4**(Suppl):101–107.

Grol R (1992). Implementing guidelines in general practice care. *Qual Health Care* **1**:184–191.

Grol R (1997). Beliefs and evidence in changing clinical practice. *BMJ* **315**:418–421.

Grol R and Grimshaw J (2003). From best evidence to best practice: Effective implementation of change in patients' care. *Lancet* **362**:1225–1230.

Grol R and Wensing M (2004). What drives change? Barriers to and incentives for achieving evidence-based practice. *MJA* **180**:S57–S60.

Hall L and Eccles M (2000). Case study of an inter-professional and inter-organisational programme to adapt, implement and evaluate clinical guidelines in secondary care. *Br J Clin Gov.* **5**(2):72–82.

JCAHC (1993). *Process Improvement Models. Case Studies in Health Care*. Oakbrook Terrace: Joint Commission for Accreditation Health Care.

Kaegi L (1997). Disseminating and testing of clinical practice guidelines move to top of meeting agendas for AHCPR and Society for Medical Decision Making. *QRB* **17**:402–412.

Kok G (1987). Theorieën over gedragsbeïnvloeding [Theories in Behavioural Change]. In: Damoiseaux V, Gerards FM, Kok GJ and Nijhuis F (Eds). *Gezondheidsvoorlichting en Opvoeding [Health Education and Information]*. Assen/Maastricht: Van Gorcum.

Kotler P and Roberto E (1989). *Social Marketing Strategies for Changing Public Behaviour*. New York: Free Press.

Langley G, Nolan K, Nolan T, *et al.* (19960). *The Improvement Guide*. San Francisco: Jossey Bass.

Lomas J (1997). *Beyond the Sound of One Hand Clapping: A Discussion Document on Improving Health Research Dissemination and Uptake*. Sydney: University of Sydney.

Lomas J and Haynes R (1988). A taxonomy and critical review of tested strategies for the application of clinical practice recommendations: From 'official' to 'individual' clinical policy. *Am J Prev Med.* **4**:77–95.

McGuire W (1981). Theoretical foundation of campaigns. In: Rice R and Paisley W (Eds). *Public Communications Campaigns*. Beverley Hills: Sage.

Mehta RH, Montoye CK, Gallogly M, *et al.* (2002). Improving quality of care for acute myocardial infarction: The Guidelines Applied in Practice (GAP) Initiative. *JAMA* **287**(10):1269–1276.

Metz J, McGrath KM, Copperchini ML, *et al.* (1995). Appropriateness of transfusions of red cells, platelets and fresh frozen plasma. An audit in a tertiary care teaching hospital. *MJA* **162**:572–577.

Mittman BS, Tonesk X and Jacobson PD (1992). Implementing clinical practice guidelines: Social influence strategies and practitioner behaviour change. *QRB* **18**:413–422.

Moulding NT, Silagy CA and Weller DP (1999). A framework for effective management of change in clinical practice: Dissemination and implementation of clinical practice guidelines. *Qual Health Care* **8**:177–183.

NHMRC (2000). *How to Put the Evidence into Practice: Implementation and Dissemination Strategies*. Canberra: National Health and Medical Research Council.

NHS (1999). Centre for reviews and dissemination. Getting evidence into practice. *Effective Health Care* **5**:1–15.

Orlandi M (1987). Promoting health and preventing disease in health care settings: An analysis of barriers. *Prev Med.* **16**(1):119–130.

Ovretveit J (1999). A team quality improvement sequence for complex problem. *Qual Health Care* **8**:239–246.

Pathman DE, Konrad TR, Freed GL, *et al.* (1996). The awareness-to-adherence model of the steps to clinical guideline compliance. The case of pediatric vaccine recommendations. *Med Care* **34**:873–889.

Prochaska JO and Velicer WF (1997). The transtheoretical model of health behavior change. *Am J Health Promot.* **12**:38–48.

Qasim A, Malpass K, O'Gorman D and Heber M (2002). Safety and efficacy of nurse-initiated thrombolysis in patients with acute myocardial infarction. *BMJ* **324**:1328–1331.

Robertson N, Baker R and Hearnshaw H (1996). Changing the clinical behaviour of doctors: A psychological framework. *Qual Health Care* **1**:51–54.

Rogers E (1983). *Diffusion of Innovations*. New York: Free Press.

Rogers E (1995). Lessons for guidelines from the diffusion of innovation. *Jt Comm J Qual Improv.* **21**:324–328.

Solomon DH, Hashimoto H, Daltroy L and Liang MH (1998). Techniques to improve physician's use of diagnostic tests: A new conceptual framework. *JAMA* **280**:2020–2027.

Spence W (1994). *Innovation. The Communication of Change in Ideas, Practices and Products*. London: Chapman and Hall.

Tuckfield A, Haeusler MN, Grigg AP, *et al.* (1997). Reduction of inappropriate use of blood products by prospective monitoring of transfusion request forms. *MJA* **167**:473–476.

Wye L and McClenahan J (2000). *Getting Better with Evidence*. London: King's Fund.

Zaltman G and Duncan R (1997). *Strategies for Planned Change*. New York: John Wiley.

Part II

Guidelines and innovations

Chapter 4

Characteristics of successful innovations

Richard Grol and Michel Wensing

KEY MESSAGES

- Guidelines, new procedures and proposals to change care processes are 'products' that must meet certain requirements to make them attractive for target groups and to promote their implementation.
- Specific characteristics of such innovations, such as compatibility with existing norms and values, the opportunity to try them out and a clear and attractive design, have a positive influence on adoption by the target group.
- Involving the target group in the development of an innovation or change proposal and offering them the opportunity to adapt it to their own situation also promote implementation.

Box 4.1 Demands that users make on guidelines (Watkins *et al*. 1999)

In a postal survey, almost 400 doctors were asked about the desirable aspects of guidelines. A total of 238 answers were classified. The positive characteristics of guidelines most often mentioned were:

Characteristic	Percentage
Sharp delineation, clarity, simple to use	24
Easy to look up, within reach when needed	18
Offers support for complex problems	15
Certainty that the guideline is good, credibility	12

These results showed the importance of a high-quality product that is comprehensible, easily accessible and offers solutions to the problems that care providers encounter in every day patient care.

INTRODUCTION

The first step in the implementation of change is the development, selection or establishment of a well-founded guideline or protocol for practical application, or the formulation of a concrete proposal or targets to improve the care provision to patients (*Figure 4.1*).

As mentioned in the Introduction, this book addresses the implementation of diverse improvements and changes in care – central and local guidelines and care protocols or pathways, well-tested procedures, techniques and programmes, changes in care processes and the improvement of practical routines (*Table 4.1*). Various types of improvements in patient care require the implementation of various types of change proposals (Cretin 1998). We discuss each of these change proposals briefly below.

Scientific literature and guidelines

Concrete insights gained from the scientific literature and (evidence-based) guidelines for practice can help care providers and patients make optimal decisions about the most appropriate action to be taken. Such

Figure 4.1 Implementation of changes

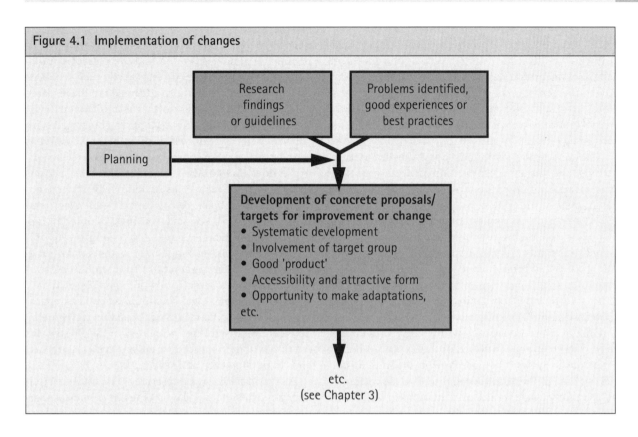

Table 4.1 Types of improvement and implementations

Improvement in	Possible proposals
Clinical decision making	(Summary of) scientific literature (Evidence-based) guidelines Risk tables and decision aids
Multi-disciplinary routines	Care protocols, plans and /or integrated care pathways Disease management systems
Efficiency in care provision	Improving care processes ('business redesign') 'Best practices'

insights are usually published in general scientific or specialist journals, or can be found in databases such as Medline or the Cochrane Library. To an increasing extent, insights are summarised from several studies by means of systematic reviews and meta-analyses. The rate of publication of new insights and techniques is so large that it is not possible for individual care providers (particularly generalists) to keep up to date (Mulrow 1994). Therefore, there is an urgent need to condense the information and to translate the knowledge into practical tools that support decision making in patient care. Within the evidence-based medicine approach, the aim is to teach care providers the skills required to review the scientific literature critically – how to ask pertinent questions, search one of the data bases and make critical appraisals of the studies available (Sackett et al. 1997). Increasingly, the consensus is that the majority of clinicians cannot or will not learn this expertise (Guyatt et al. 2000; Tomlin et al. 1999). A study by McColl et al. (1998) showed that, while a majority of the doctors they contacted had a positive view of evidence-based medicine, they preferred guidelines or practical summaries made by well-informed colleagues. Such well-designed literature analyses and guidelines can form an important aid to the implementation of optimal patient care, as long as they are of such high quality and accessibility that the target group can accept and use them easily. Guidelines are being developed on a steadily increasing scale by scientific societies, government bodies, insurance companies and patient organisations. In view of their importance, Chapter 5 focuses on the development of guidelines and protocols.

A striking development over the past few years, which is linked closely with the increasing involvement of patients and consumers in healthcare provision, is the attempts to better integrate patient preferences and opinions into clinical practice guidelines (Huttin 1997). For many decisions in healthcare, science does not give unequivocal advice. Often there are many alternatives, each with its own advantages and disadvantages in terms of the expected health gain and the risks involved. Patients attribute different values to these advantages and disadvantages. This requires designs and presentations of guidelines in which such benefits and risks are explained clearly, so that the patient – within the framework of shared decision making – can express his or her preference (*Box 4.2*).

Consequently, a steadily increasing number of guidelines are accompanied by decision aids, tables or figures that present the advantages and disadvantages of a certain approach, with the intention that such information should assist shared decision making (Edwards and Elwyn 1999).

Care protocols and clinical pathways

For a proportion of the decisions in patient care, insufficient hard evidence is available and, even when it is available, it cannot always be translated directly into recommendations for practice (Naylor 1995). In scientific research the emphasis is usually on the internal validity of the study, whereas in daily practice people are often confronted both by patient populations that lack homogeneity and by complex problems that are different from those addressed in the research studies (Starfield 1998; Knottnerus and Dinant 1997). In many cases, scientific research is concerned with concrete, clearly defined clinical actions, whereas actual practice often concerns combinations of actions or routines that comprise a series of related actions and decisions. Such series of actions as a whole are seldom the subject of research (Van Weel and Knottnerus 1999). For such routines, people in practical situations usually have more need for care protocols or care plans tailored to the patient and setting. A protocol is a management recommendation based on a programmed description of the policy (Altena *et al.* 1994). It contains clear, well-defined choices regarding the policy to be followed, based on agreements between the disciplines involved. In the English literature, synonymous terms used are 'critical pathway' and 'integrated care pathway'.

A critical pathway is described as a multidisciplinary guideline that displays a time line of clinical goals that patients should attain during a care period, along with the optimal sequence and timing of interventions by care providers to attain those goals (Huttin 1997). The term integrated care pathway was defined by Campbell *et al.* (1998) as a structured multidisciplinary care plan in which actual steps in the care of a patient with a specific clinical problem are described in detail, along with the expected outcomes for patients. In other words, it represents a structured manner in which to translate evidence-based guidelines into local protocols and decision trees. The tasks of the various disciplines, the order in which activities should take place and the time line are all laid out clearly. These plans or guidelines also contain a sort of checklist of the necessary actions that can form part of a dossier or care plan. Whereas a guideline usually makes global recommendations regarding the management of certain disorders or complaints, protocols

Box 4.2 Implementation of an evidence–based guideline for the treatment of cardiac dysrhythmia (Howitt and Armstrong 1999)

In a practice with 13,000 patients, 100 patients with cardiac dysrhythmia were selected who – according to evidence-based guidelines – would benefit from anticoagulation medication. These patients received structured information with explicit illustrations about the advantages of treatment and the decreased risk of suffering a stroke. At the same time, the risks of treatment were explained. Having considered this information, only one half of the patients chose to receive the medication recommended.

and pathways provide detailed regulations about the care in a specific setting. In this way, they form both the subject of implementation and an aid to the implementation of new knowledge, guidelines or working methods in practice.

Integrated care pathways also fit within a disease management approach to care (Hunter and Fairfield 1997). In such systems, the patient with the (chronic) disease (e.g. with diabetes, heart failure, stroke or depression) is placed in the centre and the care is built around the process that the patient goes through. This care is therefore not regarded as a series of separate episodes or fragmentary contacts, but as a continuous process built around the patient, into which evidence-based guidelines can be integrated. All care becomes part of the protocol, all actions, care outcomes and financial costs are evaluated and the patient receives tailored information (*Box 4.3*). Thus, disease management systems can also form a way to translate (scientific) insights into patient care.

Improving care processes and 'best practices'

Many improvements in care are not so much motivated by guidelines, protocols or new procedures proved value as by problems identified in care delivery that lead to errors, wastage or inefficiency. Such problems can be identified from complaints by patients, the experience of care providers or by monitoring care processes. In such instances there are rarely any ready-made solutions that say precisely how the care process should be changed. Therefore, formulating the change itself forms part of the implementation process.

People work, step by step, to analyse existing processes, search for causes of the undesirable procedure and formulate a plan to improve and evaluate their results. This is a process of bottom-up learning instead of top-down implementation (Health Council 2000). Total quality management literature, in particular, provides useful models for the improvement of care processes [e.g. the FOCUS–PDSA cycle (see Chapter 3 and *Box 4.4*)]. These match the step-by-step model employed in this book.

In the case of erroneous or inefficient care processes, people can also look for examples of more optimal working methods ('best practice'). At other institutions or practices, the care providers may have already satisfactorily solved the problem. Adopting and adapting these solutions to the situation of the new target group can potentially save much time and effort. This approach is also integrated into the 'breakthrough collaboratives' now set up in many countries.

As well as systematic reviews, evidence-based guidelines, care protocols, integrated care pathways, disease management systems and best practices, several other innovations can form the subjects of implementation, such as preventive programmes or quality-of-care methods that have proved their worth in certain settings. In all these cases, we are dealing with innovations that the target group may not necessarily be eagerly awaiting or readily willing to accept. The literature shows that it is important to consider at an early stage the likelihood of successful implementation and the possible reactions of the target group when selecting or developing a guideline or new working method. While safeguarding quality,

---

Box 4.3 Disease management protocol for geriatric patients (Wasson *et al*. 1997)

In a project aimed at elderly patients, the researchers built protocols and decision trees for the treatment of geriatric problems into a disease management system. When a patient of over 70 years of age visited the clinic for a (follow-up) consultation, he or she was first asked to fill in a short questionnaire with questions about:

- Health status, experienced symptoms;
- Quality of life;
- Use of medication, possible drug interactions;
- Preventive care received;
- Satisfaction with the information and care received.

A healthcare assistant used an optical scanning system to enter the data into the computer. On the basis of guidelines stored on the computer (in the form of algorithms), a patient-tailored letter was immediately produced that contain information about self-care activities and medication use. The doctor also received the information in an easily assessable form before seeing the patient. During the consultation, both the doctor and patient were prepared for the problems that would be discussed. The geriatric specialist could discuss any aspects of the written information in detail. The information formed a sort of homework assignment for the patient regarding medication, eye care, preventing falls, physical exercise, etc. On the basis of the data entered into the computer for a large group of patients, the doctors also received regular feedback about their patient population.

Box 4.4 Improvement of the continuity of care at a health centre (Kibbe *et al.* 1993)

Patients complained that they were not always seen by their own doctor, but were nearly always referred to someone else. This gave rise to a change project that followed a FOCUS–PDSA step-by-step plan (see Chapter 3).

1. Find what needs to be improved – the complaints patients had made over the previous 9 months were reviewed, and 75% were concerned at not being seen by their own doctor. More consultations with a patient's own doctor was agreed as the desired improvement.
2. Organise a team – a multidisciplinary group of interested professionals held 90 minute meetings every week for a period of 6 months.
3. Clarify knowledge of the process – an audit of 125 patient records, selected at random, showed that only 45% had seen their own doctor. A survey among the patients showed that they would rather wait to see their own doctor than be seen by someone else the same day. Physicians held the view that contact with a patient's own doctor should be possible in a minimum

of 70% of the cases and set this as a desirable and achievable goal.
4. Understanding the causes – problem analysis was performed by producing a cause–consequence diagram, a flowchart and a Paretogram (see Chapter 7). The largest problem lay in the system of making appointments; receptionists usually chose the route that was most practical for themselves.
5. Selecting process improvements – various processes were selected for improvement, including the appointment system, the allocation of a doctor to a patient, the working schedules of the doctors and education of the assistants and receptionists. These processes were assimilated into protocols (or pathways).

Implementation took place via redesigning the appointment system, staff training, reorganising the health centre into smaller units and relocating the units to specific, easily accessible stations.

The audit was repeated 1 year later, and showed that 70% of the patients were seen by their own doctor.

---

at the earliest possible stage developers seek ways to think in terms of optimal use of the innovation (discussed in the next three sections):

- Certain characteristics of innovations promote or hinder implementation;
- A carefully thought out and attractive form can contribute to implementation;
- Involvement of the target group and the opportunity to adapt the innovation to their working situation improves the chance of implementation.

Characteristics of innovations that promote implementation

Most importantly, the innovation, whether it is a guideline, a care protocol or a 'best practice', must be of the best possible quality. The target group must have every confidence that using the 'product' leads to the desired goal. In the health service, this usually means better care for the patients that leads to better health or better quality of life. However, other desirable goals may be cheaper or more efficiently organised care, such as a reduction in work pressure, or prevention of problems or errors in the execution of care tasks. The literature mentions a great many characteristics of innovations that might promote or hinder their actual application (e.g. Grol *et al.* 1998; Spence 1994; Wolfe 1994; Orlandi 1987; Rogers 1983, 1995;

Zaltman and Duncan 1977). An overview is given in *Table 4.2*.

Very little empirical research has explored the actual influence of such characteristics. Much of the literature is contemplative or based on other sectors of society. Below we describe in more detail a number of the above-mentioned characteristics, particularly those put forward by Rogers (1983, 1995) and frequently cited in publications – benefit, compatibility, complexity, trialability and visibility.

Benefit

Benefit is the degree to which the innovation can be seen as an improvement on existing practice. In general, a new working method is only introduced if it seems to offer advantages over the existing situation. To achieve better care outcomes for patients is usually the most important motivation for many care providers. However, other benefits, including financial or increased status for the people who apply the innovation, may be of influence, as well as increased pleasure in work or reduced work pressure. Such advantages are weighed against possible disadvantages, such as extra time commitment, money and disruption that may accompany the innovation. As the balance between the advantages and disadvantages becomes more favourable, implementation is likely to be more successful. Implementation of an innovation can, there-

Table 4.2 Characteristics of innovations that might promote or hinder their implementation

Characteristic	Description
Relative advantage and utility	Better than existing or alternative working methods
Compatibility	Consistent with existing norms and values
Complexity	Easy to explain, understand and use
Costs	Balance between cost and benefits, and level of investment necessary
Risks	Degree of uncertainty about result or consequences
Flexibility, adaptability and revisability	Degree to which innovation can be adapted to needs and/or situation of target group
Involvement	Degree to which target group is involved in development
Divisibility	Degree to which parts can be tried out separately and implemented separately
Trialability and reversability	Degree to which, without risk, an innovation can be tried out, stopped or reversed if it does not work
Visibility and observability	Degree to which other people can see and observe the results
Centrality	Degree to which the innovation affects central or peripheral activities in the daily working routine
Pervasiveness, scope and impact	How much of the total work is influenced by the innovation, how many people are influenced and how much time does it take; what is the influence on social relationships
Magnitude, disruptiveness and radicalness:	how many organisational, structural, financial and personal measures the innovation requires
Duration	Time period within which the change has to take place
Form and physical properties	What sort of innovation or change it is (material or social, technical or administrative, etc.)
Collective action	Degree to which decision making about the innovation has to be performed by individuals, groups or a whole institution
Presentation	Nature of presentation, length, clarity and attractiveness

fore, be promoted by including in the presentation a clear description of the advantages and of solutions to any possible disadvantages and limitations.

Different individuals and institutions can have widely varying opinions about the advantages and disadvantages of the same innovation. For example, a hospital may attribute great importance to following a guideline for the prevention of infections, or the correct use of antibiotics in the fight against bacterial resistance. For individual doctors or nurses, the perceived advantages might be much smaller, because they have to monitor patients more closely and provide them with more detailed information and explanation of their treatment. In addition, patients may be convinced that

they should receive antibiotics for their condition, although from a medical point of view they are of little value. When implementing a change it is important to have a clear view of the advantages and disadvantages as perceived by the people involved.

Compatibility

Compatibility is the degree to which the innovation complies with existing opinions, needs, norms, values and routines. No matter how great the advantages of a different working method might be, implementation does not run smoothly if the innovation is not consistent with existing norms and values, or the professional experience of the people in the target group (Sheldon *et al*. 1998). There are quite often mismatches between the sort of evidence or the insights that come from scientific research and the sort of evidence that care providers want to see or consider applicable to their patients (Tannenbaum 1996). Therefore, it is important to involve people from the target group (the users) in the development of a guideline or a proposal to change existing practice, so that they can understand its importance and help ensure that the new procedure or process is consistent with existing views held within the target group. Sometimes an innovation can be linked to other procedures, organisational processes or routines that people already feel positive about (*Box 4.5*).

Complexity

Complexity is the degree to which a new working method is considered to be difficult to understand and awkward to use. A complex innovation is obviously more difficult to implement, because the users have to spend a great deal of energy on learning to understand it (*Box 4.6*). The importance of complexity in the implementation of guidelines has been shown in several studies (Grol *et al*. 1998; Van Assema *et al*. 1998). A particularly important factor is how the people involved experience the complexity. One study (Van Assema *et al*. 1998), for example, investigated the national implementation of guided group visits to a supermarket in the framework of a campaign 'Watch out for fat!' The adoption of the programme by District Health Authorities was evaluated. The high level of complexity of the programme had a negative impact on its application. Programmes were less well accepted and used as the complexity of their execution was perceived to increase by the District Health Authority staff. As perceived complexity plays such a large role in the implementation of innovations, it is important to pay attention to their understandability and accessibility, by using summaries, a variety of media, clear texts or chopping proposals into pieces so that they are easier to grasp.

Trialability

Trialability is the degree to which people can try out the innovation on a small scale, without the risk of becoming overwhelmed by its consequences. Trying out an innovation on a small scale helps to demonstrate its value in people's own setting and helps them identify what is necessary to make it work. This is one way to deal with the uncertainty that every change brings with it. Trying things out is of particular importance to those who try things first. Those who follow can make use of the experience of the group that went before. The effort put in by the people who have tried out the innovation and the presentation of their experience can form a powerful support for the broader acceptance of a new practice or routine. However, not every innovation can be tried out on a small scale (e.g. if expensive equipment has to be bought).

Visibility

Visibility is the degree to which the results of a new working method are visible (observability). Showing that the new performance is both feasible in practice and quickly accomplishes the desired results can stimulate its implementation. Most people are sensitive

---

Box 4.5 Physical exercise programmes for the elderly (Wensing *et al*. 2000)

Physical exercise is known to have a positive effect on health, but the success of such 'keep-fit' programmes varies in elderly people. A large proportion of the elderly do not take any exercise at all, and many – otherwise effective – keep-fit programmes do not reach these groups. One explanation is that many elderly people do not see themselves as the sporting type and have a low opinion of sport or good physical fitness. However, they are interested in social contact with other people and like to participate in enjoyable activities. Therefore, new programmes are being developed in which contact with others and enjoyable activities are combined (e.g. dancing sessions).

Box 4.6 Characteristics of effective guidelines

Grilli and Lomas (1994) analysed of recommendations from guidelines described in 23 studies, in which the implementation of the guidelines was also reported. A total of 143 recommendations were categorised by the characteristics put forward by Rogers (1983) – complexity, trialability and visibility. The former two characteristics had a significant influence on implementation – compliance with complex recommendations was 42%, compared to 56% for non-complex recommendations. Compliance with trialable recommendations was 56%, compared to 37% for non-trialable recommendations.

to the opinions of others when making choices, particularly when they consider the other person to be exemplar or a role model. In the framework of an implementation plan it is therefore important to deploy people who have experience of the new practice, so as to show how they apply it, what experience they have with it and what results they have achieved with it so far (*Box 4.7*).

FORM AND PRESENTATION

Another important aspect of the implementation of an innovation is the way in which it is presented (*Box 4.8*). Which method should be chosen (written, audio-visual, verbal) and how understandable, accessible and attractive is the final presentation? Different forms can be used for different target users. For example, for self-study or further education, use can be made of texts that contain extensive information, whereas for direct instruction in a hospital ward a flow chart may be more convenient.

When considering the issue of clarity, the following are important points to consider:

■ Do not use language that is susceptible to multiple interpretations (Field and Lohr 1990), so avoid abstract and vague terms, use terminology consistently and avoid jargon – inclusion of a glossary of difficult terms and abbreviations is often helpful.

■ Use logical, easy to understand presentations of the recommendations or new routines, and keep them as simple as possible to allow rapid understanding. The information must be easy to access in various situations. The study by Watkins *et al.* (1999) showed the most important demand that doctors made of

---

Box 4.7 Attributes of guidelines that influence guideline use in practice (Grol *et al.* 1998; Burgers *et al.* 2003; Foy *et al.* 2002)

Based on the literature, Grol *et al.* (1998) formulated 16 attributes of recommendations that could influence the use of guidelines in practice. A panel of four experts determined the presence of these characteristics in 47 recommendations selected from 10 guidelines developed by the Dutch College of General Practitioners (NHG). Data recorded in general practices were used to determine the extent to which the recommendations were followed. The analysis showed that 17% of the variation in compliance could be explained by attributes of the recommendations. The attributes with the highest scores were 'compatible with existing norms and values', 'concrete, specific and clearly defined' and 'demanded no changes of existing routines'. Recommendations with these attributes were followed more often in practice.

In a subsequent study, Burgers *et al.* (2003), using a sample of 96 recommendations selected from 28 NHG guidelines, also found that recommendations with high compliance rates were often supported with scientific evidence, were not part of a complex decision tree and did not require new skills. For diagnostic recommendations the ease of application and the potential (negative) reactions of patients were more relevant than they were for therapeutic recommendations.

Another study in 16 gynaecology departments in Scotland (Foy *et al.* 2002) utilised 13 attributes of guidelines to examine the compliance with 42 recommendations before and after audit and feedback. Recommendations compatible with clinical values and recommendations that did not require changes to fixed routines were associated with greater compliance. However, significant changes in compliance were only found for recommendations seen as incompatible, probably because there was more scope for improvement in compliance with these recommendations.

Box 4.8 Style of consensus guidelines (Kahan *et al.* 1988)

An analysis on the presentation style of American consensus guidelines showed that the guidelines could be classified according to three dimensions:

■ Scholarly dimension – the degree to which the guidelines give a more-or-less abstract description of the scientific evidence for certain actions;

■ Discursive dimension – the degree to which the guidelines give a more-or-less complete and abstract description of the desired actions, with few concrete recommendations;

■ Didactic dimension – the degree to which the guidelines contained more-or-less straightforward recommendations that described how to act with certain patients in concrete circumstances.

According to the authors, a high score on the didactic dimension and a low score on the discursive dimension improved acceptance by care providers.

guidelines was that they must be transparent and easily accessible.

■ Adaptation of both form and language use to the everyday problems in care practice and to the way in which the people involved go about their work. This may mean that a guideline or care protocol is presented in the form of a decision tree, or a written plan that gives the chronological order of the activities that the different care providers have to perform.

■ Highlight the most essential elements of the activities of the care providers who are involved (Sanazaro 1983). Less important aspects or details are not considered. The literature on patient education shows that a message should be presented in small doses and restricted to the essential information. Important information should be repeated, because a person can only read and remember a limited number of messages at a time (Grol et al. 1991; Ley 1983).

■ Provide educational aids to promote understanding of a guideline or new working method. For example, the provision of easy-to-understand texts and programmes for further education, or the definition of indicators and criteria for audit or assessment (Box 4.9).

■ Design an attractive layout – the guideline or proposal for a new working method should immediately attract interest through its form, such as:
  – Attractive typographic layout and selective use of bold script and colours;
  – Use of summaries;
  – Restriction of the number of literature references.

In a study, 2600 doctors were asked their opinion about the best way to present guidelines. Brevity and clarity were found to be most important, while they also required the presentation of a summary of the scientific evidence behind each recommendation (Hayward et al. 1993).

For a number of years, the British Medical Journal (BMJ) has used boxes that contain the key messages in each article to increase the educational value and accessibility of their journal. It also offers, under various headings (e.g. Editor's choice, This week in BMJ), brief information about articles to stimulate the reader to delve more deeply into the article itself. Strategies such as this make the journal more accessible to readers.

INVOLVEMENT OF THE TARGET GROUP AND LOCAL ADAPTATION

The above text emphasises the importance of involving the (representatives of the) target group in the development or selection of a guideline, care protocol, preventive programme or proposal for changing care processes in practice. It is also necessary to tailor the innovation to the needs, problems encountered and work setting of those people who are intended to apply the innovation (Kotler and Roberto 1989). In addition, involvement helps the target group to consider the innovation as their own and encourages them to take responsibility for it.

When considering the question who should be involved in the development process, factors such as recognisability, representativeness and expertise are important:

Box 4.9 Summary of the Dutch College of General Practitioners guideline for acute otitis media on a plastic card supplied with the publication of the guideline

Information

■ In 90% of cases, the worst complaints are over in <3 days, follow-up unnecessary;

■ Some cases develop otorrhoea, which usually disappears spontaneously in <2 weeks;

■ Tympanic membrane perforation – no swimming with head underwater, but showering permitted;

■ After acute otitis media, hearing is often poor because of fluid development behind the tympanic membrane, which disappears spontaneously in several weeks or months.

Medication therapy

■ Symptomatic therapy – advise analgesics in all cases, with paracetamol as first choice, and, if necessary, nose drops for nasal congestion;

■ Instruct patient or parents to contact the general practitioner (GP) if course is irregular – illness deteriorates, poor fluid intake, increase in earache or no improvement after 3 days;

■ Indication for antibiotics – children <6 months of age, primary antibiotic therapy; irregular course (illness deteriorates, poor fluid intake, increase in earache); no improvement after 3 days, etc.

■ *Recognisability* – the target group must be able to identify with the developers. In a survey, medical specialists stated, for example, that they seldom used guidelines for GPs (Van Everdingen 2003). An average of less than one-quarter of the specialists attributed any value to GP guidelines, as opposed to 80–90% for the guidelines developed by their own societies. A representation of various professional groups reported that they also attributed less value to multidisciplinary guidelines of an independent national agency for guideline development (40–50% positive judgement).

■ *Representativeness* – related to the nature of the innovation and whether use is made of the experience and expertise of all the relevant parties. Who these people are varies from one innovation to another.

■ *Expertise* – the status enjoyed by the developers on the basis of their expertise and authority also influences acceptance.

CONCLUSIONS

Guidelines, care pathways, changes in care processes and care programmes are innovations that have to meet certain demands if the target group is to accept them and adopt them into their normal care routines. To this end, the people who develop the proposals for change have to start thinking at an early stage about factors in the innovation itself that promote implementation. Involvement of the target group, the perceived advantage of the procedure or care process, an attractive and easy to understand presentation can all affect uptake.

The implementation of guidelines and protocols forms one of the most important challenges in the improvement of the quality of patient care. Guidelines can be used to devise targets for improving care, as well as systems to measure and monitor actual care. In this way, the development and implementation of guidelines forms one of the gauges of quality policy in healthcare in most countries. Given that these activities encounter problems in practice, Chapter 5 addresses the matter of effective guidelines in more depth.

Recommended literature

Rogers E (1995). Lessons for guidelines from the diffusion of innovation. *Jt Comm J Qual Improv*. 21:324–328.

References

Altena HJ, Harten WH van, Westert GJ, *et al.* (1994). Protocollen in de gezondheidszorg [Protocols in Health Care]. *Med Contact* **49**:837–840.

Assema P van, Brug J, Glanz K, *et al.* (1998). Nationwide implementation of guided supermarket tours in the Netherlands: A dissemination study. *Health Educ Res*. **13**(4): 557–566.

Burgers JS, Grol RPTM, Zaat JOM, Spies TH, Van der Bij AK and Mokkink HGA (2003). Characteristics of effective clinical guidelines for general practice. *Br J Gen Pract*. **53**:15–19.

Campbell H, Hotchkiss R, Bradshaw N, *et al.* (1998). Integrated care pathways. *BMJ* **316**:133–137.

Cretin S (1998). *Implementing Guidelines: An Overview*. Report. Santa Monica: RAND.

Edwards A and Elwyn G (1999). How should effectiveness of risk communication to aid patients' decisions be judged? A review of the literature. *Med Decis Making* **19**:428–434.

Everdingen JJ van, Mokkink HGA, Klazinga NS, Grol R and Koekenbier GJS (2003). De bekendheid en verspreiding van CBO-richtlijnen onder medisch specialisten [The knowledge and distribution of CBO guidelines among medical specialists]. *TSG* **81**(8):468–472.

Field M and Lohr K (1990). *Clinical Practice Guidelines: Directions for a New Agency*. Washington: National Academic Press.

Foy R, MacLennan G, Grimshaw J, Penney G, Campbell M and Grol R (2002). Attributes of clinical recommendations that influence change in practice following audit and feedback. *J Clin Epidemiol*. **55**:717–722.

Grilli R and Lomas J (1994). Evaluating the message: The relationship between compliance rate and the subject of a practice guideline. *Med Care* **32**(3):202–213.

Grol R, Beurden W van, Binkhorst T, *et al.* (1991). Patient education in family practice. The consensus reached by patients, doctors and experts. *Fam Pract*. **8**:133–139.

Grol R, Eccles M, Maisonneuve H, *et al.* (1998). Developing clinical practice guidelines. The European experience. *Dis Man Health Out*. **4**:255–266.

Guyatt G, Meade M, Jaeschke R, *et al.* (2000). Practitioners of evidence based care. *BMJ* **320**:954–955.

Hayward R, Wilson M, Tunis B, *et al.* (1993). More informative abstract of articles describing clinical practice guidelines. *Ann Intern Med*. **118**:731–737.

Health Council (2000). *From Implementation to Learning*. Den Haag: Gezondheidsraad.

Howitt A and Armstrong D (1999). Implementing evidence-based medicine in general practice: Audit and qualitative study of antithrombotic treatment for atrial fibrillation. *BMJ* **318**:1324–1327.

Hunter D and Fairfield G (1997). Disease management. *BMJ* **315**:50–53.

Huttin C (1997). The use of clinical guidelines to improve medical practice: Main issues in the United States. *Int J Qual Health Care* **9**:207–214.

Kahan J, Kanouse D and Winkler J (1988). Stylistic variations in National Institutes of Health consensus statements 1979–1983. *Int J Technol Assess*. **4**:289–304.

Kibbe D, Bentz E and McLaughlin C (1993). Continuous quality improvement for continuity of care. *J Fam Pract.* **36**:304–308.

Knottnerus J and Dinant GJ (1997). Medicine-based evidence, a prerequisite for evidence-based medicine. *BMJ* **315**:1109–1110.

Kotler P and Roberto E (1989). *Social Marketing Strategies for Changing Public Behaviour.* New York: Free Press.

Ley P (1983). Patients understanding and recall in clinical communication failure. In: Pendleton D and Hasler J (Eds). *Doctor–Patient Communication.* London: Academic Press.

McColl A, Smith H, White P, *et al.* (1998). General practitioners' perceptions of the route to evidence-based medicine: A questionnaire survey. *BMJ* **316**:361–365.

Mulrow CD (1994). Rationale for systematic reviews. *BMJ* **309**:597–599.

Naylor CD (1995). Grey zones of clinical practice: Some limits to evidence-based medicine. *Lancet* **345**:840–842.

Orlandi M (1987). Promoting health and preventing disease in health care settings: An analysis of barriers. *Prev Med.* **16**(1):119–130.

Rogers E (1983). *Diffusion of Innovations.* New York: Free Press.

Rogers E (1995). Lessons for guidelines from the diffusion of innovation. *Jt Comm J Qual Improv.* **21**:324–328.

Sackett D, Richardson W, Rosenberg W and Haynes R (1997). *Evidence-Based Medicine: How to Practice and Teach.* London: Churchill Livingstone.

Sanazaro P (1983). Determining physicians performance. Continuing medical education and other interacting variables. *Eval Health Prof.* **2**:197–210.

Sheldon T, Guyatt G and Haines A (1998). Getting research findings into practice: When to act on the evidence? *BMJ* **317**:139–142.

Spence W (1994). *Innovation. The Communication of Change in Ideas, Practices and Products.* London: Chapman and Hall.

Starfield B (1998). Quality of care research. Internal elegance and external relevance. *JAMA* **280**:1006–1008.

Tannenbaum S (1996). 'Medical effectiveness' in Canada and US health policy: The comparative politics of inferential ambiguity. *Health Serv Res.* **31**:517–532.

Tomlin Z, Humphrey C and Rogers S (1999). General practitioners' perceptions of effective health care. *BMJ* **318**:1532–1535.

Wasson J, Jette A, Johnson D, *et al.* (1997). A replicable and customizable approach to improve ambulatory care and research. *J Ambulatory Care Manage.* **20**(1):17–27.

Watkins C, Harvey I, Langley C, *et al.* (1999). General practitioners' use of guidelines in the consultation and their attitudes to them. *Br J Gen Pract* **49**:11–15.

Weel C van and Knottnerus J (1999). Evidence-based intervention and comprehensive treatment. *Lancet* **353**:916–918.

Wensing M, Bij A van der and Laurant M (2000). *Implementation of Exercise Programmes for Older People. A Literature Review.* Den Haag: ZON.

Wolfe R (1994). Organisational innovation: Review, critique and suggested research directions. *J Manage Stud.* **31**:406–431.

Zaltman G and Duncan R (1977). *Strategies for Planned Change.* New York: John Wiley.

Chapter 5

Clinical guidelines as a tool for implementing change in patient care

Jako Burgers, Richard Grol and Martin Eccles

KEY MESSAGES

- Clinical guidelines are an important aid in translating research findings and new insights into clinical practice. However, they should not be considered as a 'magic bullet' to improve healthcare.
- Whether clinical guidelines can improve the quality of care depends on several factors, including the characteristics of the clinical guidelines.
- Characteristics that could contribute to use of clinical guidelines in practice include:
  - Have concrete aims and objectives;
  - Have sufficient scientific evidence to support most of the recommendations;
  - Have a clear structure and attractive layout;
  - Have clear and specific recommendations;
  - Take into account the norms and values of the target users;
  - Applicable in different settings.
- Clinical guidelines should be developed within a structured and co-ordinated programme by a credible central organisation. To promote their implementation, central guidelines could be used as a template for local care protocols and interdisciplinary agreements.

Box 5.1 Quality of clinical guidelines assessed

Shaneyfelt *et al.* (1999) assessed 279 clinical guidelines, published between 1985 and 1997 and retrieved via MEDLINE, using 25 criteria about the process of development, the use of scientific evidence and the methods used to formulate recommendations. None of the clinical guidelines satisfied all the criteria. On average, 43% of the criteria were satisfied. Recent clinical guidelines achieved higher scores than older ones. The length of a clinical guideline also correlated with a higher score. The type of organisation responsible for the guideline had no influence on the results.

Criteria	Guidelines that satisfied the criteria (%)
Objective of the guideline is described concretely and/or explicitly	75
Participants in the development are described	26
Patient population to which guideline is directed is described concretely	46
Desired results in patients are described specifically	40
Manner of compiling scientific evidence is specified	17

INTRODUCTION

The aim of clinical practice guidelines (hereafter referred to as clinical guidelines) is to improve patient care by providing clearly supported and appropriate recommendations for daily practice. Preferably, these are based on the best-available evidence, supplemented with clinical expertise. The definition from the Institutes of Medicine is widely accepted, 'clinical practice guidelines are systematically developed statements to assist practitioner and patient decisions about appropriate healthcare for specific clinical circumstances' (Field and Lohr 1992). This definition emphasises that clinical guidelines are an aid to daily practice, not only for healthcare professionals, but also for patients. The patient should benefit from the clinical guidelines, which should help patients take part in healthcare decisions – and they should be developed in a rigorous, systematic way.

Sometimes other terms are used. The distinction between guidelines and protocols is discussed in Chapter 4. Another term used is 'standards', which has two meanings. Firstly, according to Eddy (1992), clinical standards are recommendations for the use of interventions for which the health and economic consequences are sufficiently well known. Standards *must* be followed in all cases, while guidelines *should* be followed in most cases, depending on the individual patient, the setting and other factors. Secondly, the concept of a 'standard' is also used in the evaluation of the use of guidelines. Here, the term applies to the level of performance of a given criterion: for example, for the criterion of diastolic blood pressure, a standard could be that in 80% of all patients with hypertension this should be less than 90 mmHg (Lawrence and Olesen 1997). Standards can be set at the lowest level that should be achieved in all cases (minimum standard), the maximum that can be achieved (ideal standard) or somewhere in between to reflect optimised care (optimum standard).

PURPOSES OF CLINICAL GUIDELINES

Clinical guidelines can be developed for different purposes (*Box 5.2*), which should be clear to the target users. In general, two main purposes of guidelines can be distinguished:

- *Guidelines as professional aids.* Clinical guidelines can be regarded as a reflection of the current state of knowledge for both professionals and patients. They can be used to teach and in continuing education, and also as the basis for interdisciplinary agreements or as part of internal, professional, quality-improvement policy activities.

- *Guidelines as a means to external control.* Not only care providers and patients, but also other parties (e.g. medical insurers and governmental or federal agencies) could have an interest in clinical guidelines. For insurers, guidelines could be used in contracts or budgetary control. Governments could use guidelines in policy making or rationing healthcare (Feek 2000; Norheim 1999). From the policy makers' perspective, cost effectiveness and efficiency are at least as relevant as quality of healthcare, and clinical guidelines should primarily aim to prevent unnecessary healthcare and unnecessary costs.

To avoid misunderstandings and the possibility of subsequent professional resistance, a clinical guideline should clearly describe both its scope and purposes (Gevers and Biesaart 1999; Grol and Heerdink 1992).

Box 5.2 Opinions of physicians about the use of clinical guidelines (Grol and Heerdink 1992)

National surveys among samples of Dutch general practitioners (GPs) taken at the start of a guideline programme revealed that a majority feared guidelines would be obligatory. They considered clinical guidelines especially useful for the training of doctors, for peer review and continuing education, and for local consensus about care provisions. The use of clinical guidelines as an external control was seen as much less useful.

Clinical guidelines use	GPs thought useful or very useful (%)
Training of physicians	85
Peer review	84
Continuing education	84
Local consensus	81
Co-operation with other disciplines	68
Recertification	39
Insurance contracts	25

POTENTIAL BENEFITS AND LIMITATIONS OF CLINICAL GUIDELINES

Over the past two decades there has been a steady increase in clinical guideline activities (Burgers *et al.* 2003a; Burgers 2002; Woolf *et al.* 1999) and guideline development has become more formalised and institutionalised. Not only healthcare professionals, but also policy makers and government organisations are interested in clinical guidelines and increasingly support guideline development.

Guidelines are occasionally presented as a 'magic bullet' to resolve problems of effectiveness or efficiency of care. However, they are only one option for improving the quality of care. They are especially useful for situations in which there is uncertainty about the appropriate practice and scientific evidence can provide an answer (Woolf *et al.* 1999). In other situations, multidisciplinary protocols, integrated care pathways or changing care processes might be more suitable.

However, while it is clear that clinical guidelines can improve both the process and outcome of care (Grimshaw *et al.* 2004), it is useful to examine how exactly guidelines may contribute to improving the quality of care and the limitations that may occur in this process.

Potential benefits

Clinical guidelines can contribute to improvements in patient care in a number of ways (*Table 5.1*):
- *Improving the quality of care.* This refers to the process as well as the outcome of healthcare. An improvement of the process of care may lead to less variation in healthcare delivery. In areas with good clinical evidence it is also reasonable to expect an improvement in process to contribute to improvements in patient outcomes.
- *Improving information about optimal care.* Clinical guidelines summarise the potential benefits and limitations of procedures and interventions for defined health problems. When they are accompanied by patient versions, which explain the clinical content in lay language, they provide patients with information that may empower them to share the decision making with healthcare providers (Elwyn 2001; Woolf 1997).
- *Summary of research findings.* The development of a clinical guideline includes a systematic review of recent scientific literature, which provides individual care providers with an overview of new developments (Haynes and Haines 1998). It also highlights gaps in the current knowledge, which could be a stimulus for further research.
- *External accountability.* Clinical guidelines link care provision with a body of scientific knowledge and with professional consensus about good medical practice, which could improve the transparency of decisions. Clinical guidelines may also be used in disciplinary or judicial proceedings.
- *Basis for teaching and education.* A generally accepted and up-to-date clinical guideline offers a sound basis for training or continuing medical education. In contrast, textbooks often contain material that is too general and often out of date, whereas a clinical guideline provides specific recommendations based on recent research findings. The guideline can also be used as a point of reference for audit and the evaluation of healthcare.

Table 5.1 Potential benefits and limitations of clinical guidelines

Potential benefits	Possible limitations
Improving the quality of care	Cookbook medicine
Improving information about optimal care	Unrealistic expectations
Summary of research findings	Loss of clinical autonomy
External accountability	Professional resistance and concern for legal consequences
Basis for teaching and education	Misuse by governmental authorities
Basis for interdisciplinary co-operation	Uncertainty about cost-effectiveness
Contributing to efficient care	Hidden political motives
Setting healthcare priorities	

■ *Basis for interdisciplinary collaboration*. Many clinical guidelines cover topics that involve different disciplines, for instance low back pain (GPs, neurologists, orthopaedic surgeons, rheumatologists, rehabilitation physicians and allied professions, such as physiotherapists and psychologists). In this context a clinical guideline can serve as a basis for interdisciplinary agreements about the management of a condition or disease.

■ *Contributing to efficient care*. Ideally, clinical guidelines describe how optimal care can be offered with due consideration of the resources available. They should thus not only improve the quality of patient care, but also increase the efficiency of care. If they reduce excessive or inappropriate use of healthcare services, clinical guidelines will reduce excessive costs (Shapiro *et al.* 1993).

■ *Setting research and healthcare priorities*. Clinical guidelines can call attention to under-recognised health problems. If a systematic review of the available evidence fails to identify evidence on an important clinical area, this can be flagged to research-fund providers as a priority research topic. In addition, guidelines can, within their content, identify the needs of specific (neglected) patient populations, such as drug addicts or patients in deprived areas. Thus, they can promote distributive justice and advocate better delivery of services to those in need.

Possible limitations

Clinical guidelines may also have limitations (*Table 5.1*), such as:

■ *Cookbook medicine*. A clinical guideline usually takes a hypothetical standard patient as a point of reference and does not specifically address individual, unique patients with their own wishes and preferences. Thus, guidelines may oversimplify clinical practice and neglect its complex reality (Tonelli 1998), thereby encouraging users to apply recommendations rigidly or unthinkingly, even in situations for which departure from the clinical guideline may be desirable (Hurwitz 1999).

■ *Unrealistic expectations*. Clinical guidelines formulate the way in which optimal healthcare should be provided. Adequate application of clinical guidelines suggests a certain health gain (Woolf 1993). However, it is not clear to what extent this can be achieved in routine practice (Worrall *et al.* 1997). Many clinical guidelines are produced on the basis of results from clinical studies of selected populations in standardised settings. Results achieved in experimental studies are often not achieved in daily practice (Starfield 1998; Knottnerus and Dinant 1997), and the effect of interventions recommended in the clinical guideline cannot be predicted with certainty.

■ *Professional resistance and concern for legal consequences*. In general, healthcare professionals strive for professional autonomy. The need to follow clinical guidelines may threaten this autonomy (Tunis *et al.* 1994). Similarly, some professionals fear that clinical guidelines increase their medico-legal exposure (Hurwitz 1999). In court, the actions suggested by clinical guidelines may come to overrule those of expert clinical judgement (Garfield and Garfield 2000).

■ *Misuse by governmental authorities*. Clinical guidelines may also be used by governmental and other authorities. In France, for example, this has led to measures whereby care providers were sanctioned by reductions in their income if they failed to follow certain clinical guidelines (Durand-Zaleski *et al.* 1997). However, introducing clinical guidelines together with sanctions might harm the image of the clinical guidelines and increase professional resistance (Durieux *et al.* 2000).

■ *Uncertainty about cost-effectiveness*. The development of clinical guidelines makes large demands on resources. The cost of developing a national clinical guideline varies from 10,000 to more than 200,000 Euros (Burgers *et al.* 2003b). There are also costs for dissemination and implementation of the clinical guidelines. Whether practice guidelines can improve the cost-effectiveness of healthcare routinely has not yet been demonstrated (Haycox *et al.* 1999), but there are examples where this is the case (Mason *et al.* 2001).

■ *Political motives*. Professional groups may produce clinical guidelines to draw attention to themselves or to strengthen their position in healthcare, at the cost of other professional groups. Here, a guideline is used to mark out territory or to stake a claim to a clinical area.

SHOULD CLINICAL GUIDELINES BE DEVELOPED AT A NATIONAL OR LOCAL LEVEL?

Guidelines can be developed *de novo* at a national (central) or at a local level, and guidelines developed nation-

Table 5.2 Local and central guideline development

Level	Objective	Methods include
Central	Guidelines with a good scientific basis and broad validity	Systematic procedure with literature analysis and consensus discussions Delphi methods
Local	Local agreements Care protocols for a department or institution Emphasis on practical feasibility and support of care processes	Consensus work groups Quality teams Nominal group method Focus groups

ally can be adapted at a local level (*Table 5.2*). There are advantages and disadvantages to each.

Central approach

In the central approach (*Table 5.3*) an invited representative group of experts (including patients) from one or more relevant organisations, professional groups or associations reaches agreement on an area of healthcare. This takes place on the basis of a thorough analysis of the scientific literature, consultation with all those involved in care provision and an exchange of opinions. Recommendations with a broad or national validity are thus proposed. Such development of high-quality, valid guidelines requires specific expertise and considerable resources. It has a solid scientific basis and its broad validity brings the potential to eliminate wide variations in care (*Table 5.3*). The disadvantages are that the target group of users is almost certainly less directly involved and thus may feel less committed to follow the guideline, although

the literature is equivocal on this point (Hutchinson and Baker 1999). In addition, it is not always possible to define the desired performance precisely within central guidelines based on data from general populations, at least in part because of generic recommendations (Hutchinson and Baker 1999).

Local approach

In the local approach a local group of care providers and patients formulates the clinical guidelines. The emphasis is on producing local agreements around care processes at the departmental, practice or institutional level. The advantages of this are that it is an instructive process, and the process of acceptance and application is probably more straightforward than with central clinical guidelines. In addition, the guidelines are likely to be better focused on relevant local practice conditions (*Table 5.3*). The disadvantages or risks are that it takes a great deal of time and effort to make such clinical guidelines, that the scientific quality often leaves

Table 5.3 Advantages and disadvantages of central and local approaches to clinical guideline development (Grol 1993)

Level	Advantages	Disadvantages
Central	Scientific basis Careful procedure Wide base Uniformity New insights from research Efficient: not continually reinventing the wheel	Expensive Target group less involved Too general Not focused on specific needs and situations Can evoke anxiety and resistance Possible misuse by patients or insurers
Local	Educational Involvement in the end product Guidelines adapted to local situation Acceptation easier	Time consuming, not efficient Lack of skills No systematic literature analysis Average performance used as guidelines Different guidelines in different regions

something to be desired (*Box 5.3*), and that, in the absence of a systematic review, obsolete insights may become enshrined within the clinical guidelines.

Local translation of central clinical guidelines

Given the methodological problems with locally developed clinical guidelines, a process whereby centrally produced clinical guidelines are translated into local ones offers an approach that combines the advantages of both methods (Hutchinson and Baker 1999). At the national or central level, the available scientific knowledge is brought together in a systematic and accessible manner and all the concerned persons have been heard and all interests represented appropriately. At the local level, the central clinical guidelines can be utilised to make local guidelines or to draw-up care protocols, both of which are generally more specific and describe care in more detail (*Box 5.4*). Criteria and indicators can also be derived from these to measure the quality of care delivery (*Box 5.5*). Data on the use of local clinical guidelines and local experiences can,

in turn, feed into central clinical guideline development. Information on local clinical guidelines that have had their implementation tested in practice can be used to develop or revise clinical guidelines at the central level. In this way, central and local clinical guideline development is interlinked.

A risk of local translation of national clinical guidelines is that methodically well-substantiated guidelines are rewritten such that the evidence is reinterpreted. In areas where the evidence is weaker, there is more room for local translation of the recommendations. For example, the evidence for the effectiveness of radiotherapy and breast-sparing surgery in women with breast cancer is very extensive and difficult to interpret differently. In contrast, there is little evidence for the best model of palliative care and hence more room for local preferences (Hutchinson and Baker 1999).

It is not always necessary to translate central guidelines. Sometimes the description of the desired procedure is so clear and detailed that the guideline can be used locally as it is. However, if there is a marked difference between the two settings, translation for the

---

Box 5.3 The scientific basis of clinical guidelines (Varonen and Mäkelä 1997)

In Finland, a search among databases and journals and inquiries for institutions and organisations located 719 guidelines from the period 1989–1995 (150 national, 120 regional and 449 local). Of the national guidelines, 83% were supported by a systematic literature analysis, while only 18% of the regional guidelines and 9% of the local guidelines were.

Box 5.4 Translation of central clinical guidelines into local working agreements (guideline on 'prevention of pressure ulcers')

Central guideline	Derived local working agreements
Several identifiable and quantifiable factors increase the probability of the development of pressure ulcers	In the record of each patient older than 60 years of age in department A, the risk score for pressure ulcers must be recorded on the day of entry
These factors must be examined in each patient and expressed in a risk score	In the event of surgery in patients with an elevated risk, the risk score must be reported on the anaesthesia request form

---

Box 5.5 From clinical guideline to local improvement goals (Hutchinson and Baker 1999)

- Evidence-based guideline – myocardial infarction patients who use beta blockers have a much lower risk of dying (evidence level A2, see *Box 5.10*);
- Recommendation – all patients with a myocardial infarction must be treated with a beta blocker (recommendation level 2, see *Box 5.14*);
- Local standard or goal – 90% of all myocardial infarction patients who need symptomatic therapy use beta blockers regularly.

local situation should be considered. If a central clinical guideline for stroke advises treating patients with aspirin upon arrival at hospital, such a recommendation can simply be incorporated without change into the local clinical guidelines of a medical department. However, if the recommendation advises that a stroke service be established, a more extensive local translation that involves a multidisciplinary working group is needed.

A modified form of the methods for guideline development described in the next section can also be used to develop local clinical guidelines.

DEVELOPMENT OF EFFECTIVE CLINICAL GUIDELINES

In this section we describe the different processes in clinical guideline development that take specific account of

the need for implementation. These processes reflect the methods of evidence-based clinical guideline development commonly used internationally (*Table 5.4*). Depending on the context (e.g. central versus local clinical guideline development), certain steps can be omitted or added.

Topic selection

It is likely that the more *relevant* and *appropriate* a topic is to the resolution of problems encountered in practice, the more the clinical guideline will be accepted and used. Therefore, one should start with an analysis of problems that need to be addressed by the clinical guideline. Some problems, although either important or urgent, cannot be resolved by guidelines (NHMRC 1999), such as:

▨ Problems caused by a shortage or incorrect use of staff, beds or resources;

Table 5.4 Development of clinical guidelines for practice		
Step	Aim related to implementation	Activities to promote implementation
Topic selection	Relevance	Analysis of actual needs and problems Confirmation and definition of topic
Preparation	Create conditions for a good product	Composition of working group Technical and administrative support Work plan with aims, target group and desired outcomes
Development of draft guideline	Scientific basis, credibility	Use of existing guidelines and reviews Analysis of scientific literature Contribution of experts from practice Formulation of recommendations

Consultation	Applicability
	Broad support and general acceptance
		Pilot test in several practices and/or institutions
		Written survey in target group
		Collection of opinions, comments via:
		  consensus meetings
		  hearings
		  surveys and/or interviews

Authorisation	Official endorsement	Voting procedure in plenary meeting Official panel Independent committee Formal approval by professional organisation, governing board or directors
Design	Accessibility and attractiveness	Comprehensive, clear and attractive layout Design adapted to intended users

Evaluation and revision	Monitoring use
	
	Keeping up-to-date
		Evaluation of:
		  application in practice
		  achievement of aims
		Regular updating

■ Malpractice that results from inefficient procedures;
■ Topics in which patient preferences dominate the decisions.

In deciding whether a topic is appropriate for clinical guideline development, answers to the following questions could be useful:

■ Which aspects of the topic are especially complicated? For which questions or problems encountered by healthcare providers and patients in practice are clinical guidelines expected to provide an answer?
■ What do we know about the actual care and what are its shortcomings? How often does the problem occur and in which group? If care is inadequate, are there new methods or better techniques that require a change in care?
■ What barriers can be expected in developing guidelines for the selected topic. What can be done to overcome these?

Such systematic analysis at the beginning of the guideline development process, by healthcare providers, patients' representatives, policy makers, insurers and managers, should help to select and define suitable topics, that is to focus on the essential elements of actual problems (for examples, see *Table 5.5*). An analysis of needs could be performed via a survey, interviews or group methods (Box 5.6 gives group methods of analysis of needs). According to Lohr (1997), the selection and refinement of a topic requires a formal, systematic and reproducible approach.

Criteria for selecting a topic

Once potential topics have been identified there is a process to decide whether they are really suitable for clinical guideline development, especially from the perspective of implementation. To this end various criteria can be used (*Box 5.7*):

■ The topic should concern a *relevant* problem in daily practice. The condition or disease should occur frequently and/or clinical guidelines should have the potential to produce significant health benefits for patients. As an example, 'diabetes mellitus' is a commonly selected topic for clinical guidelines, because such a guideline on this topic may contribute to better healthcare and prevention of complications in a large patient group. One of the first UK clinical guidelines for nurses was for the management of pressure ulcers, a complicated and common problem for nurses. Other relevant considerations may be the cost of a procedure or management of a condition and the potential to make care more efficient.
■ It should be possible to *clearly define* the topic and specify the most crucial aspects of the care for which a clinical guideline is needed. This is important to conduct literature reviews as well as to develop indicators that could be used to monitor the actual care and any changes over time.
■ There is *uncertainty* or a *difference of opinion* about what care should be provided. There might be controversy within a discipline, between disciplines or between primary and secondary care providers. Such controversies need a well-founded solution. In the Netherlands the lack of agreement on the appropriate margin in the diagnostic and therapeutic excision of skin melanomas was the main stimulus to develop a clinical guideline on this topic.
■ The target group should see a *need to bring together the scientific knowledge and expertise* on this subject.

Table 5.5 Important questions from GPs in delineating subjects for guidelines (survey among 42 GPs, Hofstra *et al*. 1993)		
Subject	Patient population	Questions
Diabetes type II	>50 years of age, obese	How to lose weight, which diet, how to motivate patients? When to start medication?
Ankle sprain	Athlete, 12–30 years of age	Fractured or not? Radiograph or not? Taping or not?
Otitis media	<12 years of age	When to prescribe antibiotic? Adenoidectomy or not?
Urinary tract infection	<12 years of age	When is there an underlying abnormality? How many recurrences before referral?

Box 5.6 Methods of analysis of needs for guideline topics (Van Assema *et al*. 1992; Mills *et al*. 1988; Ramirez and Shepperd 1988, Fink *et al*. 1984)

To explore opinions and needs in a structured manner, to identify the most important bottlenecks in healthcare and to select and define a genuinely relevant topic, various group methods can be used, in which healthcare providers, patients and other interested parties participate.

■ *Interactive brainstorming*. The group members generate as many ideas as possible without immediately discarding any as being unusual or unattainable. Gradual progress is made towards good combinations of ideas. The key question is put on a flip chart (e.g., 'What are the most important problems in daily work for which guidelines could be a good tool in defining optimal care?'). Then, without discussion, as many ideas as possible are identified and written down. When there are no more ideas, the group leader and the group members work together to combine ideas. Finally, they decide the combinations that could be applicable.

■ *Nominal group method*. Individual and group work are combined in a structured way, and all members participate equally. Each begins by writing down his or her own responses to the posed question. These are assembled without discussion, written down and, if necessary, explained. The ideas put forwards are then ranked in order of preference. Each member selects the five most important ideas or topics in the entire list and indicates their relative importance. These data are utilised to select the topic.

■ *Focus-group interview*. In a structured way, the needs and perceptions about a topic are explored in a group of 6–12 people who all belong to the same profession or group (nurses, physicians or patients). First, a clear question is formulated and the method is explained. Then opinions are collected in an open discussion in which members can respond to each other. There is no interference unless the discussion deviates from the topic or the question. An open discussion is encouraged. All ideas are written down and, immediately after the meeting, a summary is made of the themes and strongest ideas held in common. This summary is subsequently presented to the members for approval.

Box 5.7 Criteria for topic selection

■ The topic concerns a relevant problem that occurs frequently, and guideline development allows improvement in health or cost reduction;
■ It is possible to define the topic and focus on the most crucial aspects;
■ There is uncertainty or difference of opinion about the best care;
■ There is a need to bring together scientific knowledge and expertise, or there are new insights;
■ Sufficient scientific evidence is available;
■ There is a real opportunity to achieve consensus on the final recommendations;
■ It is possible to formulate feasible recommendations.

This can arise from a question about new scientific insights or new procedures or techniques. It can also be raised by healthcare providers themselves when confronted with concrete problems in practice for which they need an answer. This need can be stimulated by questions from patients or by newly proposed regulations. For example, dieticians working in kidney dialysis centres began to demand a guideline when a new job-ranking system was introduced.

■ There should be *sufficient scientific evidence* available to carry on useful discussions and to draw firm conclusions. For some healthcare providers the availability of evidence is decisive for the acceptance of guidelines or innovations in care. Multidisciplinary guidelines for stroke, for instance, contain recommendations for the prescription of aspirin, which are supported by convincing empirical evidence. However, such clinical guidelines also often include recommendations formulated in the absence of supporting studies, such as for rehabilitation and psychological management.

■ There should be a *real opportunity to achieve consensus* about the final recommendations for practice. The opinions and interests of the stakeholders should not differ too much. Not only do scientific and clinical aspects play a role in estimating the chance of developing a successful clinical guideline, but so also do social, ethical and financial aspects. In particular, for clinical guidelines that cover prevention and screening a great variety of non-scientific considerations and controversies often play a role. To facilitate later successful implementation, a debate on this topic should be arranged before starting on a clinical guideline. As an example, it was the usual practice of gynaecologists to perform a caesarean section in pregnant women who carry herpes simplex virus and whose infants are at risk of herpes neonatorum – vaginal delivery in such cases was considered tantamount to malpractice. However, new scientific findings showed the risks to be small, a result that was in agreement with the clinical experiences of many gynaecologists. Thus, it was timely to develop a clinical guideline.

■ The topic should allow *feasible guidelines*, which include recommendations that can be readily applied in practice. These are clinical guidelines for which no great practical, financial or legal barriers are expected. Certainly, if the clinical guideline partly reflects actual care and experiences – based on new insights and expertise – it is more likely to be widely accepted.

Topic definition

After selecting the topic, the scope of the clinical guideline should be clearly defined. Key questions that address the important clinical issues should be formulated. A mix of healthcare providers, patients and policy makers may be consulted to formulate these questions (see *Table 5.5*).

For example, a few key questions were addressed by each of four clinical guidelines developed by the North of England guideline development project. Concerned with the available evidence for potential health benefits and cost effectiveness (Eccles *et al.* 2000), these addressed:

■ Depression – what is the most appropriate first-choice antidepressant?

■ Vascular diseases – is secondary prevention with aspirin necessary?

■ Heart failure – should angiotensin-converting enzyme (ACE) inhibitors be prescribed or not?

■ Arthritic pain – should non-steroidal anti-inflammatory drugs (NSAIDs) or paracetamol be prescribed?

The analysis of the scientific literature and formulation of recommendations was then focused on these key questions.

There is sometimes a need (e.g. for political reasons) to define a broad scope for clinical guideline development, such as 'the management of diabetes mellitus'. From the perspective of implementation, it is still a good idea to narrow the scope. For example, development of a clinical guideline on diabetes care in hospitals in the Netherlands focused on four topics: the diabetic foot, retinopathy, nephropathy and cardiovascular risks in diabetes. The prevention of complications in patients with diabetes was the main objective.

The definition of the topic should include a description of the target users (e.g. physicians, professions allied to health, nurses), the patients to whom the guideline is meant to apply (e.g. children, women, pregnant women, patients over 65 years of age, etc.) and the decisions covered by the clinical guideline.

Preparation

The next step is concerned with preparing conditions for the development of credible and feasible clinical guidelines. This requires a balanced working group that incorporates people with clinical and methodological expertise, adequate technical support and a defined and agreed work plan.

Composition of the guideline development group

The composition of the guideline development group (or working group) can influence the content of the clinical guideline and its acceptance. In local clinical guideline development, all users might be part of the group. However, in national clinical guideline development, a group of representatives needs to be convened. The status of the clinical guideline is related to the status and credibility of the people or institutions involved.

The group should include individuals from all relevant professional groups to both promote broad support for the clinical guideline and to ensure adequate discussion of its content. Therefore, most clinical guideline groups are multidisciplinary, and so are less likely to be biased (*Box 5.8*; Shekelle *et al.* 1999). For example, vascular surgeons valued carotid artery surgery more positively than a mixed group of vascular surgeons and other specialists (Leape *et al.* 1992).

The status of the organisation responsible for the clinical guideline influences its acceptance. It makes a difference whether a guideline comes from a prominent institution or an external organisation (Marriot *et al.* 2000). For example, of two almost identical nationally distributed guidelines, the one approved and distributed by a national association of internists scored much higher on credibility than the other, which was published by an insurer (Hayward *et al.* 1993).

Working groups usually consist of 6–15 people. Larger groups are more difficult to manage, unless dif-

Box 5.8 Expertise needed for clinical guideline development (Shekelle *et al.* 1999)

- Literature search and literature analysis;
- Epidemiology and biostatistics;
- Healthcare research;

- Clinical expert knowledge;
- Social group processes;
- Writing and editing of clinical guideline texts.

ferent subgroups are formed. The skills of the group leader are crucial for effective and efficient clinical guideline development.

The role of the group leader is both to ensure that the group functions effectively (the group process) and that it achieves its aims (the group task). Although clinical guideline groups are often chaired by pre-eminent experts in the topic area, they are better moderated by someone familiar with (though not necessarily an expert in) the management of the clinical condition and the scientific literature, but who is not an advocate. Such an individual acts to stimulate discussion and to allow the group to identify where true agreement exists, but not inject personal opinion into the process. This requires someone with both clinical skills and group-process skills. There is also evidence that conducting the group meetings using formal group processes rather than informal ones produces different, and possibly better, outcomes.

There is increasing recognition of the importance of good technical support. The development of high-quality and credible clinical guidelines is a complex task, for which good support is needed to carry out literature searches, organise meetings and develop draft texts.

Some clinical guidelines may also be supported by health economics. For instance, in a guideline for the drug treatment of depression the cost-effectiveness, in terms of benefits and risks, of different treatments was analysed (Eccles *et al.* 2000). Such data were considered in the formulation of the final recommendations.

It is important that patients' views and preferences inform the clinical guideline development. This better promotes broad acceptance of the clinical guideline within health service provision. However, the best way to involve patients or their representatives in clinical guideline development is not yet clear (Eccles *et al.* 1996a, 2000). While the use of balanced focus groups of patients guided by a trained facilitator to explore patients' opinions is a feasible method (van Wersch and Eccles 2001; Eccles *et al.* 2000; NHMRC 1999), equally involvement of at least two patient representatives as members of the clinical guidelines development group is a popular alternative.

Work plan

The next step is to formulate a work plan that includes the aims of the clinical guideline, the relevant aspects to be covered, the time schedule and the division of tasks and responsibilities. The target group of the clinical guideline and the desired outcomes of the recommended care should be clearly defined. A work plan describes, for example, the:

- Disease, condition or health problem;
- Patient population to whom the guideline is meant to apply;
- Healthcare setting in which the guideline can be used;
- Interventions discussed in the guideline;
- Desired outcomes (e.g. mortality, morbidity, complications, hospital admissions, quality of life and prevention of absenteeism from work);
- Range of technical tasks and who is responsible for them.

Ideally, all these aspects should be discussed before starting clinical guideline development, otherwise implicit differences of opinion between working group members could lead to confusion and conflicts. As an example of different desired outcomes, comparison of English and Dutch clinical guidelines on acute otitis media revealed that the aim of the English one was to reduce the duration of pain and distress, while the Dutch one was more orientated to the prevention of hearing problems. This explained why the English clinical guideline advocated early use of antibiotics in contrast to the Dutch one (Lawrence and Olesen 1997).

Development of draft guidelines

In developing the draft guidelines it is important to provide a proper scientific basis for the guideline, use clinical expertise optimally where scientific data are lacking or unclear and translate the scientific evidence and clinical expertise into concrete recommendations for practice.

Important steps in this process are to:

- Identify and review existing guidelines and systematic literature reviews;

- Search for scientific evidence and assess its quality and relevance;
- Involve clinical experts;
- Formulate recommendations for practice.

Each of these steps is discussed briefly in this chapter. For more details, the literature in this area should be consulted (e.g. NHMRC 1999).

Identify and review available guidelines and reviews

The first step in compiling scientific evidence for specific recommendations is to determine whether national or international clinical guidelines on the same subject have already been published or whether systematic literature analyses have already been carried out or are underway. Existing clinical guidelines can be retrieved by searching guideline databases, such as the US National Guideline Clearinghouse or the websites (*Box 5.9*) of successful clinical guideline programmes, such as NICE in England or SIGN in Scotland. In addition, the Cochrane Library can be consulted to identify whether there is a group somewhere in the world that is already reviewing the relevant literature.

Collect and evaluate scientific studies

Studies are best identified by systematic review. The usual starting point is to search a range of electronic databases, such as Medline, Cinahl, Embase and the Cochrane Library. The reference lists of identified articles may identify further studies, as may asking expert members of the clinical guideline development group. This minimises the risk of missing important information. Relevant journals can be hand searched and the 'grey' literature (not published in scientific journals) can be studied. The degree to which all of these are carried out depends on the time and resources available.

Next, the relevance and quality of the identified studies needs to be evaluated (Shekelle *et al*. 1999). A first step

is to evaluate the relevance of the study for the questions and problems and for the patient group to which the clinical guideline is directed. This can usually be achieved on the basis of the abstract, which reduces the number of studies that must be read in detail.

Having done this, for those studies identified the next step is to evaluate the content and quality of the published research and therefore of the strength of the scientific evidence. Information about the advantages, disadvantages, risks and eventual costs of the studied diagnostic and therapeutic methods and care interventions is examined. An attempt is made to categorise the risk of bias within the evidence using evidence-grading schemes. A number of different schemes are in use – they differ for preventive, diagnostic and therapeutic procedures (*Box 5.10*).

Contribution of clinical expertise and experience

Clinical guideline development cannot succeed without the contribution of experts in the field concerned. First of all, for some of the questions or choices there will be no or only conflicting evidence. It is estimated that less than half of the decisions in most disciplines are supported by good empirical studies (Buchan 2004). In the development of a clinical guideline for the management in patients with angina pectoris in England, it was found that only 21% of the recommendations could be based directly on randomised studies or meta-analyses (Eccles *et al*. 1996b). Even when there is internally valid and consistent evidence for a given clinical practice, the optimal method of proceeding is seldom immediately clear (Naylor 1995). Hence it is always necessary to call upon the collective expertise and experience of the working group. Even if evidence is found for certain care interventions, it may be in different patient populations, so it is necessary to determine whether the results can be extrapolated to those populations seen in routine care. For example, much of the evidence for practice in primary care is derived from more or less selected groups

---

Box 5.9 Websites

- US National Clearinghouse: www.guideline.gov
- NICE England: www.nice.org.uk
- SIGN Scotland: www.sign.ac.uk/
- New Zealand Guideline Group: www.nzgg.org.nz/
- NHMRC Australia: www.health.gov.au/nhmrc/

Cochrane Collaboration:

- Cochrane Library – database on disk and CD-ROM. Cochrane Collaboration, Oxford: Update Software (updated quarterly).

Box 5.10 Classification of the literature according to the strength of the evidence (CBO 2000)

For articles concerning intervention (prevention or therapy):

A1 Systematic reviews of at least a few studies on the A2 level, of which the results of independent research studies are consistent;

A2 Randomised comparative clinical research of good quality (randomised, double-blind, controlled trial of adequate scope and consistency);

B Randomised clinical trials of moderate quality or insufficient scope, or other comparative research (non-randomised, cohort studies, patient-control studies);

C Non-comparative research;

D Opinions of experts, such as the working group members.

For articles concerning diagnosis:

A1 Studies of the effects of diagnosis on clinical results in a prospective, well-defined patient group with a previously defined policy on the basis of the research test results, or medical decision-making research on the effects of diagnosis on clinical results, in which A2 level results are used as the basis and adequate attention is given to the underlying dependence of diagnostic tests;

A2 Research with regard to a reference test ...

And so on.

---

of patients recruited from secondary care settings and with different prior probability of disease. Finally, the available evidence must still be interpreted in the light of the clinical questions and problems to which the clinical guideline hopes to provide an answer.

In the discussion of the interpretation of scientific evidence, its translation into clinical guidelines and the use of opinions of experts, various problems can arise:

▪ Research findings may be used selectively, so that personal preferences still tip the balance in the end;

▪ Conclusions from the analyses of scientific literature and recommendations for practice may be distinguished inadequately (*Box 5.11*);

▪ When the working group is pressed for time, consensus may be forced;

▪ Some working group members or the chairperson may dominate the discussion with personal opinions;

▪ Discussions may be so dominated by considerations of what is achievable that research findings or new information are ignored.

By formalising and structuring the discussions as much as possible, an attempt can be made to avoid such problems. Formal consensus methods are useful for this, and allow all group members to make their contributions (e.g. a nominal group method or a Delphi method, see *Box 5.15*). For acceptance of the guideline by the target group it is important to be able to trust that the development process has proceeded very carefully and that

all the information and opinions have been considered (Sudlow and Thompson 1997). Many clinical guideline programmes now make a clear distinction in their texts between conclusions from scientific literature, the value of the evidence per individual conclusion (from A1 to D) and advice for management in practice.

Formulation of conclusions and recommendations

In formulating recommendations for practice, the scientific evidence and clinical and other expertise are brought together (*Box 5.12*). Here, in the formulation of what is seen as correct or suitable care, considerations relevant to implementation need discussing. In formulating recommendations the following issues should be considered:

▪ Nature and strength of the scientific evidence – the balance between the advantages of a given intervention and its disadvantages and risks;

▪ Generalisability or applicability of the evidence to the population with which the guideline is concerned;

▪ Costs associated with the proposed care intervention – data on cost-effectiveness;

▪ Achievability of the proposed intervention in terms of the required skill, instruments, money, time, available staff, preferences of patients and possibilities and limitations of the healthcare system (e.g. legal regulations);

▪ Opinions, norms and values, and ethical considerations of the working group members.

Box 5.11 Reproducibility of guidelines (Pearson *et al.* 1995)

Three panels, each composed of 5–7 internists, were requested to make decision diagrams for two clinical problems (dyspepsia and sinusitis). Comparison of the results of the three groups revealed that the recommendations for dyspepsia were quite similar, but those for sinusitis were extremely divergent.

Box 5.12 Development of a clinical guideline for the treatment of depression (Eccles *et al.* 2000)

In the development of a guideline for the medical treatment of depression, two important groups of antidepressives were found to have a comparable effect, only small differences in side effects, but great differences in both toxicity in overdose and cost. A key question in formulating the recommendations was therefore how much should it cost to avoid the risk of fatal overdose associated with antidepressive use? By considering the various advantages, risks, costs, etc., it was possible to arrive at a concrete recommendation.

Haycox *et al.* (1999) describe an example that suggested the introduction of a new clinical guideline on gastric complaints in England would lead to three times as many endoscopies. The question was who would pay for this and whether the healthcare system could and would afford it. With a view to implementation, a working group cannot avoid this problem. If a clinical guideline says that a patient who has a heart attack must receive thrombolysis within 30 minutes of arrival in the hospital, the entire care process after arrival must be directed to that aim. If requesting and performing an echocardiogram (ECG) routinely takes 40 minutes, it is a meaningful recommendation only if care processes can be changed accordingly.

In the interpretation of the evidence and the use of expertise, normative and cultural opinions about the desired health benefit and the acceptable risks also play an important role (Fahey 1998; Burgers *et al.* 2002). This is not bad as long as there is awareness of it and care is taken to ensure that the recommendations are in agreement with the norms and values within the target group (*Box 5.13*).

It is becoming increasingly common in clinical guidelines to include a final evaluation of the *level of evidence* for the conclusions and recommendations. In so doing the working group attempts to emphasise the degree to which the supporting studies have excluded bias (distorting factors) and the extent to which application of the recommendations leads to the intended results. For the target group, such evaluations make the recommendations transparent and lucid, which can have an important influence on acceptance and application in practice. There are different schemes to classify the level of the evidence, such as that in *Box 5.14* used by the CBO (2000).

To arrive at such a determination of the level of evidence per recommendation, preferably there should be a democratic voting procedure in the working group after extensive discussion in which all of the

Box 5.13 Guidelines for the management of an elevated risk of breast cancer (Eisinger *et al.* 1999)

An analysis of US and French clinical guidelines for the management of an elevated risk of breast cancer revealed interesting differences concerned with the interpretation of the scientific evidence in the light of the desired results and with the norms and values of the guideline developers and the target group. US clinical guidelines advise regular breast self-examination, while French ones point to the anxiety and insecurity that this can evoke in women. The US guidelines also advise an active approach by physicians with regard to the preventive removal of the associated lymph nodes, while the French ones are very reserved about the medical indications for such an intervention and advise waiting a few months before the definitive decision is made. The authors point to the cultural differences that underlie such divergent recommendations, such as the greater emphasis on autonomy for patients in the USA.

Box 5.14 Level of evidence underlying a conclusion (CBO 2000)

1 At least two independently carried out level A1 or A2 investigations, or a systematic review (A1);
2 At least two independently carried out level B investigations;
3 Research other than level B;
4 Opinions of working group members or of experts in the literature (level D).

information (evidence, costs, patient preferences, practical consequences, etc.) has been considered.

Consultation and authorisation

In the final acceptance and use of the clinical guideline, it is likely that its applicability in daily care and the users' agreement with it also play an important role. To facilitate this process the recommendations of the guideline should be tried out on a small scale and be presented to a representative group for comment and/or approval.

Testing
Useful information about the applicability of the clinical guideline can be collected from a pilot test by a few departments, practices or healthcare teams. Care providers are asked to follow the practice guideline as closely as possible. Performance is recorded and any bottlenecks experienced in applying it are reported. The reactions of patients may also be included. This testing can also be performed as a written exercise with a list of scenarios that describe typical patients, and questions that ask care providers how they would handle these patients and what problems they would anticipate in applying the clinical guideline. The results of such testing and the revisions based on these should, ideally, be incorporated as part of the dissemination strategy of the clinical guidelines. It is potentially useful for other care providers to know that colleagues have already worked with the clinical guideline, and to have information about the possible problems that might occur when it is introduced and about the possible solutions to these problems.

Consultation
To promote *wide support* for the clinical guideline and to discover possible problems in its acceptance, it is advisable to ask the ultimate target group, others involved and experts for their opinions about the guideline. This can be done in various ways (*Box 5.15*):

Box 5.15 RAND-modified Delphi Procedure (Stoevelaar *et al.* 1999; Kahn *et al.* 1988)

This method is derived from the Delphi method and was developed by the American research institute RAND and the University of California at Los Angeles (UCLA; Kahn *et al.* 1988). It is especially suitable for drawing up recommendations for clinical problems for which little scientific evidence material is available. A panel of experts forms an opinion about the appropriateness of different treatments in a large number of cases. These cases are paper patients ('vignettes') with certain diagnostic characteristics that have been shown to influence the decision whether or not to carry out a given treatment (e.g. gender, age, nature of the complaints or certain abnormal findings on physical examination). The different combinations of possible characteristics determines the number of cases. The judgement of the appropriateness of a treatment in each circumstance is determined by considering the advantages (effectiveness, rapidity and duration of the response) and disadvantages (invasiveness, side effects and complications) and is expressed on a nine-point scale (nine being the highest score for appropriateness). The panel members should, independently, score the appropriateness of the various treatment possibilities for each case. Then, in a plenary session, each individual's scores are compared with the overall scores of the other panel members. This session is to clarify any uncertainty about the definitions and procedures used. The panel members are again asked to evaluate individually all or some of the cases. In the analysis of the results attention is given to the degree of agreement and the degree of appropriateness. A treatment is considered to be 'appropriate' if the median of the scores is in the range 7–9 and less than one-third of the individual scores are in the range of 1–3. For 'inappropriate' the reverse applies. In all other cases the degree of appropriateness is 'uncertain'.

An example of the use of the RAND–UCLA method as a meaningful addition to existing guidelines was the determination of the optimal treatment of benign prostatic hyperplasia (Stoevelaar *et al.* 1999). A choice had to be made between watchful waiting, medical treatment and surgery. In the so-called grey area in which neither severe nor mild pathology is present, the indication is unclear and the scientific literature offers too little upon which to base a choice. To still be able to arrive at a conclusion, a panel of 12 urologists was asked to evaluate the appropriateness of treatment with an α-adrenergic blocker, finasteride, or surgery in 1152 cases. In 48% of the indications there was agreement among the urologists. There was a clear difference of opinion in less than 1% of the cases. An α-adrenergic blocker was advised in cases in which there had been no previous treatment, while there appeared to be practically no indications for finasteride. Surgery was recommended in 60% of the cases if treatment with an α-adrenergic blocker had not worked. In practice, these results can be included in the process of weighting a clinical decision, in which the personal preference of the patient also plays an important and perhaps decisive role. The advantage of the RAND–UCLA method is that it expresses 'expert opinion' finely differentiated in size and number; the disadvantage is that this opinion is subjective and, by definition, not shared by the entire profession.

■ *Meeting*. The clinical guideline is presented at an open meeting for comment and approval. An organised discussion is held, based on the guideline recommendations, which are explained by the working group. This can include their views on the most important conclusions and recommendations. Then the audience can express their comments, criticisms and suggestions, verbally or in writing. Such a meeting can be organised at a national level, regionally or within an institution, inviting as many of the involved disciplines as possible. To obtain comments and support for four new diabetes guidelines for hospitals in the Netherlands, regional guideline meetings were organised for interested specialists. If a working group in an individual hospital has drafted a guideline for antibiotic usage, a meeting of all the relevant departments in the hospital can be planned. A meeting offers participation, but has the potential disadvantage that those who speak loudest or those with strong opinions can dominate the discussion. Including the possibility for written comments or using a voting system can, at least potentially, mitigate this.

■ *Survey and/or interview*. A sample of users, experts and other concerned individuals (e.g. patients, insurers, policy makers and managers from the institution) receive a structured questionnaire or are interviewed about concrete recommendations for the management of care in practice. For example, the Dutch College of General Practitioners routinely present their draft guidelines to 50 members plus a small number of specialists in the area. This activity generally provides a good impression of the achievability and problems with the clinical guideline.

Authorisation

The results of the testing of the clinical guideline and the consultation process are incorporated in the new version of the guideline. The uptake of a clinical guideline can be promoted if it has the support or endorsement of a professional association or an independent institution. Such a body may have been associated with the guidelines development or may be approached after the draft is complete.

Endorsement can take a variety of forms:

■ A panel of diverse experts can be used to evaluate the results;

■ Formal approval and ratification of the clinical guideline can be requested from the parent professional organisation, patient organisations or, if it concerns an institution, from the directors or the management;

■ An independent scientific council or commission can be brought in to verify the procedure and its results;

■ The clinical guideline can also be submitted for approval to an agency especially established for this purpose (many countries have such an agency).

Such authorisation has a number of ritual characteristics (Grol *et al.* 1990). Each professional group must seek out the appropriate channel for this. Rituals are usually intended to close ranks and preserve unity, and in this sense they can be decisive in the acceptance of a clinical guideline by the users.

Design of the guideline

The next step in the development of a clinical guideline, from the perspective of implementation, is an accessible, understandable and attractive design. This concerns both the layout and the adaptation of the design to the specific situation in which the guideline must be applied. Different users, purposes, conditions and implementation strategies may need different designs (*Box 5.16*).

Box 5.16   Different designs of clinical guidelines (Cretin 1998)

Design	Suitable for
Text	Explanation of arguments for a particular procedure Explanation of controversies Detailed documentation of the literature used
Decision diagram and/or algorithm	Clarification of the logic in the decision making Quick understanding of recommendations
Tables of evidence	Results of reviews Summaries of key recommendations

For example, clinical guidelines for primary care physicians in the Netherlands are made available in the following forms:

- Publication in a professional journal with comprehensive scientific explanation of each recommendation, with references;
- Summary of the key recommendations on a plastic-laminated card, which is easy to consult in routine practice;
- Cards for practice assistants and receptionists for use in telephone contacts with patients;
- Explanatory folders and letters for patients, which give the recommendations of the clinical guideline in language patients can understand;
- At the same time, indicators and criteria are developed to evaluate whether the guidelines are followed.

For the clinical guideline to be used for education comprehensive texts that explain and substantiate the recommendations are required. In routine practice, handy, clear summaries and decision diagrams are likely to be more useful. For audit and performance review, critical elements of the clinical guideline are needed in the form of assessment criteria, and the clinical guidelines must be presented in the form of a set of indicators or a measuring instrument. For patients, the clinical guideline is summarised in lay terms. It may be helpful if different components of a guideline have distinguishing design features (e.g. different colours), and that accessible designs are also developed for the patient.

Much of this can be achieved for a clinical guideline developed at a national level. However, at a local level organisations may wish to go through a further process to format and present the clinical guidelines.

Evaluation

A final step in the development of clinical guidelines is the overall process of the evaluation of their application, their applicability and their effects in the daily provision of care, as well as revision of the guidelines on the basis of these evaluations. Relevant elements of such evaluations are:

- How well are the guidelines known and to what extent are they valued: are the recommendations read, are they discussed with colleagues, are they well understood and remembered, are they accepted and used in local consensus meetings and quality-improvement activities?

- To what extent are the recommendations applied: are they all followed; if not, which are not, and what are the problems in their application?
- To what extent are they effective: does their application lead to achievement of the objectives envisioned, such as better health, fewer complications, lower costs, better quality of life, greater efficiency and more satisfied patients?

Information that arises out of such evaluations can lead to revision of the clinical guidelines to be reintroduced, and a plan to carry this out. The results of the evaluation can raise questions about the validity and applicability of the recommendations.

The evaluation is discussed in more detail in Part VI of this book (Chapters 16–20).

Updating guidelines

While there is increasing consensus about the methods needed to develop evidence-based guidelines, less attention has been paid to the process of assessing when guidelines should be updated. The most common advice is for guidelines to include a scheduled review date. However, this could result in wasted resources if a full update is undertaken prematurely within a slowly evolving field, or if clinical guidelines in a rapidly evolving field become out-of-date before the scheduled review. Some guidelines state that they should be updated when new information becomes available, but it is unclear how this should be effected. Shekelle *et al*. (2001a) propose a set of principles and a pragmatic model for assessing whether guidelines need to be updated. They suggest that clinical guidelines may require updating because of changes in any or all of the:

- Evidence on the existing benefits and harms of interventions;
- Outcomes considered important;
- Available interventions;
- Evidence that current practice is optimal;
- Values placed on outcomes;
- Resources available for healthcare;

They suggest a two-stage method focused on dealing with changes in interventions, outcomes or performance. The two stages are to identify significant new evidence, and to assess whether the new evidence warrants a full updating of the guidelines.

A multidisciplinary group of experts review selected recommendations within the clinical guideline and are asked whether they are aware of new evidence or developments in the field relevant to the guideline recommendation and, if so, whether this evidence is sufficient to invalidate the clinical guideline recommendation. This process is supplemented by limited literature searches to guard against oversights by the experts.

The next step is an independent assessment of whether the new evidence or interventions identified are of sufficient importance to invalidate the clinical guideline recommendation. In some cases, the new information provides *prima facie* evidence that the guideline recommendation is invalid, while for other situations this assessment necessarily involves judgement, and such judgements are generally more balanced if they involve both topic experts and generalists with expertise in clinical guideline development.

Within any individual clinical guideline some recommendations are invalid while others remain current. A clinical guideline needs updating if the majority of recommendations are out-of-date, with new evidence demonstrating that the recommended interventions are inappropriate, ineffective or superseded by new interventions. However, in other cases a single, outdated recommendation may not invalidate the document.

Using this method Shekelle *et al.* (2001b) assessed the validity of 17 practice guidelines published by the Agency for Healthcare Research and Quality (AHRQ). For 13 guidelines, new evidence and expert judgement indicated that an update was required, three guidelines were judged still valid and for one guideline it was not possible to reach a conclusion. They showed that about half the guidelines were out of date 6 years after their publication and 90% were still valid after 3.6 years. They suggest that, as a general rule, guidelines should be reassessed for validity every 3 years.

QUALITY OF GUIDELINES: CRITERIA FOR GOOD GUIDELINES

High-quality guidelines can improve healthcare (Grimshaw *et al.* 2004), but low-quality guidelines may harm patient care (Shekelle *et al.* 2000). In the past few decades there has been an impressive increase in guideline development activities, which has led to an explosion of published guidelines. In some countries, such as Great Britain and the USA, physicians are confronted with multiple guidelines on the same clinical subjects (Littlejohns *et al.* 1999; Thompson *et al.* 1998; Feder 1994). While several studies have suggested that many guidelines are of poor quality (*Boxes 5.17* and *5.18*; e.g. Grilli *et al.* 2000; Littlejohns *et al.* 1999; Shaneyfelt *et al.* 1999), each used different criteria to assess guideline quality. Therefore, there is a need to identify consistently those well-developed guidelines that can contribute to optimal patient care.

Building upon an instrument developed by Cluzeau *et al.* (1994, 1997), an international appraisal instrument for clinical guidelines was developed and validated by an international consortium of experienced clinical guideline developers: the Appraisal Instrument for Guidelines Research and Evaluation (AGREE instrument). The purpose of the AGREE Instrument is to provide a systematic framework for assessing key

---

Box 5.17 Quality of guidelines appraised

Grilli *et al.* (2000) evaluated 431 guidelines developed by associations of medical specialists, published between 1988 and 1998 and retrieved via MEDLINE. For the evaluation they used three criteria – description of the type of professionals involved in the development of the guideline, description of the method of literature search and explicit grading of the evidence in support of the main recommendations. Only 5% met all the criteria, and 54% did not meet any criterion. The most recent clinical guidelines scored significantly better with regard to the description of the method of literature search and to the grading of recommendations.

Criterion	Guidelines that met the criterion (%)
Description of type of professionals involved in guideline development	33
Description of method of literature search	13
Grading of evidence supporting the recommendations	18

Box 5.18 Quality of guidelines assessed (Littlejohns *et al.* 1999)

45 national and local guidelines with recommendations for the management of depression in primary care were identified. These were assessed by six independent experts with regard to the method of development, reliability, applicability, clarity and flexibility. There appeared to be differences in the content of the guidelines and the way in which the recommendations were presented. Most guidelines used the recommendations of well-known organisations such as the Royal College of Psychiatrists and the Royal College of General Practitioners. The authors suggest that the most cost-effective way to produce guidelines is to provide a high-quality, national evidence-based guideline that could be used as a template for local adaptation and local healthcare protocols.

components of clinical guideline quality, including the process of development and the reporting of that process. The items cover the methodology as well as the clarity and applicability of the clinical guideline. Previous drafts of the instrument were field-tested in two rounds on 100 clinical guidelines from 11 countries with 264 appraisers (AGREE Collaboration 2003). Acceptability of the instrument was high – 95% of the appraisers found the instrument easy to apply and perceived it to be useful for judging the quality of clinical guidelines. Reliability was satisfactory for most domains: Cronbach's alpha ranged from 0.64 to 0.88, and inter-rater reliability (i.e. intra-class correlations) ranged from 0.57 to 0.91 with four appraisers per guideline. The criteria are presented in *Box 5.19* with a short explanation (for more details see www.agreecollaboration.org).

Box 5.19 Appraisal of Guidelines for Research and Evaluation (AGREE) Instrument

Scope and purpose

1 The overall objective(s) of the clinical guideline is (are) specifically described.

For example, the prevention of long-term complications of patients with diabetes mellitus, or the rational prescribing of antidepressants.

2 The clinical question(s) covered by the clinical guideline is (are) specifically described.

For example, how many times per year should the HbA1c be measured in patients with diabetes mellitus, or are selective serotonin reuptake inhibitors (SSRIs) more cost-effective than tricyclic anti-depressants (TCAs) in the treatment of patients with depression.

3 The patients to whom the clinical guideline is meant to apply are specifically described.

For example, a guideline on diabetes mellitus only includes patients with non-insulin-dependent diabetes, or a guideline on screening of breast cancer only includes women between 50 and 70 years of age.

Stakeholder involvement

4 The clinical guideline development group includes individuals from all the relevant professional groups.

They could be members of the working group or could be involved at another stage of the development process.

5 The patients' views and preferences have been sought.

For example, information could be obtained from patient interviews, literature reviews or patients could be involved in the clinical guideline development group.

6 Target users of the clinical guideline are clearly defined.

The target group refers to healthcare providers (e.g., doctors, nurses or other disciplines) who must apply the guideline in practice.

7 The clinical guideline has been piloted among target users. This concerns testing the feasibility and applicability of the guideline in practice.

Rigour of development

8 Systematic methods were used to search for evidence.

For example, by using electronic databases such as Medline, Embase and the Cochrane Library.

9 The criteria for selecting the evidence are described clearly. Both the inclusion and exclusion criteria, as well as the reasons for these criteria, should be described.

10 The methods used to formulate the recommendations are described clearly.

This concerns how final decisions are arrived at (e.g. using a voting system or formal consensus procedures such as the Delphi technique).

11 Health benefits, side effects and risks were considered in formulating the recommendations.

For example, in the management of breast cancer these may include survival and quality of life against side effects and risks of chemotherapy or radiation.

12 There is an explicit link between the recommendations and the supporting evidence.

Each recommendation should be linked with a list of references on which it is based.

13 The clinical guideline was reviewed externally by experts prior to its publication. *(cont.)*

Box 5.19 (*cont.*) Appraisal of Guidelines for Research and Evaluation (AGREE) Instrument

Reviewers are not members of the development group, but are experts in clinical and methodological aspects of the guideline. Representatives of patient organisations may also be included as reviewers.

14 A procedure for updating the clinical guideline is provided.

For example, by providing a time scale, or by a standing panel that regularly receives updated literature searches.

Clarity and presentation

15 The recommendations are specific and unambiguous.

The recommendations should concretely and precisely indicate which management is appropriate in which situation and in what patient group. If there is insufficient evidence, it should be stated that there is uncertainty about the best management.

16 The different options for management of the condition are presented clearly.

For example, in the management of depression (a) TCAs, (b) SSRIs, (c) psychotherapy or (d) combination of drug and psychotherapy.

17 Key recommendations are easily identifiable.

For example, by summarising them in a box, by bold type or underlining, or by presenting them as flow charts.

18.The guideline is supported with tools for application.

For example, a summary document, education packages, patient leaflets or computer support.

Applicability

19 The potential organisational barriers to applying the clinical guideline were discussed.

For example, by recommending stroke units co-ordinate the care of stroke patients.

20 The potential cost implications of applying the recommendations were considered.

For example, the need for more specialised staff, new facilities or expensive drug treatment, which may have implications for healthcare budgets.

21 The clinical guideline presents key review criteria for monitoring and/or audit purposes.

Adherence to the guideline can be measured using review criteria and compared to predefined standards of care (e.g. the HbA1c should be lower than 8.0 in 90% of diabetes patients).

Editorial independence

22 The clinical guideline is editorially independent from the funding body.

The clinical guideline should include an explicit statement that the interests of the funding body have not influenced the final recommendations.

23 Conflicts of interest of clinical guideline development members are recorded.

Members of the development group should have declared whether they have any conflict of interest, such as participating in research funded by a pharmaceutical company.

CONCLUSION

To aid the successful introduction of clinical guidelines or protocols in daily practice, their development should, where possible, take into consideration their ultimate implementation from the very beginning. Attention to this should ideally be incorporated into the development procedures. This includes attention to:

- Relevance – guidelines must provide an answer to questions that occupy the concern of care providers and patients;
- Credibility – systematic development and careful, transparent procedures;
- Bias – involvement of the target group in the development;
- Applicability – attention to not only the scientific basis, but also to the applicability to patient groups with which the target group is involved and to the consequences of application in terms of resources, materials, facilities and patients;
- Accessibility – neat, clear and attractive design;
- Integration in normal care processes – efforts need

to be made to incorporate the guidelines in local care protocols, disease management systems and systems for monitoring care.

Recommended literature

AGREE Collaboration. Appraisal of Guidelines for Research and Evaluation (AGREE) Instrument. www.agreecollaboration.org.

Grimshaw J, Eccles M and Russell I (1995). Developing clinically valid practice guidelines. *J Eval Clin Pract*. 1:37–48.

Hutchinson A and Baker R (1999). *Making Use of Guidelines in Clinical Practice*. Abingdon: Radcliffe Med Press.

Shekelle P, Woolf S, Eccles M, *et al*. (1999). Developing guidelines. *BMJ* 1999;**318**:593–596.

References

AGREE Collaboration (2003). Development and validation of an international appraisal instrument for assessing the quality of clinical practice guidelines: The AGREE project. *Qual Saf Health Care* **12**:18–23.

Assema P van, Mesters I and Kok G (1992). Het focus-interview: Een stappenplan [The focus-interview: A stepwise approach]. *TSG* **70**:431–437.

Buchan H (2004). Gaps between best evidence and practice: Causes for concern. *MJA* **180**:S48–S49.

Burgers JS (2002). Twenty-five years of clinical guideline development: Strengths, limitations and questions. In: Burgers JS, *Quality of Clinical Practice Guidelines*, pp. 15–41. Thesis. Nijmegen: Nijmegen University.

Burgers JS, Bailey JV, Klazinga NS, Van der Bij AK, Grol R and Feder G, for the AGREE Collaboration (2002). Inside guidelines: Comparative analysis of recommendations and evidence in diabetes guidelines from 13 countries. *Diabetes Care* **25**(11):1933–1959.

Burgers JS, Cluzeau FA, Hanna SE, Hunt C, Grol R, and the AGREE Collaboration (2003a). Characteristics of high quality guidelines: Evaluation of 86 clinical guidelines developed in ten European countries and Canada. *Int J Technol Assess Health Care* **19**(1):148–157.

Burgers JS, Grol R, Klazinga NS, Mäkelä M, Zaat J, for The AGREE Collaboration (2003b). Towards evidence-based clinical practice: An international survey of 18 clinical guideline programmes. *Int J Qual Health Care* **15**(1):31–45.

CBO (2000). *Richtlijnontwikkeling binnen het Kwaliteitsinstituut voor de Gezondheidszorg [Guideline Development in the Quality Institute for Health Care]*. Utrecht: CBO.

Cluzeau F, Littlejohn P and Grimshaw JM (1994). Appraising clinical guidelines: Towards a 'Which' guide for purchasers. *Qual Health Care* **3**:121–122.

Cluzeau F, Littlejohns P, Grimshaw JM, *et al.* (1997). *Appraisal Instrument for Clinical Guidelines. Version 1*. London: St George's Hospital Medical School.

Cretin S (1998). *Implementing Guidelines: An Overview*. Report. Santa Monica: RAND.

Durand-Zaleski I, Colin C and Blum-Boisgard C (1997). An attempt to save money by using mandatory practice guidelines in France. *BMJ* **315**:943–946.

Durieux P, Chaix-Couturier C, Durand-Zaleski I and Ravaud P (2000). From clinical recommendations to mandatory practice. The introduction of regulatory guidelines in the French healthcare system. *Int J Technol Assess Health Care* **16**:969–975.

Eccles M, Clapp Z, Grimshaw J, *et al.* (1996a). North of England evidence-based guidelines development project: Methods of guideline development. *BMJ* **312**:760–762.

Eccles M, Clapp Z, Grimshaw J, *et al.* (1996b). Developing valid guidelines: Methodological and procedural issues from the North of England evidence-based guideline development project. *Qual Health Care* **5**:44–50.

Eccles M, Mason J and Freemantle N (2000). Developing valid cost effectiveness guidelines: A methodological report from the North of England evidence-based guideline development project. *Qual Health Care* **9**:127–132.

Eddy DM (1992). *A Manual for Assessing Health Practices and Designing Practice Policies: The Explicit Approach*. Washington: American College of Physicians.

Eisinger F, Geller G, Burke W, *et al.* (1999). Cultural basis for differences between US and French clinical recommendations for women at increased risk of breast and ovarian cancer. *Lancet* **353**:919–920.

Elwyn G (2001). *Shared Decision Making. Patient Involvement in Clinical Practice*. Thesis. Nijmegen: Nijmegen University.

Fahey T (1998). Assessing heart disease risk in primary care. *BMJ* **317**:1093–1094.

Feder G (1994). Management of mild hypertension: Which guidelines to follow? *BMJ* **308**:470–471.

Feek CM (2000). Rationing healthcare in New Zealand: The use of clinical guidelines. *MJA* **173**:423–426.

Field MJ and Lohr KN (1992). *Institute of Medicine. Guidelines for Clinical Practice. From Development to Use*. Institute of Medicine. Washington, DC: National Academy Press.

Fink A, Kosecoff J, Chassin M, *et al.* (1984). Consensus methods: Characteristics and guidelines for use. *Am J Public Health* **74**:979–783.

Garfield FB and Garfield JM (2000). Clinical judgement and clinical practice guidelines. *Int J Technol Assess Health Care* **16**:1050–1061.

Gevers JKM and Biesaart MCIH (1999). Medische beslissingen, kostenoverwegingen en richtlijnen voor medisch handelen: Kanttekeningen vanuit het recht [Medical decisions, cost considerations and guidelines for medical performance: Aspects of law]. *Ned Tijdschr Geneeskd.* **143**:2629–2632.

Grilli R, Magrini N, Penna A, *et al.* (2000). Practice guidelines developed by specialty societies: The need for a critical appraisal. *Lancet* **355**:103–106.

Grimshaw JM, Thomas RE, MacLennan G, *et al.* (2004). Effectiveness and efficiency of guidelines dissemination and implementation strategies. *Health Technol Assess* **8**(6):1–84.

Grol R (1993). Development of guidelines in general practice. *Br J Gen Pract.* **43**:146–151.

Grol R and Heerdink H (1992). De bekendheid met en acceptatie van standaarden onder huisartsen (The familiarity and acceptance of guidelines among general practitioners). *Huisarts Wet.* **35**:101–104.

Grol R, Everdingen J van, Kuipers F, *et al.* (1990). Consensus over consensus. Een kritische beschouwing van de procedure van CBO-consensusontwikkeling [Consensus over consensus. A critical reflection on the CBO consensus development]. *Ned Tijdschr Geneeskd* **134**:1186–1189.

Haycox A, Bagust A and Walley T (1999). Clinical guidelines: The hidden costs. *BMJ* **318**:391–393.

Haynes B and Haines A (1998). Barriers and bridges to evidence based clinical practice. *BMJ* **317**:273–276.

Hayward RSA, Wilson MC, Tunis SR, *et al.* (1993). More informative abstracts of articles describing clinical practice guidelines. *Ann Int Med.* **118**:731–737.

Hofstra M, Boshuizen E, Grol R, *et al.* (1993). *Aansluiting van Nascholing op het Kennissysteem van huisartsen [Linking CME to knowledge of GPs]*. Nijmegen: WOK.

Hurwitz B (1999). Legal and political considerations of clinical practice guidelines. *BMJ* **318**:661–664.

Hutchinson A and Baker R (1999). *Making Use of Guidelines in Clinical Practice*. Abingdon: Radcliffe Medical Press.

Kahn KL, Kosecoff J, Chassin MR, *et al.* (1988). Measuring the clinical appropriateness of the use of a procedure. Can we do it? *Med Care* **26**:415–422.

Knottnerus J and Dinant GJ (1997). Medicine-based evidence, a prerequisite for evidence-based medicine. *BMJ* **315**:1109–1110.

Lawrence M and Olesen F (1997). Indicators of quality in health care. *Eur J Gen Pract* **3**:103–108.

Leape L, Park R, Kalhan J, *et al*. (1992). Group judgements of appropriateness: The effect of panel composition. *Qual Assur Health Care* **4**:151–159.

Littlejohns P, Cluzeau F, Bale R, *et al*. (1999). The quantity and quality of clinical practice guidelines for the management of depression in primary care in the UK. *Br J Gen Pract* **49**:205–210.

Lohr K (1997). *The Quality of Practice Guidelines and the Quality of Health Care*. Paper. WHO meeting on guidelines in health care practice. Tübingen, Germany.

Marriot S, Palmer C and Lelliot P (2000). Disseminating health care information: Getting the message across. *Qual Health Care* **9**:58–62.

Mason J, Freemantle N, Nazareth I, Eccles M, Haines A, Drummond M and the Evidence-based OutReach (EBOR) Trialists (2001). The economics of influencing the behaviour of health professionals: Findings of the EBOR trial. *JAMA* **286**:2988–2992.

Mills G, Pace R and Peterson B (1988). *Analysis in Human Resource Training and Organization Development*. Reading: Addison-Wesley.

Naylor CD (1995). Grey zones of clinical practice: Some limits to evidence-based medicine. *Lancet* **345**:940–942.

NHMRC (1999). *A Guide to the Development, Implementation and Evaluation of Clinical Practice Guidelines*. Canberra: National Health Medical Research Council.

Norheim OF (1999). Healthcare rationing – are additional criteria needed for assessing evidence-based clinical practice guidelines? *BMJ* **319**:1426–1429.

Pearson S, Margolis C and Davis S (1995). Is consensus reproducible, a study of an algorithmic guideline development process. *Med Care* **33**(6):643–660.

Ramirez A and Shepperd J (1988). The use of focus groups in health research. *Scand J Prim Care* **1**(Suppl):81–90.

Shaneyfelt TM, Mayo-Smith MF and Rothwangl J (1999). Are guidelines following guidelines? The methodological quality of clinical practice guidelines in the peer-reviewed medical literature. *JAMA* **281**:1900–1905.

Shapiro DW, Lasker RD, Bindman AB, *et al*. (1993). Containing costs while improving quality of care: The role of profiling and practice guidelines. *Ann Rev Public Health* **14**:219–241.

Shekelle P, Woolf S, Eccles M, *et al*. (1999). Developing guidelines. *BMJ* **318**:593–596.

Shekelle PG, Kravitz RL, Beart J, *et al*. (2000). Are nonspecific practice guidelines potentially harmful? A randomized comparison of the effect of nonspecific versus specific guidelines on physician decision making. *Health Serv Res.* **34**:1429–1448.

Shekelle P, Eccles MP, Grimshaw JM and Woolf SH (2001a). When should clinical guidelines be updated. *BMJ* **323**:155–157.

Shekelle PG, Ortiz E, Rhodes S, *et al*. (2001b). Validity of the Agency for Healthcare Research and Quality clinical practice guidelines: How quickly do guidelines become outdated? *JAMA* **286**:1461–1467.

Starfield B (1998). Quality of care research. Internal elegance and external relevance. *JAMA* **280**:1006–1008.

Stoevelaar HJ, McDonnell J, Beek C van de, *et al*. (1999). Passende behandeling bij benigne prostaathyperplasie [Appropriate performance in benign prostatic hyperplasia]. *Ned Tijdschr Geneeskd* **143**:2425–2429.

Sudlow M and Thompson R (1997). Clinical guidelines: Quantity without quality. *Qual Health Care* **6**:60–61.

Thompson R, McElroy H and Sudlow M (1998). Guidelines on anticoagulant treatment in atrial fibrillation in Great Britain: Variation in content and implications for treatment. *BMJ* **316**:509–513.

Tonelli MR (1998). The philosophical limits of evidence-based medicine. *Acad Med* **73**:1234–1240.

Tunis SR, Hayward RSA, Wilson MC, *et al*. (1994). Internists' attitudes about clinical practice guidelines. *Ann Intern Med* **120**:957–963.

Varonen H and Mäkelä M (1997). Practice guidelines in Finland: Availability and quality. *Qual Health Care* **6**:75–79.

van Wersch A and Eccles M (2001). Involvement of consensus in the development of evidence-based guidelines: Practical experiences from the North of England evidence-based guideline development programme. *Qual Health Care.* **10**:10–16.

Woolf SH (1993). Practice guidelines: A new reality in medicine, III: Impact on patient care. *Arch Intern Med.* **153**:2646–2655.

Woolf SH (1997). Shared decision-making: The case for letting patients decide which choice is best. *J Fam Pract.* **45**:205–208.

Woolf SH, Grol R, Hutchinson A, *et al*. (1999). Potential benefits, limitations, and harms of clinical guidelines. *BMJ* **318**:527–530.

Worrall G, Chaulk P and Freake D (1997). The effects of clinical practice guidelines on patient outcomes in primary care: A systematic review. *Can Med Assoc.* **156**:1705–1712.

Part III

Diagnostic analysis

Chapter 6

Determinants of effective change

Michel Wensing and Richard Grol

KEY MESSAGES

- Implementation should be based on an adequate analysis of the target group, the setting in which change is planned and the determinants of change.
- This analysis is to answer the following questions:
  - Who is involved? Which interests are relevant?
  - What is current practice? Which improvements are needed?
  - What are the barriers and facilitators for change in different subgroups?
  - Which subgroups can be distinguished in the target group and at what stages of change are these subgroups?
- Barriers and facilitators can relate to the individual care provider (knowledge, attitude, motivation for change and personal characteristics), the social setting (care providers and patients) or the organisational and financial system (organisation, resources, financial structure, personnel and logistics).

Box 6.1 Implementation of a stroke guideline 2000 (Hooi *et al.* 2000)

A multidisciplinary guideline on stroke, developed in the Netherlands, contained a large number of global and concrete recommendations. One of these recommendations was:

> There are indications that improved and intensified organisation of care (a regional stroke service) results in more effective care provision and therefore better functional health outcomes. Care delivery in follow-up organisations (revalidation centres, nursing homes, primary healthcare) should meet the same high standards as does the stroke unit in the hospital. Continuing education of care providers is crucial to maintain a high level of quality.

A multidisciplinary working group of physicians, nurses and allied health professionals identified the following barriers to the implementation of these recommendations:

- Doubts about the adequacy of this recommendation;
- Lack of clarity about the definitions of a stroke unit and stroke service;
- Co-ordination and transfer of patients is currently poor;
- Lack of specific expertise at many sites;
- Some patients prefer an organisation that is not part of a stroke service;
- Problems related to beds being occupied by 'wrong' patients;
- Problems related to the financial structures.

Facilitators for change included:

- A well-run unit was seen as satisfying for all care providers;
- Continuing education of care providers;
- Feasible protocols and arrangements;
- Sufficient places for patients in various organisations;
- A co-ordinator;
- Flexible financial structures;
- Adequate organisation and communication.

INTRODUCTION

The second step in the model for implementation (*Figure 6.1*) includes an analysis of:

- The context of implementation – who is involved and the interests they have;
- Current practice and aspects that need to be improved;
- Barriers and incentives for change, and specific factors within different subgroups;
- Characteristics of the target group and subgroups within it.

A wide range of factors can influence the success of strategies used to implement innovations. In a study in primary care, physicians were asked to follow guideline recommendations for the management of serum cholesterol in the primary and secondary prevention of heart disease (Van der Weijden *et al.* 1998). There proved to be a problem of both underuse and overuse of tests. They gave as reasons for not following the recommendations that:

- They doubted the value of cholesterol screening in specific subgroups of patients;
- Prevention did not have a high priority for them, because they did not want to interfere actively with patients' lives;
- The recommended care was very complex and time consuming, because, for instance, the serum cholesterol measurements had to be performed three times;
- They often performed serum cholesterol measurements when patients requested them, even if this was against the guideline;
- Following the guideline would increase the workload considerably and demand extra staff.

Factors such as these are legitimate if they prevent the implementation of ineffective or harmful activities. However, when dealing with the introduction of effective clinical practices, such factors may be seen as barriers to successful implementation.

A good 'diagnostic analysis', an analysis of actual performance and the target group and setting, is crucially important in every approach to improving patient

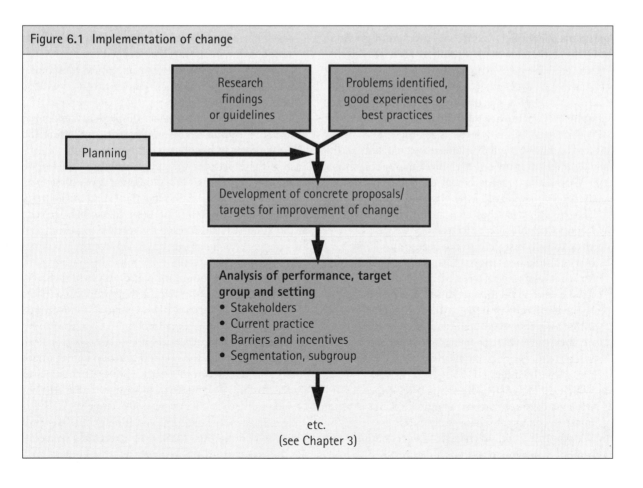

Figure 6.1 Implementation of change

care, because implementation strategies are more likely to be effective if they focus directly on problems in care provision and factors that influence change (Grol 1997). In the example of the cholesterol guideline above, scientific information is needed to convince general practitioners (GPs) of the value of screening, as well as patient education to influence patients' requests for care. Additional strategies could be used to enhance the implementation, such as the use of respected colleagues who are opinion leaders in the field of cholesterol management to draw attention to the guideline. Furthermore, some factors can modify the effect of implementation strategies (effect modifiers). A strategy to implement the cholesterol guideline may be more effective in larger group practices than in small practices, because it is easier to buy desk-top test facilities and train a practice nurse to perform tests in larger practices. If this is correct, 'practice size' is an effect modifier. Effect modifiers can be measured before, during or after the application of an implementation strategy (see also Chapter 18).

Factors considered in such a diagnostic analysis may be derived empirically, for instance through open-ended questions in interviews with care providers or previous studies on guideline implementation. Alternatively, the factors may be derived from theories on behaviour change that have been developed in various disciplines, such as psychology, economics and sociology (see Chapter 2). A better use of theory in implementation projects is seen by many experts as crucial for a better understanding of implementation processes and for the development of more effective implementation strategies. This chapter focuses, however, on the more empirically driven methods to assess barriers for change.

This chapter describes what should be included in a 'diagnostic analysis'; it discusses:

- How to gain insight into the background and context of implementation – who wants what change for what reason, who has what interest and who has what role in the implementation process?
- What is current practice – to what extent does it differ from the recommended performance or best practice, and where is change most needed?
- What are the barriers and facilitators for change with respect to the intended change?
- Which characteristics does the target group have – which subgroups can be distinguished and in what phase of change are these subgroups?

In Chapter 7 the methods used to collect and interpret information on these questions are addressed.

GAINING INSIGHT INTO THE BACKGROUND AND CONTEXT OF IMPLEMENTATION

A systematic approach to implementation starts with the identification of those people and organisations that are involved in the change process, and of their interests and objectives. A so-called social map of the situation is constructed. In the example of cholesterol management, an analysis of relevant people and organisations may include:

- GPs, who want to provide appropriate medical care and, at the same time, maintain a good doctor–patient relationship;
- Patients, who may want to reduce their risk of cardiovascular disease and therefore may be prepared to change their life style and take medication;
- Professional organisations of physicians, which set standards for the appropriate medical care of cholesterol problems, and local groups of physicians may also have set standards in this clinical area;
- Cardiologist, internists and organisations for cardiovascular disease, who have developed clinical guidelines for the treatment of cardiovascular disease, as well as internists and cardiologists in the hospitals to which the GPs refer patients;
- Pharmacists and various pharmaceutical companies, who want to generate a financial profit as well as improve other outcomes;
- Government and insurance companies, who aim to improve public health while also controlling the public costs of healthcare.

Each of these parties can support or inhibit the implementation of the cholesterol guideline, depending on its interests and objectives. It is inevitable that the interests and objectives of different parties will conflict. This can be illustrated by considering the relative importance to the various players of the dimensions of the effectiveness of a clinical intervention, its efficiency, the equity of provision across a population and individual choice. Patients might wish to maximise their individual choice of a treatment irrespective of how good it is, how much it costs and with little consideration to the opportunity costs incurred for other members of a population. Clinicians, who care for a population of patients, might value effectiveness and equity above efficiency and choice. Authorities and financiers might value efficiency and equity over effectiveness and choice.

This is seen, for example, with respect to the prescription of antibiotics (*Table 6.1*). There may be a conflict between appropriate care and cost control, or a

Table 6.1 Determinants of unnecessary use of antibiotics

Determinant	Physicians	Patients and public
Lack of education	Suboptimal approach to diagnosis and treatment; lack of knowledge of natural course of viral diseases	Lack of knowledge of viral versus bacterial infections
Experience	Fixed routines in antibiotic prescribing	Previous knowledge that antibiotics appeared effective
Expectations	Idea that patients want antibiotics; idea that satisfaction depends on prescribing	Idea that specific conditions make antibiotics necessary
Resources	Time pressure	Wish to return to work soon

conflict between the objectives of the society at large and those of individual care providers and patients. In the example of cholesterol management, government or financiers and professional organisations may put pressure on physicians to reduce the number of cholesterol tests performed and the number of prescriptions issued for lipid-lowering medications. However, physicians may continue to carry out tests and prescribe medication to maintain an effective doctor–patient relation in the longer term. From the perspective of the individual physician, this can be a rational approach that helps to achieve his or her aims.

Thus, it is important to build an overview of the relevant people and organisations involved in the implementation process and, on the basis of this, to identify those who should be involved in the process and in the development of appropriate implementation strategies.

CURRENT PRACTICE AND HOW IT MATCHES THE PROPOSED PERFORMANCE

The next step in the analysis is to measure the current practice and compare how it matches, or not, the desired routines. This is important because time and resources for implementation activities are limited and it is not efficient to target implementation activities on areas of practice that are already acceptable. An all-inclusive measurement of current practice is usually too complex to be possible, so a limited number of crucial aspects of care should be selected for the measurement, such as key recommendations in a clinical guideline or those aspects of care that cause most problems to patients. The type of innovation determines which aspects are relevant. Relevant aspects of care for asthma patients might, for example, include available (diagnostic) facilities, the organisation of care (delegation to nurses, arrangements in the practice or hospital department), drug manage-

ment, patient education and communication (shared decision making). It is important that the crucial aspects of the guideline or new routine be reflected in the data collected. *Table 6.2* presents the rates of performance of a number of aspects of care that relate to a guideline for low back pain in primary care – these were derived from the key recommendations in that guideline. The development of indicators that give valid information of current practice is described in Chapter 16.

A wide range of data collection methods may be used and all have their advantages and disadvantages. Examples include the manual or electronic abstraction of data from medical records, the (prospective) documentation or monitoring of activities by care providers or patients, and documentation of activities by an observer. Methods can be relatively simple or extensive and complex, depending on the aims of the exercise and practicalities of the situation. In many cases, simple measurements can provide useful information on current practice. It is a good principle to take small but representative samples, to incorporate the measurement as much as possible into daily routines and to measure processes and outcomes of care as well as the costs of care provision (Nelson *et al*. 1998). More information and examples are presented in Part VI of this book.

The measurement of current practice identifies where it does not match the patterns of care proposed by a guideline, best practice or new procedure. For instance, a study in primary care showed that current practices adhered reasonably to guidelines for low back pain, but that they deviated on specific aspects, such as advising the regular use of analgesics in the acute phase or the referral to physiotherapy (*Table 6.2*; Schers *et al*. 2000). The implementation strategy subsequently developed defined specific targets to improve prescribing and referrals to physiotherapy.

Table 6.2 Management of low back pain in primary care (n = 937 patient contacts; Schers *et al*. 2000)

	Proportion of contacts at which action was performed (%)		
	Acute (0–6 weeks)	Subacute (6–12 weeks)	Chronic (>12 weeks)
Advice to take bed rest	7	5	4
Advice to resume activities despite pain	79	70	73
Counselling about pain and disability	NA	70	73
Information on pain and psychosocial problems	NA	44	56
Prescribing analgesics	55	20	38
Instruction to take medication according to fixed schedule	63	42	64
Referral to physiotherapy	22	64	44
Referral to secondary care	0.3	3	7

Based on such data it is possible to identify what changes in current practice are needed and which aspects of care the implementation strategy should target. These may include:

- To start a completely new routine, for instance the use of a new technology or drug, such as the use of angiotensin-converting enzyme (ACE) inhibitors in patients with heart failure;
- To stop a current routine, for instance to stop prescribing an ineffective medication (no diazepam in cases of low back pain);
- To reduce specific routines, for instance to reduce the number of lumbar spine radiographs for low back pain;
- To adapt specific routines, for instance increase one routine and reduce another, such as advise patients to use pain killers for low back pain continuously during a specified period and not only when in pain.

It is recommended that a valid assessment be made of the aspects of care that need to be changed most and to link concrete targets to these aspects.

BARRIERS AND INCENTIVES FOR CHANGE

In this section we describe factors that may enhance or inhibit implementation. If the context, setting, persons and organisations involved are known, if the most important problems in current practice are clear and targets for change defined, next barriers and incentives for change should be analysed in more detail. Some of the factors will be generic (they influence many implementation processes), while others will be specific to the specific change being implemented. In most cases several factors are relevant.

Factors related to individual care providers

Competence

The use of a guideline or new technology often requires specific knowledge and skills, so the presence or absence of these competence factors can determine the success of the implementation in some cases. Self-assessment of competence and performance by care providers is often not very accurate (Allen and Rashid 1998). A study showed that physicians prescribed diazepam much more often than they had estimated themselves (Rosser 1983), and when Montano and Phillips (1995) compared physician self-report data with both chart audit and patient survey, the latter two proved to be strongly correlated while the relationships between physician self-report and the other two were much weaker.

In terms of variation in performance (and thus skills), in a classic study from 1934 a group of paediatricians assessed the need for tonsillectomy in 389 children; tonsillectomy was deemed necessary in 45% of the children. The 55% of children for whom it was felt tonsillectomy had not been indicated were then assessed again, but by a different group of paediatricians. On this occasion tonsillectomy was again thought to be indicated in 46% of these non-indicated cases (Bakwin 1945). Similar results were found in a replication of this study (Ayanian and Berwick 1991).

An important prerequisite for the implementation of innovations is the skill to find and understand new insights. Professionals have different styles of finding information. A survey study among 1041 Norwegian physicians showed that 98% had participated in courses and conferences in the previous 12 months and that

80% felt they had received useful information (Nylenna *et al.* 1996). In professions for which continuing education is voluntary, however, a large proportion of the professionals may not be reached by courses and conferences. 100 British physicians were interviewed about the reasons for change in their clinical routines (*Table 6.3*). The most important reasons reported were changes in the organisation of practice, participation in continuing education and contacts with colleagues. Consultants were more strongly influenced than GPs by medical journals and scientific conferences. Continuing education was the main reason for change in 17% of the cases and mentioned in 37% of all changes. Clinical guidelines were rarely mentioned as a reason for change (<1%). This may, of course, be different in other groups of healthcare workers.

Attitudes and opinions

An individual's attitude towards an innovation is, of course, a factor that may influence the implementation of that innovation. When considering the features of an innovation, individuals usually consider characteristics such as complexity (how difficult it is to do), visibility of any improvement (how obvious any change is and how quickly it will occur) and the potential for testing it on a small scale (see Chapter 4). Although many care providers have an overall positive attitude towards clinical guidelines or protocols, some have specific concerns about a reduction of clinical freedom, the scientific evidence behind the recommendations and the possible (mis)use of guidelines for cost containment or legal purposes, for instance after complaints from patients (*Table 6.3*; Gupta *et al.* 1997; Hayward *et al.* 1997; James *et al.* 1997; Newton *et al.* 1996; Siriwardena 1995; Grol 1990). Acceptance of guidelines seems to be better if the guidelines were developed by professional organisations rather than by external organisations, such as the government or insurers (Hayward *et al.* 1997; Newton *et al.* 1996). Such considerations may be unclear for other innovations, such as protocols, pathways or best practices. Some care providers argue that many clinical guidelines or pathways take a rather linear approach to decision making, which is not representative of real consultations with patients (Tomlin *et al.* 1999; Woolf *et al.* 1999; Tonelli 1998), in which often a general recommendation has to be tailored to an individual patient, taking into account the patient's age, sex and health status. Furthermore, the decisions not only depend on medical knowledge, but also on the patient's needs and preferences (see Chapter 5).

It is, however, unclear to what extent attitudes and opinions influence adherence to a proposed new routine. A study on preventive procedures showed, for instance, that performance of the procedures was related only weakly to the stated wish to perform more preventive

Table 6.3 Reasons for change (1080 reasons for 361 changes mentioned by 100 physicians; Allerly *et al.* 1997)

Reasons for changing practice	Number of times mentioned:
Organisation of practice and/or healthcare policy making	193
Continuing education	182
Contact with colleagues	141
Patients' wishes	104
Availability of new technology	101
Economic factors	93
Clinical experiences	85
Pharmacological innovations	56
Personal contacts	39
Pharmaceutical industry	36
Waiting lists	32
Medical law suits	17

Table 6.4   Opinions of 160 British physicians on recommendations for management of asthma (Armstrong *et al*. 1994)

Management	Evident (%)	Useful (%)	Controversial (%)
House dust mite in pillows and sheets is the most important cause of asthma in children	17	33	50
Asthma patients should not smoke	83	13	4
Oral corticosteroids should be prescribed for longer periods only after consultation with a pulmonary specialist	17	28	55
Breathing exercises have little value for asthma patients	16	24	60

activities, the need to support preventive practices or the perceived support by the management (Solberg *et al.* 1997). Care providers' opinions regarding desired behaviour may be better associated with performance than with general attitudes regarding guidelines or new routines. Theories on behaviour change (see Chapter 2) and research in health education suggest that the associations between attitude and opinions on appropriate healthcare and actual behaviour are influenced by factors such as social norms, self-efficacy and practical barriers.

Motivation for change

Several motivational factors can be relevant to the achievement of change (*Box 6.2*), so a plan for implementation should address these. Dissatisfaction with one's performance can induce a process of change (Geertsma *et al.* 1982). Such dissatisfaction may be caused by a gap between a professional's objectives and actual practice, or by receiving negative comments from others. Individuals differ, of course, with respect to their experience and tolerance of such gaps. In many cases the motivation to change grows gradually under the influence of experiences in practice or (repeated)

information about a specific (deviating) routine. Sometimes a specific event, such as a serious error or incident (e.g. the death of a patient caused by medication interaction), leads to a sudden strong motivation to change performance (Armstrong *et al.* 1996).

Individual characteristics

A professional's behaviour is also related to age, gender and other characteristics (*Box 6.3*). Some studies show, for instance, that older physicians perform more diagnostic tests (Winkens 1994; Kristiansen and Hjortdahl 1992), but other studies show the opposite (Winkenwerder *et al.* 1993; Woo *et al.* 1985). Physicians who are members of professional organisations are often more positive about clinical guidelines and other innovations (Grol and Wensing 1995; Siriwardena 1995; Nelsen *et al.* 1994; Grol 1990). The professional discipline also influences the management of a clinical problem. For instance, internists order a wider range of diagnostic tests for three non-acute cardiology problems than cardiologists (Glassman *et al.* 1997), and GPs order diagnostic tests more often than cardiologists (Young *et al.* 1987).

Psychological characteristics are also relevant – the tendency to accept risk explains some of the variation in both

Box 6.2 Motivations of care providers to change their behaviour (Scott 1997)

- Income – amount of income and financial problems;
- Leisure time – number of hours worked, duties at weekends and during the night, burden for the family and social life, and not wanting to work at home;
- Burden of work – number of consultations per hour, number of urgent calls and home visits, amount of administrative work and unrealistic expectations of patients;
- Ethical code – concerns about complaints from patients, concerns about making the correct diagnosis, the extent to which one can really help the patient and the extent to which self-care can be enhanced;
- Societal motivations – to participate as a care provider in activities outside direct patient care;
- Status recognition from colleagues – no negative publicity, support from colleagues;
- Intellectual satisfaction – wanting to apply available knowledge and skills, or to read the professional literature;
- Autonomy – freedom to determine, and to be responsible for, their own routines and activities, with no external control.

Box 6.3 Characteristics of physicians and patients related to adherence with 29 clinical guidelines (Spies and Mokkink 1999)

A study with 200 GPs, who recorded their clinical activities over several months, showed that:
- National clinical guidelines are applied more often in older patients (>52 years of age);
- Guidelines are applied more often in male than female patients;
- Older GPs apply the guidelines more often;
- Male GPs and GPs in solo practices apply the guidelines more often;
- GPs who use the summary sheets of the guidelines also used the guidelines more often.
- The differences between subgroups was, however, small (3–5%).

diagnostic test ordering and referral to other care providers (Zaat and Eijk 1992; Holtgrave *et al*. 1991). The estimation of probabilities and coping with risks is an important aspect of patient care. These characteristics may be related to the type of healthcare system and opinions as to what is appropriate care – GPs in Belgium were, for instance, less prepared to accept risks than GPs in the Netherlands (Grol 1990). The confidence in one's own performance is often a predictive factor for specific activities (Maibach and Murphy 1995).

Factors related to the social setting

Patients

Patients' age, sex and socioeconomic status are relevant to clinical decisions. For instance, young men are more likely to receive a diagnosis of coronary heart disease than are young women (Clark *et al*. 1991). Patient characteristics can stimulate or inhibit change of professional routines. Furthermore, many professionals have subjective preferences for different categories of patients. Some studies show that many physicians prefer young patients (Tarbox *et al*. 1987; Keeler *et al*. 1982), which may reduce the time they devote to improving the care of older patients. In a study of 720 physicians (Schulman *et al*. 1999), case histories of patients with chest pain were presented. The physicians thought that women were less likely to have heart disease than men were, and would refer female patients less often for cardiac catheterisation. Black patients were less likely to be referred when compared to white patients. The study concluded that a patient's sex and ethnicity influenced the physician's management. Furthermore, patients often have specific ideas about appropriate healthcare or preferences that differ from those of care providers. For instance, patients and GPs have differing priorities with respect to primary care (*Table 6.5*). Such opinions determine where and when individuals seek healthcare and also whether they follow the advice and instructions given by the care provider.

Table 6.5 Priorities of patients and GPs with respect to primary care (Jung *et al*. 1997)

Priorities[a]	Patients (n = 455)	GPs (n = 263)
More important for patients		
It should be possible to make an appointment with a GP at short notice	4	17
GP should tell me everything I want to know about my illness	5	23
It should be possible to see the same GP at each visit	17	33
GP should be willing to check my health regularly	23	38
More important for GPs		
GP should work according to accepted knowledge about good general practice care	10	5
GP should take a personal interest in the patient as a person and his or her life situation	30	15
There should be good co-operation between a GP and his or her staff	20	4
GP should give the patient written information about surgery hours, telephone number of the practice, etc.	38	21

[a]Ranked numbers in a set of 38 priorities: 1 = most important, 38 = least important.

The effect of patients' opinions on healthcare and change in performance are partly mediated through the care providers' interpretation of these opinions. Professionals may change their behaviour because of their ideas about what patients think. Physicians in the Netherlands mentioned the following reasons for deviating from their own views on appropriate care (Veldhuis *et al*. 1998): the need to be nice (42% of deviations), the wish to avoid conflict with the patient (30%) and a lack of mutual trust (10%). Perceived problems with adherence to the guideline for ankle injury resulted mainly from patients' behaviour and wishes (Grol *et al*. 1991).

Other studies show that some physicians ordered diagnostic or preventive tests primarily to reassure the patient or – the opposite – did not order tests because of the inconvenience for the patient (Van Boven *et al*. 1994; Resnicow *et al*. 1989). 21 GPs and 567 patients were asked, before their consultation, to state their expectations of having a diagnostic test performed or receiving medication. In those patients who expected to receive a diagnostic tests (laboratory test, radiographs, etc.), the likelihood of receiving one was four times higher (odds ratio 4:1) than in those patients who did not expect to receive one. Similarly, if they expected medication, the likelihood was 2.5 times higher (odds ratio 2:5; Van Velsen *et al*. 2000). US GPs referred patients with heart failure to a cardiologist more often if they lived further away from the practice and they prescribed different medication to patients of lower and higher socioeconomic status. In so doing they deviated consciously from an evidence-based guideline for heart failure (James *et al*. 1998).

Another study showed that the likelihood of prescribing medication was three times higher (odds ratio 2:9) if the patient expected a prescription. However, the likelihood was 10 times higher (odds ratio 10:1) if the physician thought that the patient expected a prescription, regardless of the accuracy of this estimation (Cockburn and Pit 1997).

Colleagues

Many care providers are influenced heavily by opinions of colleagues in their direct environment. In a British–US study several hundreds of hospital physicians were interviewed. The results showed that many physicians actively observed their colleagues and many discussed new insights and routines with their colleagues. Actual practice changed only when there was a local consensus on the appropriate routines, rather than by scientific publications or the marketing of a technology by manufacturers (Greer 1988). The most important conditions for implementation proved to be local communication about the risks and benefits of the new procedure, the availability of local demonstration and education, and positive expectations of relevant individuals. Another study showed that physicians in rural areas in the USA used flexible sigmoidoscopy more often if another physician in the local community also used this technique (Nelsen *et al*. 1994).

There is often a local opinion leader in a department or group of professionals – a professional who can influence colleagues' opinions regarding the new procedures. Opinion leaders are individuals consulted by colleagues for information and advice and who set an example with their performance (Stross 1996). This requires that they be technically competent as well as a dedicated member of the local group (Greer 1988). They are not necessarily those who are the first to implement new routines. Studies in medical and paramedical settings show that opinion leaders can be identified by members of a department or practice and such opinion leaders can be used to disseminate new knowledge in specific settings, although the results of studies that evaluated this strategy are not uniform and the effects are usually small (*Box 6.4*; Lomas *et al*. 1991; Hong *et al*. 1990).

Box 6.4 Local opinion leaders in nursing (Hong *et al*. 1990)

A quality-improvement project was started in a hospital to reduce the number of urinary tract infections caused by the inadequate use of catheters. Local opinion leaders were identified by asking nurses from several departments about individuals with a lot of expertise in this area, who would be able to provide education and who had sufficient authority to influence others. Everyone was invited to mention three people and the person mentioned most often was identified. These opinion leaders were recruited to implement new guidelines on urinary tract infections. In group A, opinion leaders gave a lecture of 30 minutes for all nurses and demonstrations in small groups of 6–10 nurses. In this group 77% of nurses' actions were according to the guidelines. In group B opinion leaders only gave the lecture, and 64% of the nurses' actions met the guidelines. In a control group no lecture or demonstration was provided, and guideline adherence was 52%.

Factors related to the system

Organisation and structure

A crucial pre-condition for the implementation of new routines is, of course, that the necessary facilities and materials are available. For instance, practices that had facilities for diagnostic imaging used this four times as much as practices that had to refer to other settings for it (Hillman *et al.* 1990). Physicians mentioned 'a lack of facilities' as one of the most important barriers to preventive screening (Resnicow *et al.* 1989).

A study on diabetes care showed that, while a diabetes team was available in many hospitals in the Netherlands, the number of disciplines (internist, diabetes nurse, dietician, podiatrist and surgeon) in it was often limited and insufficient to allow adherence to guidelines in the clinical area (Dijkstra *et al.* 2000). Furthermore, a protocol was available in many cases, but it was often not followed (*Table 6.6*). When a patient was actually seen by a diabetes nurse, care proved to be more in line with evidence-based guidelines than when the patient was seen by a medical specialist only (Dijkstra *et al.* 2004).

A number of specific organisational characteristics have been shown to influence the likelihood of change. An example is the rate at which patients are seen – the higher this rate, the less the appropriate diagnostic tests are ordered (Brook *et al.* 1990; Davis and Yee 1990; Chassin *et al.* 1987). In teaching hospitals diagnostic tests were used more appropriately than in non-teaching hospitals (Brook *et al.* 1990; see Box 6.5 for an example).

Formal procedures can have a major impact on current practice. For instance, having to obtain permission for each test order (Novich *et al.* 1985) and having only a small number of tests on the test order form (Zaat and Eijk 1992) resulted in a lower number of tests ordered.

Financial resources and reimbursements

It is plausible that negative and positive financial consequences of implementation inhibit or enhance, respectively, the change process. Indeed, care providers thought that targeted financial incentives can provide an important contribution to the implementation of guidelines (Hayward *et al.* 1997; Mansfield 1995; Siriwardena 1995; Grol 1990). An Australian study showed that physicians think that implementation can be improved by information on the financial consequences of guideline adherence (Gupta *et al.* 1997). In addition, some care providers think that clinical guidelines are mainly aimed at cost control – particularly so in the USA and Canada (James *et al.* 1997; Gupta *et al.* 1997; Ferreir *et al.* 1996; Weingarten *et al.* 1995; Tunis *et al.* 1994). It is not clear to what extent this feeling is actually a barrier to implementation.

The reimbursement system can also influence care provision, at least in the USA (*Box 6.6*). Fee-for-service systems usually have more care activities than managed care or prepaid systems (Hellinger 1996). Thus, it seems more difficult to reduce specific activities in a fee-for-service system compared to a system with fixed payments. The financial conditions in a local setting are also relevant to healthcare professionals. For instance, a rehabilitation centre was used more often if the referring clinicians owned the centre (Mitchell and Sass

---

Table 6.6 Organisation of diabetes care in 106 hospitals in the Netherlands (Dijkstra *et al.* 2000)

Factor	Number of hospitals
Diabetes team available	97
Diabetes team meets once a month or more often	71
There is a written protocol	77
Diabetes team uses the written protocol	17
There are special surgeries for diabetes patients	72
Self-monitoring booklets for patients are available	85

Box 6.5 Mortality after myocardial infarction (Chen *et al.* 1999)

In this study, 60 top hospitals (mostly teaching hospitals) in the USA were compared with 4600 other hospitals with respect to mortality within 30 days of myocardial infarction. The data referred to 150,000 patients. The mortality was 15% in the top hospitals, but 18% in the other hospitals. More detailed analysis of the routines in the hospitals showed that top hospitals made better and more frequent use of evidence-based guidelines for the prescription of aspirin and beta-blockers.

1995). Targeted financial payments, for instance for preventive care, may change practice routines also (Langham *et al*. 1995). A fixed budget per year has proved to be associated with the implementation of guidelines (Salisbury *et al*. 1998), and a lower number of medication prescriptions and referrals (Gosden and Torgerson 1997).

SEGMENTATION IN THE TARGET GROUP

Within any group that is going to use a proposed practice, such as a guideline, new procedure or new technology, it is likely that different 'segments' exist and can usefully be identified. These are subgroups that may be in different phases of change and therefore may experience different problems and needs for change. Chapter 3 describes a number of theoretical frameworks for segmenting a target group. Empirical studies provide some support for this distinction into different segments, but there are a range of taxonomies that differ slightly from each other. For example, a study of 1400 physicians on adherence to guidelines for vaccination (Pathman *et al*. 1996) suggested the following groups:

- Physicians who did not know the guidelines;
- Physicians who knew the guidelines, but did not accept or use them;
- Physicians who knew and accepted the guidelines, but did not use them;
- Physicians who knew and accepted the guidelines and followed them with some patients;
- Physicians who knew and accepted the guidelines and followed them with almost all patients.

In other words, there were no physicians who used the guidelines, but did not accept them. The model that Pathman *et al*. (1996) developed was able to account for about 90% of the physicians.

A study of physicians' attitudes towards the guidelines of the Dutch College of General Practitioners in the beginning of the 1990s (Grol 1992) identified three groups of physicians:

- A group of College members, who worked in group practices and who were involved in the education of trainee GPs or medical students (group A);
- A mixed group (group B);
- A group of GPs who were not College members, worked in solo practices and who were not involved in education (group C).

Group A was better informed about the guidelines than group C and had more positive views about them (*Table 6.7*).

In Chapter 3 we present a number of phases or steps in a change process that an individual, group or

---

Box 6.6 Hospital volume and healthcare outcomes (Effective Health Care Bulletin 1996)

A large number of observational studies suggest that poor health outcomes (principally mortality) related to specific clinical procedures are associated with low volumes of these procedures. It might be that 'practice make perfect' (experience leads to better outcomes) or that high-volume hospitals attract better clinicians or support staff ('selective referral effect').

This implies that hospital volume may be a potentially powerful moderator of the effectiveness of implementation strategies. A systematic review suggests, however, that the best research did not confirm the general association between volume and quality, although in some specialities there appear to be quality gains associated with increased hospital or clinician volume.

Table 6.7 GPs' opinions on College guidelines (*n* = 339; Grol 1992)

Attribute	GPs showing the attribute (%)		
	Group A (*n* = 43)	Group B (*n* = 238)	Group C (*n* = 54)
Positive attitude regarding College	86	76	67
Positive attitude regarding guidelines	65	56	34
Positive attitude regarding use of guidelines	84	60	44
Well informed about			
Guideline on ankle injury	98	83	52
Guideline on urinary tract infections	100	89	57

organisation has to take before implementation and integration of the new routines can be achieved (*Table 6.8*). Different subgroups in a target group are often in different phases of the change process and in each of the phases other problems may influence the actual implementation. Absence of these problems, of course, facilitates change.

CONCLUSIONS

It is important to gain a clear insight into the target group and setting for implementation. Without this, the risk is that ineffective interventions are used or that implementation activities focus on aspects of patient care that are not crucial. There are often clear differences between individuals and groups of care providers, practices and hospitals with respect to their motivation to use new procedures, the way they should be approached and their barriers and incentives for change. Therefore, it is important to perform an adequate analysis of the situation, rather than to start immediately with implementation activities. The situation should be analysed from the perspective of the organisations, care providers and patients who are involved. This should make it possible to develop an effective strategy or implementation plan that includes:

Table 6.8 Barriers for implementation of guidelines and innovations (Grol and Wensing 2004)

Steps	Examples of potential barriers
Orientation	
Know the innovation Interest, involvement	No reading, no continuing education Little contact with colleagues Little need for innovation, not perceived as relevant Lack of insight into gaps in own performance
Insight	
Understand the innovation Insight into own routines	Lack of specific knowledge No understanding of the new information Forget the precise information Reject gaps in own performance Defensive attitude
Acceptance	
Positive attitude Intention to or decision to change	Perceive more disadvantages than advantages Doubts about scientific evidence Doubts about trustworthiness of developers No involvement in development process Expect problems for the implementation Lack of confidence in own skills to implement
Change	
Adoption in practice Confirmation of value	Practical barriers (time, money) Lack of skills to perform innovation No opportunity to experiment on a small scale First experiences are not positive Patients or colleagues do not co-operate, and respond negatively Negative side effects
Maintenance	
Integration in routines Integration in organisation	Relapse into old routines Forget new insights Lack of resources No support from (top) management

Table 6.9 Barriers and incentives

Element	Possible factors
Individual care provider	
Competence	To be informed, knowledge and skills for use, insight into own routines, ability to learn new insights
Attitude	Opinions on the innovation and its feasibility in practice
Motivation for change	Dissatisfaction with current routines
Personal characteristics	Age, gender, membership of professional organisations, self-efficacy and learning style
Social setting	
Patients	Needs and preferences, personal characteristics and perceptions of wishes of the patient
Care providers	Opinions of colleagues, opinion leaders and professional network
System	
Organisation and/or structure	Structural conditions, volume, bounded rationality, interests and resources
Financial reimbursement	Fee for service or fixed payment system, financial interest and targeted financial incentives

- Analysis of the background, context and parties involved;
- Analysis of the aspects of care that need to be changed most;
- Detailed documentation of the barriers and incentives for change – these may relate to the care providers, the patients, the social network and the organisational setting and the system (*Table 6.9*), and often several factors are relevant;
- Identification of segments in the target group, such as younger versus older care providers, that experience different barriers and facilitators.

Recommended literature

Cabana M, Rand C, Power N, *et al.* (1999). Why don't physicians follow clinical practice guidelines. *JAMA* **282**:1458–1465.

Grol R and Wensing M (2004). What drives change? Barriers to and incentives for achieving an evidence-based practice. *MJA* **180**:S57–S60.

Oxman AD and Flottorp S (1998). An overview of strategies to promote implementation of evidence-based health care. In: Silagy C and Haines A. *Evidence-Based Practice in Primary Care*, Ch 8, pp. 91–109. London: BMJ Books.

References

Allen J and Rashid A (1998). What determines competence within a general practice consultation? Assessment of consultation skills using simulated surgeries. *Br J Gen Pract.* **270**:1046–1051.

Allerly LA, Owen PA and Robling MR (1997). Why general practitioners and consultants change their clinical practice: A critical incident study. *BMJ* **314**:870–874.

Armstrong D, Fry J and Armstrong P (1994). General practitioners' views of clinical guidelines for the management of asthma. *Int J Qual Health Care* **6**:199–202.

Armstrong D, Reyburn H and Jones R (1996). A study of general practitioners' reasons for changing their prescribing behaviour. *BMJ* **312**:949–952.

Ayanian JZ and Berwick DM (1991). Do physicians have a bias toward action? A classic study revisited. *Med Decis Making* **11**:154–158.

Bakwin H (1945). Pseudodoxia pediatrica. *N Engl J Med.* **232**:691–697.

Boven C van, Dijksterhuis PH and Lamberts H (1994). Defensief handelen door huisarts bij aanvullend onderzoek [Defensive behaviour of general practitioners in test ordering]. *Huisarts Wet.* **37**:473–477.

Brook RH, Park RE, Chassin MR, *et al.* (1990). Predicting the appropriate use of carotid endarterectomy, upper gastrointestinal endoscopy, and coronary angiography. *N Engl J Med.* **323**:1173–1177.

Chassin MR, Kosecoff J, Park RE *et al.* (1987). Does inappropriate use explain geographic variations in the use of health care services? A study of three procedures. *JAMA* **258**:2533–2537.

Chen J, Radford MJ, Wang Y, *et al.* (1999). Do 'America's best hospitals' perform better for acute myocardial infarction? *N Engl J Med.* **340**:286–292.

Clark JA, Potter DA and McKinlay JB (1991). Bringing social structure back into clinical decision making. *Soc Sci Med.* **32**:853–866.

Cockburn J and Pit S (1997). Prescribing behaviour in clinical practice: Patients' expectations and doctors' perceptions of patients' expectations – a questionnaire study. *BMJ* **315**:520–523.

Davis PB and Yee RL (1990). Patterns of care and professional decision making in a New Zealand general practice sample. *NZ Med J*. **103**:309–312.

Dijkstra RF, Braspenning JCC, Uiters E, *et al*. (2000). Perceived barriers to the implementation of diabetes guidelines in hospitals in The Netherlands. *Neth J Med*. **56**:80–85.

Dijkstra R, Braspenning JCC, Huijsmans Z, *et al*. (2004). Patients and nurses determine variation in adherence to guidelines at Dutch hospitals more than internists or settings. *Diabetes Med*. **21**:586–591.

Effective Health Care Bulletin (1996). *Hospital Volume and Health Care Outcomes, Costs and Patient Access*. York: NHS Centre for Reviews and Dissemination, University of York.

Ferreir BM, Woodward CA, Cohen M, *et al*. (1996). Clinical practice guidelines. New to practice family physicians' attitudes. *Can Fam Phys*. **42**:463–468.

Geertsma RH, Parker RC and Krauss S (1982). How physicians view the process of change in their practice behaviour. *J Med Educ*. **57**:752–761.

Glassman PA, Kravitz RL, Petersen LP, *et al*. (1997). Differences in clinical decision making between internists and cardiologists. *Arch Intern Med*. **157**:506–512.

Gosden T and Torgerson DJ (1997). The effect of fundholding on prescribing and referral costs: A review of the evidence. *Health Policy* **40**:103–114.

Greer AL (1988). The state of the art versus the state of the science. *Int J Technol Assess Health Care* **4**:5–26.

Grol R (1990). National standard setting for quality of care in general practice: Attitudes of general practitioners and response to a set of standards. *Br J Gen Pract*. **40**:361–364.

Grol R (1992). Implementing guidelines in general practice. *Qual Health Care* **1**:184–91.

Grol R (1997). Beliefs and evidence in changing clinical practice. *BMJ* **315**:418–421.

Grol R and Wensing M (1995). Implementation of quality assurance and medical audit: General practitioners' perceived obstacles and requirements. *Br J Gen Pract*. **45**:548–552.

Grol R and Wensing M (2004). What drives change? Barriers to and incentives for achieving an evidence-based practice. *MJA* **180**:S57 S60.

Grol R, Claessens A, Velden J van der, *et al*. (1991). Kwaliteit van zorg bij enkeldistorsie: Invoering van een standaard [Quality of care for sprained ankle: Implementation of a guideline]. *Huisarts Wet*. **34**:30–34.

Gupta L, Ward JE and Hayward SA (1997). Clinical practice guidelines in general practice: A national survey of recall, attitudes and impact. *MJA* **166**:69–72.

Hayward RSA, Guyatt GH, Moore KA, *et al*. (1997). Canadian physicians' attitudes about and preferences regarding clinical practice guidelines. *Can Med Assoc J*. **156**:1715–1723.

Hellinger FJ (1996). The impact of financial incentives on physician behavior in managed care plans: A review of the evidence. *Med Care Res Rev*. **53**:294–314.

Hillman BJ, Joseph CA, Marry MR, *et al*. (1990). Frequency and costs of diagnostic imaging in office practice: A comparison of self-referring and radiologist-referring physicians. *N Engl J Med*. **323**:1604–1608.

Holtgrave DR, Lawler F and Spann SJ (1991). Physicians' risk attitudes, laboratory usage, and referral decisions: The case of an academic family practice center. *Med Decis Making* **11**:125–130.

Hong SW, Ching TY, Fung JPM, *et al*. (1990). The employment of ward opinion leaders for continuing education in the hospital. *Med Teacher* **23**:209–217.

Hooi J, Weijden T van der and Grol R (2000). *Aanbevelingen voor de Implementatie van de 'Richtlijn Beroerte 2000' [Recommendations for Implementation of the Guideline Stroke 2000]*. Rapport van de werkgroep Implementatie, CBO Richtlijn Beroerte [Report of the Implementation Committee, CBO Guidelines for Stroke]. Maastricht : WOK.

James PA, Cowan TM, Graham RP, *et al*. (1997). Family physicians' attitudes about and use of clinical practice guidelines. *J Fam Pract*. **45**:341–347.

James PA, Cowan TM and Graham RP (1998). Patient-centred clinical decisions and their impact on physician adherence to clinical guidelines. *J Fam Pract*. **46**:311–318.

Jung HP, Wensing M and Grol R (1997). What makes a good general practitioner: Do patients and doctors have different views? *Br J Gen Pract*. **47**:805–809.

Keeler EB, Solomon DH, Beck JC, *et al*. (1982). Effect of patient age on duration of medical encounters with physicians. *Med Care* **20**:1101–1108.

Kristiansen IS and Hjortdahl P (1992). The general practitioner and laboratory utilization: Why does it vary? *Fam Pract*. **9**:22–27.

Langham S, Gillam S and Thorogood M (1995). The carrot, the stick and the general practitioner: How have changes in financial incentives affected health promotion activity in general practice? *Br J Gen Pract*. **45**:665–668.

Lomas J, Enkin M, Andersson GM, *et al*. (1991). Opinion leaders versus audit and feedback to implement practice guidelines. Delivery after previous caesarean arthritis. *JAMA* **265**:2202–2207.

Maibach E and Murphy DA (1995). Self-efficacy in health promotion research and practice: Conceptualization and measurement. *Health Educ Res*. **10**:37–50.

Mansfield CD (1995). Attitudes and behaviours towards clinical guidelines: The clinicians' perspective. *Qual Health Care* **4**:250–255.

Mitchell JM and Sass TR (1995). Physician ownership of ancillary services: Indirect demand inducement or quality assurance? *J Health Econ*. **14**:263–289.

Montano DE and Phillips WR (1995). Cancer screening by primary care physicians: A comparison of rates obtained from physician self-report, patient survey, and chart audit. *Am J Pub Health* **85**:795–800.

Nelsen DA, Hartley DA, Christianson J, *et al*. (1994). The use of new technologies by rural family physicians. *J Fam Pract*. **38**:479–485.

Nelson EC, Splaine ME, Batalden PB, *et al*. (1998). Building measurement and data collection into medical practice. *Ann Intern Med*. **128**:460–466.

Newton J, Knight D and Woolhead G (1996). General practitioners and clinical guidelines: A survey of knowledge, use and beliefs. *Br J Gen Pract*. **46**:513–517.

Novich M, Gillis L and Tauber AI (1985). The laboratory test justified. An effective means to reduce routine laboratory testing. *Am J Clin Path*. **84**:756–759.

Nylenna M, Aasland OG and Falkum E (1996). Keeping professionally updated: Perceived coping and CME profiles among physicians. *J Cont Educ Health Prof*. **16**:241–249.

Pathman DE, Konrad TR, Freed GL, *et al.* (1996). The awareness-to-adherence model of the steps to clinical guideline compliance. The case of pediatric vaccine recommendations. *Med Care* **34**:873–889.

Resnicow KA, Schorow M, Bloom HG, *et al.* (1989). Obstacles to family practitioners' use of screening tests: Determinants of practice? *Prev Med*. **18**:101–112.

Rosser W (1983). Using the perception–reality gap to alter prescribing patterns. *J Med Educ*. **58**:728–732.

Salisbury C, Bosanquet N, Wilkinson E, *et al.* (1998). The implementation of evidence-based medicine in general practice prescribing. *Br J Gen Pract*. **48**:1849–1851.

Schers H, Braspenning J, Drijver R, *et al.* (2000). Low back pain in general practice: Reported management and reasons for not adhering to the guidelines in the Netherlands. *Br J Gen Pract*. **50**:640–644.

Schulman KA, Berlin JA, Harless W, *et al.* (1999). The effect of race and sex on physicians' recommendations for cardiac catheterization. *N Engl J Med*. **340**(8):618–626.

Scott A (1997). *Agency, Incentives and The Behaviour of General Practitioners: The Relevance of Principal Agent Theory in Designing Incentives for GPs in the UK*. Aberdeen: Departments of Public Health and Economics, Aberdeen University.

Siriwardena AN (1995). Clinical guidelines in primary care: A survey of general practitioners' attitudes and behaviour. *Br J Gen Pract*. **45**:643–647.

Solberg LI, Brekke ML and Kottke TE (1997). How important are clinician and nurse attitudes to the delivery of clinical preventive services. *J Fam Pract*. **44**:451–461.

Spies TH and Mokkink HGA (1999). *Toetsen aan Standaarden. Het Medisch Handelen van Huisartsen in de Praktijk Getoetst. Eindrapport [Assessment of Guidelines. Medical Care of General Practitioners Assessed in Practice. Final Report]*. Nijmegen/Utrecht: Werkgroep Onderzoek Kwaliteit/Nederlands Huisartsen Genootschap [Centre for Quality of Care Research/Dutch College of General Practitioners].

Stross JK (1996). The educationally influential physician. *J Cont Educ Health Prof*. **16**:167–172.

Tarbox AR, Connors GJ and Faillace LA (1987). Freshman and senior medical students' attitudes toward the elderly. *J Med Educ*. **62**:582–591.

Tomlin Z, Humphrey C and Rogers S (1999). General practitioners' perceptions of effective health care. *BMJ* **318**:1532–1535.

Tonelli M (1998). The philosophical limits of evidence-based medicine. *Acad Med*. **73**:1234–1240.

Tunis SR, Hayward RSA, Wilson MC, *et al.* (1994). Internists' attitudes about clinical practice guidelines. *Ann Intern Med*. **120**:956–963.

Veldhuis M, Wigersma L and Okkes I (1998). Deliberate departures from good general practice: A study of motives among Dutch general practitioners. *Br J Gen Pract*. **48**:1833–1836.

Velsen M van, Weijden T van der, Hasselt C van, *et al.* (2000). *Vage Klachten in de huisartspraktijk. Prevalentie en Determinanten van Beleid [Vague Symptoms in General Practice. Prevalence and Determinants of Management]*. Maastricht: WOK.

Weijden T van der, Grol RPTM, Schouten BJ, *et al.* (1998). Barriers to working according to cholesterol guidelines. A randomized controlled trial on implementation of national guidelines in 20 general practices. *Eur J Public Health* **8**:113–118.

Weingarten S, Stone E, Hayward R, *et al.* (1995). The adoption of preventive care practice guidelines by primary care physicians. Do actions match intentions? *J Gen Intern Med*. **10**:138–144.

Winkens R (1994). *Improving Test Ordering in General Practice. The Effects of Feedback*. Proefschrift. Maastricht: Maastricht University.

Winkenwerder W, Levy BD, Eisenberg JM, *et al.* (1993). Variation in physicians' decision-making thresholds in management of a sexually transmitted disease. *J Gen Intern Med*. **8**:369–373.

Woo B, Cook F, Weisberg M, *et al.* (1985). Screening procedures in the asymptomatic adult. Comparison of physicians' recommendations, patients' desires, published guidelines, and actual practice. *JAMA* **254**:1480–1484.

Woolf SH, Grol R, Hutchinson A, *et al.* (1999). Potential benefits, limitations, and harms of clinical guidelines. *BMJ* **318**:527–530.

Young MJ, Fried LS, Eisenberg J, *et al.* (1987). Do cardiologists have higher thresholds for recommending coronary arteriography than family physicians? *Health Serv Res*. **22**:623–635.

Zaat JO and Eijk JT van (1992). General practitioners' uncertainty, risk preferences, and use of laboratory tests. *Med Care* **30**:846–854.

Chapter 7

Methods to identify implementation problems

Michel Wensing and Richard Grol

KEY MESSAGES

- An adequate method used to identify barriers and incentives for change is a combination of a detailed study of a small number of cases to discover the relevant factors and larger scale studies to assess the relevance of the different factors in a larger group of professionals, organisations and patients.
- Semi-structured interviews, focus group interviews and (non-) participating observation may be useful for detailed studies of a small number of cases.
- Case-specific questionnaires and large-scale clinical data can be used to assess the relevance of different factors.
- However, insight into the practical usefulness of different methods remains limited.

Box 7.1 Barriers to adherence to acute low back pain guidelines (Schers *et al*. 2001)

Guidelines for non-specific acute low back pain recommend conservative management (no radiographs and no referral to a physiotherapist) for the first several weeks after the start of the problem and suggest it is very rarely appropriate to refer to a specialist. Analgesics may be prescribed, but it is important to use these regularly and not only when the pain is present (time contingent instead of pain contingent). It is important to stay physically active and take no additional bedrest. Shortly after a consultation with their general practitioner (GP), 20 patients with low back pain were interviewed. The GPs were also interviewed (separately). In the semi-structured interviews of about half-an-hour all phases of the consultation were discussed in relation to the elements of the guidelines listed above. The interviews were performed by two trained interviewers, audiotaped and then analysed. They focused on actual behaviour, routines and possible barriers to the implementation of the guideline. The categories used to describe and organise the statements, ideas and experiences of doctors and patients were developed during the coding process. A general distinction was made between statements on behaviour, opinions regarding healthcare (guidelines and expectations of care) and motivations. About half of the back pain patients had taken bedrest in the past (behaviour), but none had found that it helped. Most were satisfied with the advice of their GP to stay active, but some had doubts about this (opinion). The doubt was based on ideas of possible damage to their back by physical movement (motivation). GPs said that they routinely gave the advice to stay active (behaviour). They all agreed with this aspect of the guideline (opinion). One GP did not provide the advice, though, because he thought that the patient already knew this or was not prepared to receive it (motivation).

INTRODUCTION

Chapter 6 describes the importance of a diagnostic analysis, and how it aims to gain insight into the background and context of the implementation, current practice, segments of the target group and stage of change, and the barriers (*Box 7.2*) and incentives for change. This chapter describes a range of methods that may be used to collect data on these factors. Methods to document current practice are described in more detail in Chapter 16. Most methods have been derived from scientific research, but simple variants can also be used for (low budget) implementation projects. Methods to collect data are discussed first, followed by methods to analyse these data.

Box 7.2   Systematic literature review of studies of the barriers to adherence to guidelines (Cabana *et al.* 1999)

This overview of studies focused on the perceived barriers to the implementation of clinical guidelines. After an analysis of databases and other sources, 76 studies were found in which at least one barrier to the use of clinical guidelines was described – these comprised five qualitative studies and 120 surveys with structured questions, of which 58% concerned only one type of barrier. From these, 293 potential barriers were derived. The average percentages of respondents that perceived a barrier were:

- 55% were not aware of the guideline;
- 57% were not aware of the exact content;
- Between 6 and 68% reported little self-efficacy;
- 13% reported no positive expectation of the result;
- 42% reported lack of motivation to change;
- Between 5 and 17% reported external factors, such as time and resources.

SURVEY METHODS

Postal questionnaire surveys of care providers have often been used to gain insight into the problems and needs around a specific change. A relatively small investment is needed to survey large numbers of care providers and patients. It is important to pay attention to the development of the questionnaire – are the questions clear and one-dimensional, do they provide answers to what is being asked and are all the important topics included? Piloting of such questionnaires is recommended.

However, such surveys are not without limitations. It may be unclear to what extent individuals can report adequately on their behaviour and to what extent perceived factors do indeed influence their behaviour. In general, the association between opinions and actual behaviour is limited. Additionally, it is not possible to ask specific follow-up questions about underlying motivations, as can be done in an oral interview. A postal questionnaire survey is particularly appropriate to gather data from large numbers of care providers or patients about the extent to which they perceive specific factors as important.

Questionnaires on guidelines

There are many questionnaires on opinions towards clinical guidelines, which vary in scope (*Box 7.3*). Some cover guidelines in general, while others cover one specific guideline or even specific recommendations within a guideline. Questions on guidelines in general can give an impression of the attitudes of care providers, but concrete questions regarding the use of specific recommendations probably give information more strongly associated with actual behaviour in practice. The questions can refer to different themes, such as awareness and knowledge of the guideline or recommendations, the opinions and attitudes towards the guideline and problems and needs with respect to implementation (*Box 7.4*).

Case-specific questionnaires

The perceived barriers to and need for change in professional practice are probably more valid if the questions in a questionnaire refer to specific situations in which the new activities have or have not been per-

Box 7.3   A questionnaire on the attitude to guidelines (Newton *et al.* 1996)

A British study focused on guidelines for asthma, radiology and diabetes. The questionnaire included:

- Three knowledge questions (answered on a five-point scale from 'never heard of' to 'very much knowledge of');
- 13 questions on guidelines in general (answered on a five-point scale from 'very much agree' to 'very much disagree'), such as 'guidelines limit clinical autonomy';
- Seven questions on possible barriers to implementation (answered on a five-point scale from 'lot of pressure' to 'little pressure');
- Eight questions on the expected effectiveness of methods to enhance the use of the guideline (answered on a five-point scale from 'very likely that this helps me to follow the guideline' to 'not likely at all').

Box 7.4 Questionnaire for perceived barriers to change (Peters *et al.* 2003)

Comparison of barriers to change across different innovations and settings requires a standardised measurement instrument. A validated questionnaire was developed to identify perceived barriers to change, and then applied in 12 different implementation studies in the Netherlands. Literature analyses and focus groups with implementation experts were used to identify possible barriers to change. Validation studies were performed to test psychometric characteristics of the questionnaire. A study on the prevention of cardiovascular diseases in general practice (n = 329 GPs) showed that perceived barriers, as measured with the questionnaire, explained 39% of the self-reported clinical performance. The questionnaire includes questions on characteristics of the innovation, the care provider, the patient and the context. The questions on patients and contexts particularly focused on the implementation of preventive activities. As examples, findings from three studies are presented below (percentages).

	Prevention of cardiovascular diseases (n = 190 GPs)	Management of lower urinary tract symptoms in men (n = 40 GPs)	Management of anaemia in pregnant women (n = 160 midwives)
Innovation characteristics (%)			
Compatibility	8	83	8
Time investment	52	75	7
Specificity, flexibility	12	70	15
Didactic benefit	11	53	2
Attractiveness	15	68	4
Care provider characteristics			
Attitude, role perception	15	78	6
Knowledge and motivation	13	80	9
Doubts about the innovation	27	80	17
Lifestyle, working style	40	28	12
Education	15	–	–
Involvement	2	55	13
Patient characteristics			
Age	17	–	–
Ethnicity	68	–	–
Financial situation, socioeconomic status	52	–	–
Number of patient contacts	62	–	–
Health status	58	–	–
Motivation to change	25	–	8
Context characteristics			
Group norms, socialisation	18	58	24
Reimbursement, insurance system	61	68	4
Laws, regulations	34	–	10
Opening hours of practice	27	38	–
Supporting staff	70	–	–
Facilities	22	–	–
Practice building	38	–	–

Box 7.5 Reasons to order diagnostic tests (Van Boven *et al*. 1997)

During 1 year, 16 physicians registered all episodes of care in which diagnostic tests were ordered. They recorded on a list their reasons for ordering the test. Furthermore, they indicated whether they thought that their decision was defensive or not.

Reasons mentioned included follow-up of symptoms, confirmation of a diagnosis, screening and vaccination, to exclude malignancy, to exclude other illness, patient request and to reassure the patient.

formed (*Box 7.5*). An interesting method, therefore, is to interview care providers or patients shortly after a specific action or event. This is often time-consuming, as experiences are collected prospectively over a period of time. An alternative may be to ask for experiences in the recent past (such as the previous month), but a disadvantage of this method is that the memory of the respondent may be unreliable. The case-specific questionnaire is most useful when the relevant patients present, or events occur, frequently so that much data can be collected in a short period of time.

Questionnaires on determinants

Theories of change suggest a large number of potential determinants of change, partly supported by scientif-

ic research (Chapter 2). Examples of these factors are age and sex, use of information channels, learning style and learning needs, self-efficacy regarding a specific area, team climate or the availability of opinion leaders. Standardised questionnaires have been developed and validated to measure these factors.

It is outside the range of this chapter to provide a comprehensive overview of the available questionnaires. The relevance of these questionnaires depends on both the actual influence of the measured factor on the behaviour and on the validity of the questionnaire (*Boxes 7.6* and *7.7*). Measuring a wide variety of determinants of change may be less relevant in small-scale quality-improvement projects, but in scientific research on determinants of change it is important to obtain a comprehensive insight into such factors.

Box 7.6 Prescribing antibiotics for patients with a sore throat (Walker *et al*. 2001)

The theory of planned behaviour was used to investigate the strength of intention to prescribe antibiotics, and to identify the salient beliefs associated with this intention. A 66-item postal questionnaire was distributed to a random sample of GPs ($n = 126$, 68% response rate). The majority ($n = 69$, 55%) intended to prescribe antibiotics for less than half of their patients with sore throats. The variables specified in the theory of planned behaviour predicted 48% of the variance in intention, with past behaviour adding a further 15%. GPs who intended to prescribe were more likely to agree that antibiotics reduce the risk of minor complications and

the time taken for a sore throat to resolve, and are cost effective. Physicians who intended to prescribe antibiotics were less concerned about the problem of increasing antibiotic resistance than physicians who did not prescribe. Physicians who intended to prescribe were more likely to agree that they were inclined to prescribe for patients of a lower social class, that they would prescribe if a patient specifically asked for an antibiotic and that they would prescribe to avoid missing something. They were also more likely to believe that patients would finish a course of prescribed antibiotics.

Box 7.7 Measurement of self-efficacy (Lee and Bobko 1994)

The belief that you can perform a specific task (self-efficacy) is an important psychological determinant for the implementation of that task. Self-efficacy is related to a specific activity and is not the same as self-confidence or sense of control in general (concepts that are more general features and less predictive of actual behaviour). The measurement of a concept such as self-efficacy requires a set of statements on factors that

make the particular activity difficult. These factors are related to the specific activity and can be identified by means of individual interviews or focus-group interviews. In relation to each factor, it is important to ask about both the ability to perform elements of the activity (using yes-or-no questions) and the level to which the individual is convinced of this ability (answering on scales ranging from 'not at all' to 'extremely').

INTERVIEW METHODS

Individual interviews

Face-to-face or telephone interviews with care providers and patients can provide insight into the context of an innovation and the experiences of it. Their advantage, compared to postal questionnaire surveys, is that it is possible to ask in-depth and follow-up questions about underlying reasons, but their disadvantage is that both the performance and analysis of interviews is usually more time consuming. Thus, it is often possible to perform only a limited number of interviews, so that the findings may not apply generally. Furthermore, conducting interviews requires training and preparation. In many small implementation projects 'conversations' rather than 'interviews' are used. These conversations are often valuable, so consideration should always be given to including these in implementation activities, with or without more detailed analysis of the barriers to and incentives for change (*Box 7.8*).

Group interviews

The idea of group interviews is that the communication between group members helps to identify issues that would not have been discovered in individual interviews. There are many positive experiences with the group-interview method, but the organisation of meetings with busy clinicians can be difficult or almost impossible. A range of techniques have been developed, which differ with respect to the level and the type of communication between group members (see Chapter 5 for a more detailed description of the methods):

- Brainstorming – a technique to generate ideas on a specific topic. The most important rules are that as many different ideas as possible be identified, that extreme or unpractical ideas be allowed and that no criticism is allowed during the session.
- Focus group interviews – 4–12 participants exchange ideas with expert supervision on 2–4 topics (Morgan 1988). This type of group interview is useful mainly to explore specific topics in-depth through open-ended questions (*Box 7.9*).
- Nominal group technique – to generate and categorise ideas. Participants perform individual tasks, such as the generation of ideas and categorisation of alternatives. These individual tasks alternate with exchange and discussion in the group.
- Delphi-technique – a procedure to achieve consensus on a specific topic, such as the most important implementation problems, or to clarify different viewpoints. Participants may be anonymous. The participants are surveyed in two or more rounds and receive feedback on the answers of others. The procedure may end with a group meeting to determine the final consensus or viewpoints (*Box 7.10*).

Box 7.8 Barriers to quality improvement in GPs (Grol and Wensing 1995)

A random sample of 120 GPs was used and the GPs were interviewed, using both open-ended and closed questions. The open-ended questions focused on barriers and needs in relation to quality improvement in general and four activities in particular – use of clinical guidelines, data collection and quality assessment, quality circles and/or professional collaboratives, and continuing education based on audits. The interviewers made notes during the interviews from which they produced a report of one or two pages of A4 per interview. To classify the barriers, a taxonomy was developed by the researcher. This was tested in some interviews, improved and tested again. The final taxonomy was used independently by two researchers to classify the barriers that had been mentioned. The taxonomy contained the following categories of barriers:

- Knowledge and skills of the physician – lack of specific skills, difficulty with changing fixed routines, insufficient information on quality improvement or no idea how to start;
- Lack of motivation – fear of assessment and criticism by others, resistance to change, doubts on the effectiveness of quality improvement and fear that the activities would lead to poor patient care;
- Criticism of quality improvement – criticism of assessment and re-accreditation, national guidelines, involvement of insurers, patients and/or government, continuing education programmes and the high speed of developments in the area of quality improvement;
- Resistance in the environment – negative attitudes with regard to quality improvement among colleagues, no support from patients and a negative attitude among medical specialists;
- Organisational and practical problems – lack of time, problems in the locum group, the practice organisation and the organisation of continuing education, and lack of financial support.

Box 7.9 Focus-group interviews with diabetes teams and diabetes patients (Dijkstra *et al.* 2002)

The Dutch Diabetic Federation, a patient organisation, developed and distributed a 'diabetic record' to enhance the implementation of its guidelines on diabetes. This is a small book that summarises the guidelines and can be used by the patients to document the course of their symptoms over time. Focus-group interviews were conducted with 29 patients and four diabetes teams from four hospitals to assess whether this diabetes record could provide a contribution to the implementation of the guidelines. The record was distributed and the participants given information on its purpose and content. Subsequently, a semi-structured discussion was held on the content, dissemination method, applicability and responsibility for completing the record. The interviews were audiotaped and transcribed. A coding scheme was developed and applied by two assessors independently:

- Most patients and teams did not understand the aim of the patient-held record;
- Most patients were positive about its content, but felt parts of it were too difficult;
- Patients varied in their willingness to use the record, but most physicians were negative;
- Most physicians thought that the diabetes nurse was the central person to complete the record.

Box 7.10 Barriers to the management of urinary tract infections and sore throat (Flottorp and Oxman 2003)

The aim of the study was to identify barriers to implementing evidence-based guidelines for urinary tract infection and sore throat in general practice in Norway, and to tailor interventions to address these barriers. A pragmatic combination of qualitative research methods was used. Those involved in the process of developing the guidelines were asked specifically to comment upon factors that could influence the implementation of the guidelines. An international group of implementation experts had a brainstorming session on possible barriers. Two focus-group interviews with patients and one focus-group interview with GP assistants were also conducted. A pilot study was performed in five practices to obtain feedback on factors that influenced the implementation of the guidelines. In an intervention study GPs and assistants discussed barriers in small groups. Finally, the researchers had informal interviews throughout the project. A checklist of 12 barriers to change was developed during this process. Barriers were categorised according to practice environment (financial disincentives, organisational constraints, perception of liability, patient expectations), prevailing opinion (standards of practice, opinion leaders, medical training, advocacy), knowledge and attitudes (clinical uncertainty, sense of competence, compulsion to act, information overload).

DIRECT OBSERVATION

Direct observation of behaviours and situations is a powerful method used to identify problems in current practice and to understand both the context and the relevance of different factors. Chapters 16 and 17 focus in more detail on methods used to collect data on actual practice. However, the influence of factors on a process of change cannot be observed directly, but has to be deduced from data analysis. This requires a comparison between individuals or situations in which the change is successful with individuals or situations in which the change is problematic. This comparison focuses on the question of which factors that differ between the two situations can be assumed to be (possible) determinants of the change. There are different observation methods.

Self-registration of behaviour

Self-registration is a data collection method that involves, for example, completing a (specially designed) registration form directly after contact with a specific patient or in other specific situations. Another example would be a (structured) diary completed by a patient. While there is an issue about how accurately people can observe their own behaviour, prospective self-recording can be used to register activities or features (e.g. thoughts) that cannot be recorded by others. Depending on the level of detail requested, self-registration can be time consuming and therefore difficult to implement. However, in a small implementation project simple registration methods that focus on central issues can provide valuable or necessary information. It is important to conduct self-registration as soon after the activity as possible. When the data are recorded as a survey instrument some time away from the event, the accuracy of the data appears to fall.

Medical records

Medical records are another source of data about practice. These data can be relatively easy to collect, although obtaining written informed consent from patients can be time consuming. In addition, not all aspects of care are well recorded and not all the available data are valid and reliable (*Box 7.11*). Data on clinical performance, such as ordering a diagnostic test or the prescription of a drug, are often well recorded (particularly if a financial reimbursement is related to the activity). In contrast, details of patient education are often poorly recorded. In a comparison of physician self-report with both chart audit and patient survey, the latter two correlated highly, but the relationship between physician self-report and either of the others

was much weaker (Montano and Phillips 1995). Similar problems were demonstrated with British GPs caring for older patients with hypertension, so it has been suggested that such questionnaire methods of collecting activity data should not be used (Eccles *et al.* 1999).

Participating and non-participating observation

A trained observer can observe specific events or activities in a specific setting and can either participate in the normal activities (participant observation, *Boxes 7.12* and *7.13*) or remain 'outside' (non-participant observation). There is a risk that the presence of the observer influences the activity being observed and that the observer thus loses his or her independence.

Box 7.11 Comprehensiveness and accuracy of different methods (Spies *et al.* 2004)

In 176 consultations with seven GPs relating to 15 different health problems, three data collection methods were used: self-registration by physicians directly after a consultation, direct observation of consultations and chart audit. Clinical behaviour was assessed through the use of explicit criteria, for which data on both medical activities and patient characteristics were collected. It turned out that self-registration provided 95% of all information, direct observation 72% and chart audit 40%. The consistency between self-registration, on the one hand, and direct observation and chart audit, on the other, was (as far as data were available) good, but not perfect (kappa 0.73 and 0.86, respectively). The conclusion was that self-registration provided the most comprehensive data, which were highly consistent with the data from medical records or direct observation of the consultation, as far as this could be assessed.

Box 7.12 Participant observation of treatment of hyperlipidaemia (Diwan *et al.* 1997)

Participant observation in a Swedish healthcare setting was used for 2 years to document the exchange of information that related to hyperlipidaemia. In the first 3 months observations were made and care providers were interviewed. Next, 40 physicians who participated in a programme to prevent cardiovascular diseases were observed over 1.5 years. There was no pre-defined observation scheme but, for example, contacts with nurses were observed, detailed records were made of all observations and contacts with nurses were audiotaped. It was found that most care providers started enthusiastically with the screening and education, but they had increasing doubts over time. They felt that some patients became very anxious after screening, while others ignored the results and maintained their lifestyle. The physicians also thought that they already knew how to treat hyperlipidaemia. The nurses thought this arrogant – they had a major desire for information on the (non-medical) treatment of the problem.

Box 7.13 Observation of three hospital departments to document medical errors (Andrews *et al.* 1997)

Trained observers participated in all activities in three hospital departments (including grand rounds, patient transfers and case discussions) and registered all incidents and undesired events that were discussed or became clear during these situations. A classification scheme was developed to code the data. A total of 1047 patients were monitored, of which 18% encountered a serious incident, mostly caused by individual errors. The study was intensive and time consuming, although it showed more incidents than other methods would have done. Nevertheless, the authors say the study probably underestimated the problem.

Furthermore, observation is time consuming and expensive, so that its utility is limited. However, it can provide information that cannot be collected in a different way, as when the observed activities are not written down and cannot be recorded by the participants themselves.

Routinely collected data

In healthcare many data are collected routinely on treatment, such as medication prescriptions, referrals and diagnostic tests. Such data can also be collected for a specific implementation study and used to analyse the variation of care (*Box 7.14*). It is preferable to first design an explanatory model that is tested on the available data (Denig and Haaijer-Ruskamp 1998). This method is particularly useful to assess the relevance of factors that have been identified in small-scale (qualitative) research.

ANALYSIS

Data on the problems or barriers to change often do not immediately show a clear picture of the factors that can be used to plan implementation activities. The data have to be organised and analysed before conclusions can be drawn. It is useful to use the tools for analysis that are applied in total quality management. Most of these tools are simple. They can be used to prioritise the relevance of factors (paretogram), organise the causes of a problem (fish-bone diagram) or document a care process (flow chart, activity table and Gant chart). Some examples are given below, but more information can be found in manuals on total quality management (e.g. Berwick *et al.* 1990). An example of continuous monitoring by means of statistical process control is given in Chapter 18.

Paretogram

A paretogram is based on the assumption that a limited number of causes explain a large proportion of problems (*Box 7.15*). For example, it is claimed that 80% of the problems result from 20% of the causes, so it is efficient to focus implementation activities on this 20%. A paretogram shows the causes in decreasing order of frequency. The vertical axis shows the totals or percentages. Instead of the frequency of occurrence, it is also possible to sequence on the basis of relevance as perceived by the experts or individuals who are involved.

Fish-bone diagram

A fish-bone diagram (*Box 7.16*) groups the possible causes of a situation into a number of categories to produce a simple cause-and-effect diagram. Usually, the consequences are located on the right-hand side of the diagram (e.g. the use of a guideline or other innovation). Next, different groups of causes are identified, such as men, means, materials and methods (the four Ms). Depending on the type of problem other categories may be used. The causes are located on the left of the diagram, organised according to category.

Box 7.14 Care use for patients with low back pain (Rossignol *et al.* 1996)

In a prospective cohort study in Canada, data were collected on 2147 patients with low back pain. The analysis focused on a description of care and the factors associated with it. For instance, imaging tests were performed more often in patients with a specific diagnosis, patients from rural areas and patients with physically demanding work. Referrals to a specialist were more often made for patients with a specific diagnosis, but less often in patients from rural areas and patients with physically demanding work.

Box 7.15 Analysis of causes of unnecessarily long sickness leave in Slovenia (Kersnik 1999)

The paretogram (opposite page) shows that the first four causes are the most relevant, so that improvement activities should focus mainly on these four causes. In Slovenia, GPs are responsible for medical treatment in the case of sick leave. They should report cases of sick leave within 30 days to special commissions of experts, who have to give approval. As it was felt that many people used sick leave unnecessarily, cases that deviated from the standard (lack of data on the patient or medical condition, unclear start date for sick leave, unclear reasons for sick leave, etc.) were analysed in more detail.

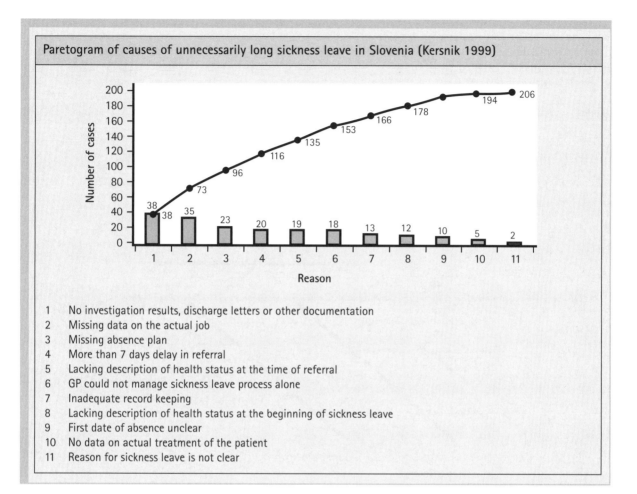

Paretogram of causes of unnecessarily long sickness leave in Slovenia (Kersnik 1999)

1   No investigation results, discharge letters or other documentation
2   Missing data on the actual job
3   Missing absence plan
4   More than 7 days delay in referral
5   Lacking description of health status at the time of referral
6   GP could not manage sickness leave process alone
7   Inadequate record keeping
8   Lacking description of health status at the beginning of sickness leave
9   First date of absence unclear
10 No data on actual treatment of the patient
11 Reason for sickness leave is not clear

Flow chart

A flow chart visually depicts the sequence of steps in a process (*Box 7.15*. It can depict the process of care provision and show points at which deviations may occur from the desired course. Some clinical guidelines use the format of a flow chart and those that do not can often be translated easily into this format. Implementation should focus on the points at which deviations occur. It is also useful to link barriers and facilitators to specific steps in the care-delivery process. Another possible use is to redesign a complete care

Box 7.16 Reduction in the delay of thrombolysis in patients with myocardial infarction at an intensive care unit in a community hospital (Bonetti *et al.* 2000)

There is sufficient proof that the prognosis of patients with myocardial infarction is improved if they receive thrombolysis as quickly as possible after suffering a myocardial infarction. There is consensus that patients should be treated within 30 minutes of arrival at the department. An audit of 16 consecutive patients showed that the average time was 57 minutes, with outliers of up to 90 minutes. In a multidisciplinary meeting all the causes were documented (see fish–bone diagram, page 118).

General problems identified were poor communication channels, too many individuals at the bedside, crucial individuals arriving too late and delays in receiving laboratory results. Processes were redesigned to change this situation (see table). The new protocol was discussed in educational sessions, with all the relevant people involved. After implementation of this, an evaluation was performed: in 16 patients the average was 32 minutes, with less variation than previously.   (*cont.*)

Causes for delay in thrombolysis for patients who suffered a myocardial infarction (ICU, intensive care unit)

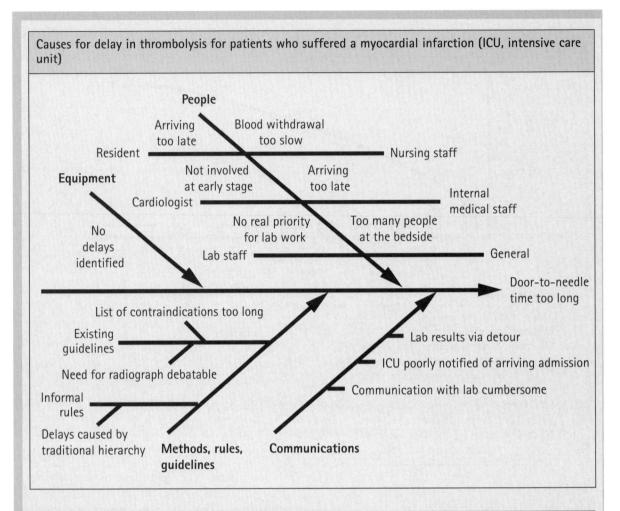

Redesigned process to improve time to thrombolysis

Timing	Physicians' tasks	Nurses' tasks
10 minutes	Patient's history	Record admission time
	Short examination	Obtain 12-lead echocardiograph (ECG)
	Interpretation of ECG	Aspirin, oral or intravenous (IV)
		Placement of first IV line
		Draw blood for serum cardiac markers, haematology, chemistry and lipid profile
10 minutes	Rule out contraindications	Placement of second IV line
10 minutes	Staff physician decides about thrombolysis	Prepare and administer thrombolytics
	Record 'door-to-needle time'	

The conclusion was that the diagnostic analysis and the design of the fish-bone diagram helped to develop a successful implementation plan.

Box 7.17 A flow diagram for hospital discharge (Berwick *et al.* 1990)

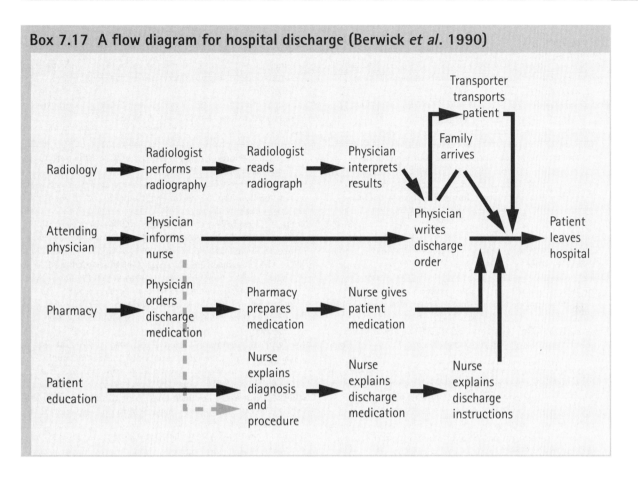

process. There are a wide range of techniques to make flow charts, but the core idea is always that the figure should be read from left to right or from top to bottom and that the blocks represent activities or events.

CONCLUSIONS

This chapter provides a brief overview of methods used to identify and analyse problems in the delivery of care and the barriers to and incentives for change. If the available budget allows, it is valuable to perform both detailed studies, to identify relevant factors, and large-scale studies, to assess their relevance in a larger group. For in-depth studies consider using interviews with individuals or groups, or (non-)participating observation. Large-scale studies may use written surveys or routine databases of clinical activities. Surveys are probably most useful if these refer to specific experiences, so case-specific questionnaires comprise an interesting method. However they are targeted, they should be administered as close to the point of the activity as pos-

sible. Small-scale improvement projects can also benefit from a good diagnostic analysis. Monitoring of (barriers in) care delivery and the implementation of change using simple instruments is often a precondition for a successful change.

There are a range of simple techniques for the analysis and presentation of factors (e.g. paretograms, fish-bone diagrams and flow charts). There is, however, little scientific research on the value of different methods for the implementation of innovations or new ways of working.

Recommended literature

Grol R, Baker R and Moss F (2003). *Quality Improvement Research. Understanding the Source of Change.* London: BMJ Books.

Oxman AD and Flottorp S (1998). An overview of strategies to promote implementation of evidence-based health care. In: Silagy C and Haines A. *Evidence-Based Practice in Primary Care*, Ch 8, pp. 91–109. London: BMJ Books.

Wensing M, Laurant M, Hulscher M and Grol R (1999). Methods for identifying barriers and facilitators for implementation. In: Thorsen T and Mäkelä M. *Changing Professional Practice*, pp. 119–132 Copenhagen: DSI.

References

Andrews L, Stocking C, Krizek T, *et al.* (1997). An alternative strategy for studying adverse events in medical care. *Lancet* **349**:309–313.

Berwick D, Godfrey B and Roessner J (1990). *Curing Health Care*. San Francisco: Jossey-Bass.

Bonetti PO, Waeckerlin A, Schuepfer G, *et al.* (2000). Improving time-sensitive processes in the intensive care unit: The example of 'door-to-needle time' in acute myocardial infarction. *Int J Qual Health Care* **12**(4):311–317.

Boven K van, Dijksterhuis P and Lamberts H (1997). Defensive testing in Dutch family practice. Is the grass greener on the other side of the ocean? *J Fam Pract*. **44**:468–472.

Cabana M, Rand C, Power N, *et al.* (1999). Why don't physicians follow clinical practice guidelines. *JAMA* **282**:1458–1465.

Denig P and Haaijer-Ruskamp FM (1998). Descriptief besliskundig onderzoek op het gebied van voorschrijfgedrag [Descriptive decision-making research on prescribing behaviour]. *Huisarts Wet*. **41**:274–279.

Dijkstra R, Braspenning J and Grol R (2002). How to implement a diabetes passport in hospital care. *Pat Educ Couns*. **47**:137–177.

Diwan VK, Sachs L and Wahlstrom R (1997). Practice–knowledge–attitudes–practice: An explorative study of information in primary care. *Soc Sci Med*. **44**:1221–1228.

Eccles M, Ford G, Duggan S and Steen N (1999). Are postal questionnaire surveys of reported activity valid: An exploration using general practitioner management of hypertension in older people. *Br J Gen Pract*. **49**:35–38.

Flottorp S and Oxman AD (2003). Identifying barriers and tailoring interventions to improve the management of urinary tract infections and sore throat: A pragmatic study using qualitative methods. *BMC Health Serv Res*. **4**:3.

Grol R and Wensing M (1995). Implementation of quality assurance and medical audit: General practitioners' perceived obstacles and requirements. *Br J Gen Pract*. **45**:548–552.

Kersnik J (1999). Management of sickness absence: A quality improvement study from Slovenia. *Qual Health Care* **8**:262–265.

Lee CL and Bobko P (1994). Self-efficacy beliefs: Comparison of five measures. *J Appl Psychol*. **79**:364–369.

Montano DE and Phillips WR (1995). Cancer screening by primary care physicians: A comparison of rates obtained from physician self-report, patient survey, and chart audit. *Am J Pub Health* **85**:795–800.

Morgan DL (1988). *Focus Groups as Qualitative Research*. Sage University Paper Series on Qualitative Research Methods 160. Beverly Hills: Sage.

Newton J, Knight D and Woolhead G (1996). General practitioners and clinical guidelines: A survey of knowledge, use and beliefs. *Br J Gen Pract*. **46**:513–517.

Peters MAJ, Harmsen M, Laurant MGH and Wensing M (2003). *Ruimte voor Verandering? Knelpunten En mogelijkheden voor Verbetering in de Patiëntenzorg [Room for Improvement? Barriers to and Opportunities for Improvement of Patient Care]*. Nijmegen: Centre for Quality of Care Research.

Rossignol M, Abenhaim L, Bonvalot Y, *et al.* (1996). Should the gap be filled between guidelines and actual practice for management of low back pain in primary care. The Quebec experience. *Spine* **21**:2893–2899.

Schers H, Wensing M, Huijsmans S, Van Tulder M and Grol R (2001). Low back pain management in primary care. *Spine* **26**:E348–E353.

Spies TH, Mokkink HGA, de Vries Robbé P and Grol R (2004). Which data source in clinical performance assessment? A pilot study comparing self-recording with patient records and observation. *Int J Qual Health Care* **16**:65–72.

Walker AE, Grimshaw JM and Armstrong EM (2001). Salient beliefs and intentions to prescribe antibiotics for patients with a sore throat. *Br J Health Psychol*. **6**:347–360.

Part IV

Interventions and strategies

Chapter 8

Selection of strategies

Richard Grol and Michel Wensing

KEY MESSAGES

- Numerous interventions (strategies and measures) can be used to change behaviour or implement innovations. The following can be differentiated:
  - Professional-oriented strategies;
  - Patient-oriented strategies;
  - Financial measures;
  - Organisational measures;
  - Legal regulations and/or rules.
- In selecting interventions as much consideration as possible should be given to:
  - Results of the 'diagnostic analysis' of both the target group and the implementation setting (see Chapters 6 and 7);
  - Existing knowledge of effective implementation and of the results of well-designed research and systematic reviews in the field of implementation strategies;
  - Phases in the actual process of implementation and change (a distinction between dissemination, implementation and maintenance of change).

Box 8.1 Intervention mapping (Bartholomew *et al.* 1998; Van Bokhoven *et al.* 2003)

An example of a structured, stepwise method to arrive at a selection of interventions, linked to the relevant factors, comes from the health promotion field, the so-called Intervention Mapping method. It offers a method to process results from a diagnostic analysis of a concrete programme for change and thus also appears to be suitable for the development of interventions to implement changes in healthcare. The following steps are usually taken:

- Problem analysis – the problems in delivery of care are described in terms of the behaviour(s) to be changed and the aims to be achieved;
- Determinants of the action to be taken – the factors that influence the action are listed;
- Matrix of programme objectives and determinants – factors that influence the action to be taken and the programme objectives are set against each other in a matrix, into the cells of which are placed the resulting behavioural elements necessary to change a given factor – this matrix is the 'Intervention Map' and the basis of the subsequent development of the intervention;
- Strategies – search for potentially suitable strategies to change the various determinants (e.g. via brainstorm sessions or analysis of the literature);
- Programme – concrete work methods are sought among the strategies and individual work methods are combined into a logical programme, a draft version of which is first tried out on a small scale;
- Evaluation plan – checking whether and how the objectives are achieved.

INTRODUCTION

In the previous chapters we consider the development of an initial proposal to change and improve patient care and the analysis of the target group and the setting in which the changes must take place. We argue that the proposal for change must be well supported, preferably developed with those involved, and must be presented in an accessible, clear and attractive form. With the aid of either simple or more detailed analyses, an understanding of the target group and the setting for the implementation is sought. To what extent, in which areas of activity and by whom is the greatest deviation from the guideline or new procedure, and what are the most important factors that can promote or hinder decreasing this deviation? These factors can be many and varied. They can involve the expertise, attitudes or personal characteristics of care providers. They can be related to the characteristics or behaviour of patients, colleagues and others in the social network of the care provider. And they can involve the organisational, financial or structural aspects of the work environment. Care providers, practices and institutions can differ on any or all of these points. An individualised, tailored

approach to the target group in the introduction of innovations is therefore usually desirable.

Ideally, strategies or measures that correspond as closely as possible to the results of the diagnostic analysis are chosen and enacted (e.g., intervention mapping in *Box 8.1*). While this may seem logical, it is often not the case in practice. People may become attached to a single, familiar intervention, such as refresher courses or financial measures, which they apply in all situations. Underlying such a choice are implicit ideas concerning the most important bottlenecks in implementation (such as a lack of knowledge) that may not be uniformly true. Therefore, the first question to be addressed in this chapter is how to select or design a set of strategies for change that can be optimally linked to the specific features of the innovation, the target group and the setting (*Figure 8.1*).

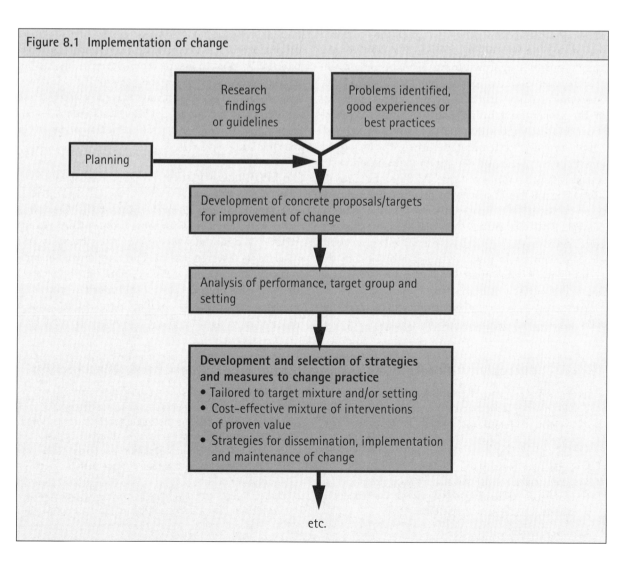

Figure 8.1 Implementation of change

Research findings or guidelines

Problems identified, good experiences or best practices

Planning

Development of concrete proposals/targets for improvement of change

Analysis of performance, target group and setting

Development and selection of strategies and measures to change practice
- Tailored to target mixture and/or setting
- Cost-effective mixture of interventions of proven value
- Strategies for dissemination, implementation and maintenance of change

etc.

Table 8.1 Strategies and their effectiveness: a review of reviews (Bero *et al.* 1998)

Usually effective	Sometimes effective and sometimes not	Of little or no effect	Effectiveness unknown
Outreach visits	Audit and feedback	Educational materials	Financial stimuli
Decision support, reminders	Efforts of opinion leaders	Courses, conferences	Administrative or organisational interventions
Interactive education	Local consensus meetings		
Multifaceted interventions	Patient-oriented interventions		
Mass media interventions			

The next question to be addressed in this chapter is, "Which strategies and measures are suitable to use in the implementation?" Which have proved their value and effectiveness and appear to be able to guide behaviour in the right direction, given the analysis of the target group and the setting, and given the indicated incentives and barriers to change? In recent years a large number of rigorous studies have become available that address the effectiveness of strategies to influence clinical management. These are collected together in the Cochrane Library. The Cochrane Effective Practice and Organisation of Care Group (Bero *et al.* 1998) organises systematic literature studies on the effectiveness of methods to implement guidelines or introduce changes in healthcare. At the same time, an increasing number of systematic reviews can be drawn upon to understand the effectiveness of interventions (*Table 8.1*). In short, there is a reasonable body of knowledge in this field; an overview of what we know about effective change in patient care is provided in the second part of this chapter. In Chapters 9–14 we present results of research in this field in more detail.

We start, however, by providing different methods and models used to classify strategies for changing practice.

CLASSIFYING STRATEGIES FOR CHANGING PRACTICE

In the literature there are many different methods, strategies and measures to introduce innovations, guidelines, best practices or new procedures into clinical practice. These vary greatly, from sending printed material by post to giving financial rewards for the desired behaviour or reorganising a multidisciplinary care process. There are various ways to classify these strategies and measures in a logical manner. A few of the ways to describe and arrange them is reviewed in this chapter.

The EPOC classification

We start with the classification of the Cochrane Effective Practice and Organisation of Care Group (EPOC). A detailed overview of the strategies and measures is given in *Box 8.2*. The components of such a classification can be debated, particularly because the strategies included are sometimes not mutually exclusive (e.g. the use of local opinion leaders can also be a way of educating a target group). Nevertheless,

---

Box 8.2 Overview of the strategies and measures in EPOC (Thorsen and Mäkelä 1999)

Interventions orientated towards health professionals

a. *Distribution of educational materials.* Distribution of published or printed recommendations for clinical care, including clinical practice guidelines, audiovisual materials and electronic publications. The materials can be delivered personally or through mass mailings.

b. *Conferences.* Participation of healthcare providers in conferences, lectures, workshops or training sessions outside their own practice settings.

I.   Small-group conferences (active participation);
II. Big-group conferences (passive participation).

c. *Local consensus processes.* Inclusion of participating providers in discussion to ensure that they agree that the chosen clinical problem is important and that the approach to manage the problem is appropriate.

d. *Outreach visits.* Use of a trained person who meets with providers in their practice settings to provide information.

The information given may include feedback on the providers' performance.

e. *Local opinion leaders.* Interventions using providers nominated by their colleagues as 'educationally influential'. How the opinion leaders were identified (by their colleagues) and how they were recruited should be stated explicitly.

f. *Patient-mediated intervention.* Any intervention to change the performance of healthcare providers in which information was sought from or given directly to patients by others (e.g. direct mailings to patients, patient counselling delivered by others, materials given to patients or placed in waiting rooms).

g. *Audit and feedback.* Any information on or summary of clinical performance in healthcare over a specified period of time. The information may be given in a written or oral format, and it may also include recommendations for clinical action. Information on provider performance may have been obtained from medical records, computerised databases, observation or patients.
I. Internal audit (i.e. audit performed by the providers themselves);
II. External audit (i.e. the providers are given data on their performance obtained by others).
The following interventions should not be included in the audit and feedback:
I. Provision of clinical information that does not directly reflect provider performance and is collected by the investigators directly from patients (e.g. scores on a depression instrument).
II. Feedback from individual patient's health record, or in an alternative format (e.g. computerised).

h. *Reminders.* Any intervention, manual or computerised, that prompts the healthcare provider to perform a clinical action. The following interventions are included:
I. Computerised decision support (use of an active knowledge system that uses two or more items of patient data to generate case-specific advice);
II. Concurrent reports (targeted at providers at the time of an encounter to remind them of the desired actions for individual patients);
III. Inter-visit reminders (targeted at providers between visits when there is evidence of suboptimal care for specific patients, such as when a test is abnormal and the appropriate follow-up is not found in the medical record);
IV. Enhanced laboratory report (laboratory report after an abnormal result and targeted at providers, which includes additional information about specific follow-up recommendations);
V. Administrative support (follow-up appointment system or stickers on charts);
VI. Implicit reminders (predictive values for abnormal

test results without an explicit recommendation for action).

i. *Tailored interventions.* Use of personal interviewing, group discussion ('focus groups') or a survey of targeted providers to identify barriers to change and the subsequent design of an intervention to address the identified barriers.

j. *Peer review.*

k. *Combined strategies.* Specify the combination using the above classification of interventions, if applicable.

l. *Other.*

Financial interventions
a. *Provider-directed interventions.*
I. Fee-for-service (provider is paid a fixed amount for the number and type of services delivered);
II. Capitation (provider is paid a set amount per person in the target population per time unit to provide specific care);
III. Provider salaried service (provider is paid a basic salary to provide specific care);
IV. Provider incentives (individual provider is given direct or indirect financial rewards or benefits for specific actions);
V. Institution incentives (institution or groups of providers are given direct or indirect financial rewards or benefits for performing specific actions);
VI. Provider grant or allowance (individual provider is given direct or indirect financial rewards or benefits that are not tied to specific actions);
VII. Institution grant or allowance (institution or groups of providers are given direct or indirect financial rewards or benefits that are not tied to specific actions);
VIII. Provider penalty (individual provider receives direct or indirect financial penalties for inappropriate action);
IX. Institution penalty (institution or groups of providers receive direct or indirect financial penalties for inappropriate action);
X. Changes in formulary (additions or removals from reimbursable available products);
XI. Other.
b. *Patient-directed interventions.*
I. Premium;
II. Co-payment;
III. User fee;
IV. Patient incentives;
V. Patient grant or allowance;
VI. Patient penalty;
VII. Other.

Organisational interventions

These may include changes in the physical structures of healthcare units, in medical record systems or in ownership.

a. *Structural interventions.*

I. Changes in the settings and/or site of service delivery (e.g. moving a family planning service from a hospital to a school);

II. Telemedicine (providing means of communication and case discussion between distant health professionals);

III. Changes in medical records systems (e.g. changing from paper to computerised records);

IV. Other changes in arrangements to maintain or retrieve information (e.g. patient tracking system);

V. Other changes in physical structure, facilities and equipment;

VI. Changes in scope and/or nature of services (e.g. introducing day surgery);

VII. Changes in presence and organisation of quality management mechanisms;

VIII. Changes in ownership and/or affiliation status of hospitals and other facilities;

IX. Other structural changes in organisation excluding staff (specify).

b. *Staff-oriented interventions.*

I. Revision of professional roles (changes in role content between health professionals, as 'professional substitution' or 'boundary encroachment' – e.g. nurse midwives provide obstetrical care or pharmacists provide drug counselling that were formerly provided by nurses and physicians, respectively);

II. Multidisciplinary teams (health professionals of different disciplines work together as a team to care for a patient or population);

III. Case management (one professional takes responsibility for co-ordinating care given to one patient by several providers and/or units);

IV. Other integration of services (follow-up mechanisms to co-ordinate a patient's care across organisational or unit boundaries, sometimes called 'seamless care');

V. Skill mix interventions (change in numbers, types or qualifications of staff);

VI. Interventions to improve provider satisfaction with the conditions of work or its material and/or psychological rewards (e.g. intervention to 'boost moral');

VII. Other.

c. *Patient-oriented interventions.*

I. Interventions to facilitate individual patient participation (e.g. decision support tools for patients);

II. Interventions to facilitate patient group participation (e.g. focus groups, patient panels);

III. Other.

Regulatory interventions

Regulatory interventions are any intervention that aims to change health-service delivery or costs by regulation or law. These interventions may overlap with organisational and financial interventions, or one intervention may contain elements from several categories.

a. *Changes in medical liability.*

b. *Management of patient complaints.*

c. *Accreditation.*

d. *Licensure.*

e. *Other.*

this is a widely used taxonomy and helpful in thinking through the available range of interventions.

Facilitating versus controlling methods

When introducing innovations, a distinction can be drawn between those methods that are primarily educational or facilitating, and those that involve more direction and control. It is possible to rank existing measures on a scale that ranges from educational and facilitating methods to controlling and compulsory methods (*Figure 8.2*).

Within this framework a distinction is first made between voluntary and involuntary methods. Involuntary methods involve external compulsion and obligation, such as that produced by regulations

that can be enforced by economic sanctions. If the process of change is approached via the voluntary activities of the target group, then a distinction can be made between methods that are aimed at stimulating the intrinsic motivation of care providers and teams, and methods that make use of external incentives and motivation. Utilising intrinsic motivation implies an effort to increase expertise by means of individual or group education, instruction and information, or by offering support and encouragement in the accomplishment of the change. The practice routines to be changed can also be influenced directly by collecting data about them and providing feedback in a variety of ways, by reminding care providers of the desired approach while they are doing the work, by offering help (e.g. computerisation) in making appropriate

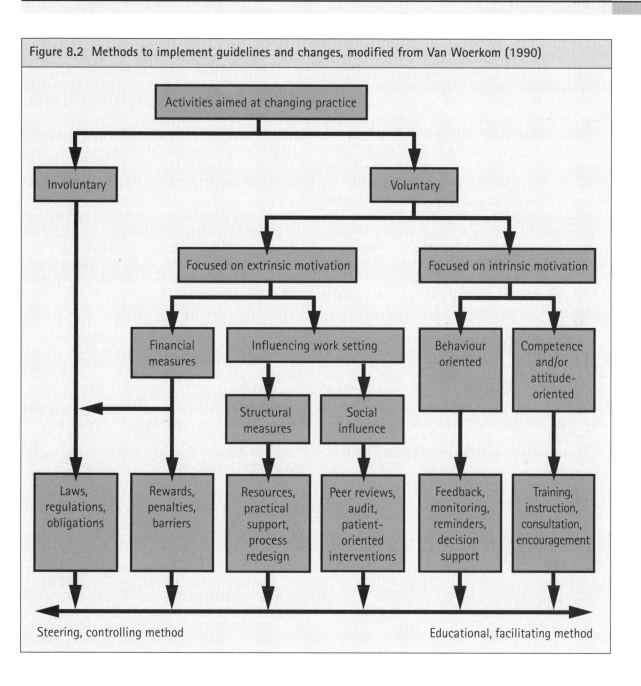

Figure 8.2 Methods to implement guidelines and changes, modified from Van Woerkom (1990)

decisions or by offering help in experimenting with new procedures or care processes.

Extrinsic motivation can involve the use of financial or material incentives for 'good behaviour', making use of organisational measures to promote the application of a new procedure or the redesign of multidisciplinary care processes. This can also involve using social pressure to change performance by the interaction with colleagues, the input of an opinion leader or informing patients about the desired practice.

The assumption is that different segments of the target group respond to different measures, some being more responsive to facilitating interventions while others need external pressure and supportive methods (see *Table 8.3*).

INTERVENTIONS IN THE DIFFERENT PHASES OF CHANGE: THE TARGET GROUP'S PERSPECTIVE

Another way to arrange, plan and describe strategies and interventions to implement change is to take the perspectives of the target group and link these to the different phases in the change process that individuals and groups have to go through (Grol and Wensing 2004; see Chapter 3). Those who are not familiar with or are not interested in the innovation require a different approach to those who are familiar with it, but do not believe that it can be accomplished successfully. If one is willing, but encounters major problems in establishing the change in the care process in one's own team or practice, yet another approach is needed. Since different subgroups are usually in different phases of the process of change, a combination of different strategies may be desirable. Examples of the possible interventions are given in *Table 8.2*. Gradually, the strategies change from a focus primarily on the dissemination of an innovation to a focus on the actual implementation and embedment of the innovation in normal practice routines.

The different steps in the change process, and the possible strategies and interventions that relate to the steps, are discussed below.

Parallel to this process of change of individuals and groups, it is useful to distinguish between:

■ Dissemination. Activities to inform the target group of the innovation, and to ensure that they understand what it consists of and that they have a positive attitude towards it. The results of the dissemination can be described in terms of being informed, having knowledge of and having a positive attitude towards a guideline or a new procedure.

■ Implementation. Activities for the actual application of the innovation and to ensure that it obtains a permanent place in the routines and in the organisation. The results of implementation lie in the actual use and the continuing application of the new procedures.

Table 8.2 Interventions and implementation strategies in different phases of the change process

Steps and possible barriers to change	Possible strategies and interventions
Orientation	
Not familiar (does not read literature, has no contact with colleagues) No interest (no need for change, does not think it is relevant)	Distribute brief messages via all types of channels, approach key figures and networks Attention-catching brochure, personal approach and explanation, confrontation with own performance
Insight	
No knowledge or understanding (information too complex or extensive) No insight or overestimation of own performance	Appropriate instruction materials, concise messages, information based on problems in practice, regular repetition Simple methods of audit, peer review and feedback
Acceptance	
Negative attitudes (sees disadvantages, doubts about developers or feasibility, inadequate attraction) Not prepared to change (doubts about success and own possibilities)	Adapt innovation to wishes of target group, local discussion and consensus, discuss resistance and clear scientific arguments, involve key individuals and opinion leaders Demonstrate feasibility through colleagues, inventory of bottlenecks and seeking solutions for these, change plans to include feasible objectives
Change	
Has not started (no time, materials or ability; does not fit with existing care procedures) Insufficient success (negative reactions)	Extra resources, support, training in skills, redevelopment of care processes, bringing in temporary support or consultants Information materials for patients, plan with feasible objectives
Maintenance	
Not integrated in routines (relapse, forgetting) Not embedded in organisation (not supported)	Monitoring, feedback and reminder systems, integration into care plans and protocols Provide resources, support from top management, organisational measures, rewards, payment for certain tasks

Orientation

Promote awareness of the innovation

Care providers must first come into contact with an innovation and become aware that it is available. This can fail simply because those concerned do not read the book or journal in which the information is published or do not attend courses. They may read selectively and only take in information that confirms their own ideas. Hence, other ways are needed (via the mass media or personal contacts) to inform care providers who are not reached via the usual channels. In particular, a personal, attractively designed mailing and the involvement of colleagues and key figures from the individual's surroundings, who could make direct contact, are appropriate strategies.

Stimulate interest and involvement

The implementation must also be such as to arouse the interest of those in the target group. They must be stimulated in a way that makes them want to know more. This can be difficult if the subject is not seen as relevant and if the design of the information is not attractive or does not make it readily understood, so the reader does not feel encouraged to explore it further. Equally problematic is when the information is not presented from the perspective or interests of the target group and is thus not recognised as being applicable or relevant to daily practice. The manner in which information is presented should address these issues, which can be accomplished by sending attractive brochures or by discussion of the problems in care delivery during meetings of the care providers concerned. Also, an enthusiastic report about the innovation by those who have already worked with it can be helpful.

Insight

Create understanding

The target group must not only be interested in the new procedures or proposal for improvement, but must also understand what it involves and the arguments behind it. Care providers should know exactly what is expected from them and why it is important. This can be a problem if they do not have enough background knowledge or experience to understand the information. A presentation that is too technical, too abstract or too detailed can also be a hindrance to understanding. Finally, what is learned can also be quickly forgotten. While it is important to provide succinct information

and instructional materials or well-organised and short presentations in courses and to deal with the translation of the central message into everyday practice, to prevent the information from being forgotten it must also be repeated. This may need to happen many times and be offered in such a way (printed, computerised) that knowledge can be refreshed very quickly.

Develop insight into own routines

To achieve change it is often not sufficient for the individual to know exactly what must be done and how it must be done. Individuals must also examine their own performance and see where improvement is needed. They should see where their routines differ from a guideline or proposal for change and accept that a change is necessary or desirable. Many care providers overestimate their own performance or are not prepared to reflect critically on their own way of working, as this may be threatening. Manageable and acceptable methods are necessary to help them over this. Simple recording and feedback methods that relate to the performance of the practice, self-assessment tools, peer review methods and simple systems for continuous monitoring of the care can be used to detect possible problems in care delivery.

Acceptance

Develop a positive attitude to change

At this stage individuals in the target group must carefully evaluate the advantages and disadvantages of the new way of working and decide their attitude to the innovation. As mentioned above, this evaluation may be negative if individuals see more disadvantages than advantages (in terms of effectiveness, demands or financial consequences), if they consider the change unfeasible in their own work setting, if they doubt the scientific basis of the proposed change or if they doubt the credibility or expertise of those who developed the innovation. The change may also be refused if it is seen as having originated elsewhere and the target group does not feel that it has been involved sufficiently in the development. This evaluation process cannot be handled easily in written materials; to discuss the arguments for and against the innovation is a more efficient way to address these issues. Resistance should be discussed seriously and openly, the arguments for the change must be demonstrated adequately and the opportunity should be offered to adapt the process of change to the situation and needs of the target group. For this, respected peers and colleagues can be brought in who have already had a positive experience with the innovation and can describe its advantages, as well as its possible limitations.

Create positive intentions or decisions to change

If an opinion about the change has been formed, the next step is a firm resolution to carry it through in practice. It is possible to be in favour of a change and yet be unable to see exactly how things can or should be other than the way they are, or to have little confidence in one's own ability to really begin to do otherwise. Specific problems of resistance may also be anticipated from patients, colleagues, directors or financiers, or problems may be foreseen in the organisation or resources needed for the change, which would make implementation difficult. The expected problems in introducing the change should therefore be considered carefully (see Chapters 6 and 7) and specific solutions to these problems must be sought. This might include a demonstration of the new procedure (as best practice) on the basis of experience elsewhere. Thus, those who will have to use it can see that it is feasible. Furthermore, the change can be divided into simple, manageable steps that, taken in succession, offer the assurance that they are all feasible. A plan for the change with achievable objectives can be a useful aid (see Chapter 15).

Change

Try out change in practice

Next is the step to the real change in the way of working. The essential step here is to actually try out the innovation, the pathway or the new programme and see whether its introduction is possible. The necessary skills may be lacking and therefore specific training may be needed. Equally, a trial period may reveal organisational problems that have yet to be resolved. Local organisations and the temporary help of experts can support people through this. What is important is that the change be tried out without great risks and consequences before widespread, and irreversible, implementation.

Confirm benefit and value of change

A limited trial must convince the target group that the change is possible and that it brings the anticipated advantages. If not, the return to the former ways of working will be rapid. Collecting data and providing feedback about the achieved improvements, as well as documenting any positive reactions from patients, can support the motivation to continue during this phase.

Maintenance

Integrate new practice into routines

If it is found to be useful, the new procedure has to be fitted into the existing care protocols or pathways, care plans and work routines. It is well recognised that after a change people can fall back into former ways of working. After a vacation, for example, one forgets how things were or precisely how they have to be done.

It is possible that the change may not have exactly the result that was expected. Appropriate strategies may be needed to assist through such a period and to stabilise the change. Increasingly, sustainability is seen as an important criterion of effective implementation. One can consider regular monitoring and feedback on the desired method, reminders about its application or rewards for the achievement of agreed objectives. It can be important to revise the entire care process of which the new procedure is now a part, and to incorporate the change into the multidisciplinary care processes in a practice or hospital.

Embed new practice into the organisation

The final step is for the new procedure to be incorporated completely into, and be supported by, the care organisation so that its continuing application is possible. This might mean that it becomes a component of the reimbursement system, of budget agreements, of the policy of the institution or of contracts. In general the organisational, structural and financial conditions must be such that they support embedment of the new procedure into the organisation or practice. This requires attention to the organisational culture, the involvement of administrators, managers and directors in the innovation, and co-operation between disciplines and departments.

SUBGROUPS WITHIN THE TARGET GROUP

As noted in earlier chapters, *subgroups* within the target group can differ with regard to needs, characteristics, and barriers and incentives to change. Some groups may not understand or may oppose a specific change in routines, while other groups may struggle to master the new procedure. Different subgroups may thus need different approaches (*Box 8.3*). In previous chapters a distinction is made between 'innovators', the 'middle majority' and 'laggards' (Rogers 1983). It has been suggested that different groups have different motives for change and thus require a different approach (*Table 8.3*).

Box 8.3 Tailoring interventions to barriers to improve the management of urinary tract infections and sore throat (Flottorp and Oxman 2003)

To identify the barriers to implementation of evidence-based guidelines for urinary tract infection and sore throat in primary care an interactive process was followed in which various methods were used – a review of the literature on barriers, a large panel of physicians involved in the development or the testing of the guidelines in practice, brainstorming in an international workshop of implementation researchers, two focus groups of patients and one with assistants in primary care practices, a pilot study in five practices using the guidelines and, finally, small group discussions at interactive courses on the guidelines. A large number of barriers were identified, of which the following were deemed the most common and relevant:

- Loss of income incurred when applying the recommended telephone consultations;
- Change of routines from normal visits to an increased use of telephone consultations is complex for all involved;
- Fear of overlooking serious disease through telephone consultations and delegating tasks to assistants;
- Patients expect tests for these conditions;
- Lack of time to prepare for new routines.

Interventions were specifically tailored to these main barriers, such as an increased fee for telephone consultations, computer-based decision support with checklist and warning signals, patient information on appropriate performance, brief versions of guidelines, computer-based reminders and incentives for participation (see Chapters 3 and 7).

Innovators may be served adequately by clear, scientifically sound information obtained via journals and qualified refresher courses. Those in the middle majority, in general, are not completely satisfied with such sources. They are more likely to respond to influences in their own social network, such as the opinion of respected peers or colleagues who introduce the new procedures or insights and translate them into their own local situation. The middle majority is also sensitive to the social pressure that arises out of activities with their colleagues (quality circles, team discussion, mutual agreements, collaboratives, small-scale education in which opinion leaders introduce new guidelines or new working methods, local consensus meetings, etc.). Those in the third group, the so-called laggards, are relatively insensitive to these social influences, partly because they are inclined to do their own thing. They have to be won over by an extra effort in the form of practical support or material rewards, or if necessary by pressure, such as a statement of the official standpoint or formal regulations by responsible leaders (managers or the Board or Directors) or formal organisations.

THE EFFECTIVENESS OF DIFFERENT STRATEGIES AND INTERVENTIONS

A large number of different strategies and interventions are aimed at implementing changes in patient care. Some focus on individual professionals, some on patients, some on groups or teams and some on specific aspects of the organisation of care. To select the best strategy for the change at hand, it is recommended that the scientific literature on effective change in patient care be used. The growing body of original studies and systematic reviews about the effectiveness of different interventions can help to select appropriate change strategies. We dis-

Table 8.3 Approach to different groups in the introduction of innovations (Rogers 1995; Grol 1992; Green et al. 1989)

	Innovators	Middle majority	Laggards
Motivation to change	Intrinsic, seeing the advantages	Belonging to group, relation to others	Extrinsic, coercion, economic pressure
Effective influence	Aimed at cognition	Aimed at attitude, motivation	Aimed at behaviour
Methods	Appropriate information, credible sources, written methods	Personal sources, opinion leaders, activities with colleagues, feedback from colleagues	Regulations and agreements, rewards and sanctions, help with practical problems, clear leadership

cuss the evidence for these strategies in the next chapters in detail. Here, a global overview of the results of 54 reviews is presented (Grol and Grimshaw 2003). The main conclusions from this overview are:

■ Change is possible when a well-designed intervention is used – most interventions studied had an effect (average of about 10% change for main targets), but no single intervention seemed to be superior for all circumstances and settings;

■ Generally, there is more evidence on professionally oriented interventions (such as education, feedback or reminders) than on organisation- or patient-oriented interventions, and economic evaluations of implementation strategies are scarce – the methodology of many studies is poor;

■ Different types of change seem to require different types of interventions, but as yet we lack a clear understanding of the likely effectiveness of different interventions for different changes in different settings.

A global summary of the effectiveness of different interventions is presented in *Table 8.4.*

Table 8.4 Overview of strategies for implementation and conclusions of reviews (Grol and Grimshaw 2003)

Strategy	Number of reviews[a]	Number of studies	Conclusions
Educational materials	9	3–37	Mixed effects
Conferences, courses	4	3–17	Mixed effects
Interactive small group meetings	4	2–6	Mostly effective, but limited numbers of studies
Educational outreach visits	8	2–8	Particularly effective for prescribing and/or prevention
Use of opinion leaders	3	3–6	Mixed effects
Education with different educational strategies	8	5–63	Mixed effects, dependant on combination of strategies
Feedback on performance	16	3–37	Mixed effects, most effective for test ordering
Reminders	13	4–68	Mostly effective, particularly for prevention
Computerised decision support	5	11–98	Mostly effective for drug doses and prevention
Introduction of computers in practice	2	19–30	Mostly effective
Substitutions of tasks	7	2–14	Pharmacists: effective for prescribing Nurses: mixed effects
Multiprofessional collaboration	5	2–22	Effective for a range of different chronic conditions
Mass media campaigns	5	22	Mostly effective
Total quality management (continuous quality improvement)	1	55	Limited effects, mostly single-site non-controlled studies
Financial interventions	6	3–89	Fundholding and budgets effective, mainly on prescribing
Patient-mediated interventions	7	2–14	Mixed effects: reminding of patients effective in prevention
Combined interventions	16	2–39	Most reviews: more effective than single interventions, but not confirmed in recent reviews

[a]Number of reviews that included studies addressing the interventions.

Single or multifaceted interventions?

Many (often the majority) of the interventions used to implement change in patient care were multifaceted. Quite a number of reviews (16) addressed the question – single or multifaceted interventions – specifically. Some of these (e.g. Hulscher *et al.* 1999; Solomon *et al.* 1998; Wensing *et al.* 1998; Oxman 1995) stated that combined interventions, which address specific barriers to change, are more effective than single interventions. This finding was not confirmed in a systematic EPOC review of 235 evaluations of guideline implementation strategies (Grimshaw *et al.* 2004). This review used an explicit analytical approach to derive a single effect size (e.g. proportion of patients who received the appropriate treatment) for each study and summarised the median effect across studies for each intervention. Single interventions proved to be equally effective or sometimes even more effective than combined interventions. The lack of an enhanced effect from combined interventions was also found in a recent review of audit and feedback (Jamtvedt *et al.* 2003). Dijkstra *et al.* (2004), in an analysis of a subset of studies on changing hospital care, also found a larger effect size for single interventions (odds ratio 2.23) than for multifaceted interventions (odds ratio 1.77).

However, studies that tested the effectiveness of different strategies to engage practitioners in prevention and life-style changes (smoking, alcohol use) showed better outcomes for multifaceted interventions. An unpublished report of a meta-analysis of 24 programmes to support primary care health providers in the treatment of tobacco dependence showed that programmes that combined professional and organisational elements were significantly more effective than either alone. An unpublished review of studies that tested the effectiveness of programmes to engage primary care physicians in the identification and management of alcohol problems showed that multifaceted programmes were more effective than single-faceted programmes.

So, the evidence as to whether single or combined strategies should be used is as yet unclear. The right choice of interventions and measure probably depends on the topic, the setting, the target group and the problems encountered. Sometimes single approaches may do the job, and in other cases a more complex interventions is needed. A rigorous analysis of the problem, target group and setting has to be the basis of the ultimate selection. More information on this issue is given in Chapter 14.

A further consideration is the cost, and the efficiency, of the interventions. It is reasonable to suppose that multifaceted interventions cost more to deliver and therefore, for a given effect, are less efficient. When there is a limited budget for implementation, the choice of strategy is also influenced by considerations of efficiency. There may be occasions for which it is more cost effective to use a less costly, but also less effective, intervention rather one that is more costly, but only marginally more effective. These issues are discussed further in Chapter 20.

CONCLUSIONS

In this chapter a wide variety of interventions, strategies and methods to implement a guideline or new procedure are considered. They are arranged according to their central activity, to whether they are more facilitating or controlling and to the change process that the target group has to go through, and by subdivisions of the target group. In selecting the strategy and in planning the implementation, it is important to work creatively and to arrive at a cost-effective mixture of measures and activities that, preferably, have been found to be effective in a similar situation. A global overview of different strategies suggests that none is superior for all circumstances. In the following chapters the status of scientific knowledge about different strategies is reviewed in more detail. Starting with a chapter about dissemination strategies (Chapter 9), we then consider:

- Educational interventions (Chapter 10);
- Feedback and reminders (Chapter 11);
- Organisational and financial measures (Chapter 12);
- Patient-oriented interventions (Chapter 13);
- Combined interventions (Chapter 14).

Together, these chapters should offer sufficient reference points to allow readers to make an informed choice about implementation activities.

Recommended literature

Grimshaw JM, Shirran L, Thomas R, *et al.* (2001). Changing provider behavior. An overview of systematic reviews of interventions. *Med Care* **39**:S2–S45.

Grol R and Grimshaw J (2003). From best evidence to best practice: Effective implementation of change in patient care. *Lancet* **362**:1225–1230.

References

Bartholomew LK, Parcel GS and Kok G (1998). Intervention mapping: A process for developing theory- and evidence-based health education programs. *Health Educ Behav.* **25**:543–563.

Bero L, Grilli R, Grimshaw JM, *et al.* (1998). Closing the gap between research and practice: An overview of systematic reviews of interventions to promote implementation of research findings by health care professionals. *BMJ* **317**:465–468.

Bokhoven MA van, Kok G, van der Weijden T (2003). Designing a quality improvement intervention: A systematic approach. *Qual Saf Health Care* **12**:215–220.

Dijkstra RF, Wensing M, Thomas RE, *et al.* (2004). *Relationship between Organisational Characteristics and the Effects of Clinical Guidelines on Medical Performance at Hospitals, a Meta-analysis.* Unpublished report. Nijmegen: WOK.

Flottorp S and Oxman AD (2003). Identifying barriers and tailoring interventions to improve the management of urinary tract infections and sore throat: A pragmatic study using qualitative methods. *BMC Health Serv Res.* **3**(1):3.

Green L, Gottlieb N and Parcell G (1989). Diffusion theory extended and applied. In: *Advances in Health Education and Promotion*, Vol. 3. Greenwich: JAI Press.

Grimshaw JM, Thomas RE, MacLennan G, *et al.* (2004). Effectiveness and efficiency of guideline dissemination and implementation strategies. *Health Technol Assess.* **8**(6):1–84.

Grol R (1992). Implementing guidelines in general practice care. *Qual Health Care* **1**:184–191.

Grol R and Grimshaw J (2003). From best evidence to best practice: Effective implementation of change in patient care. *Lancet* **362**:1225–1230.

Grol R and Wensing M (2004). What drives change? Barriers and incentives for achieving evidence-based practice. *MJA* **180**:557–560

Hulscher MEJL, Wensing M, Grol RPTM, van der Weijden T and van Weel C (1999). Interventions to improve the delivery of preventive services in primary care. *Am J Public Health* **89**(5):737–746.

Jamtvedt G, Young JM, Kristoffersen DT, Thomson O'Brien MA and Oxman AD (2003). Audit and feedback: Effects on professional practice and health care outcomes (Cochrane Review). The Cochrane Library, Issue 3. Oxford: Update Software.

Oxman AD (1995). No magic bullets. A systematic review of 102 trials of interventions to help health care professionals deliver services more effectively or efficiently. *Can Med Assoc J.* **153**(10):1423–1431.

Rogers E (1983). *Diffusion of Innovations.* New York: Free Press.

Rogers E (1995). Lessons for guidelines from the diffusion of innovation. *Jt Comm J Qual Improv.* **21**:324–328.

Solomon DH, Hashimoto H, Daltroy L and Liang MH (1998). Techniques to improve physicians' use of diagnostic tests. *JAMA* **280**(23):2020–2027.

Thorsen T and Mäkelä M (1999). *Theory and Practice of Clinical Guidelines Implementation.* DSI Rapport 99.05. Copenhagen: DSI Danish Institute for Health Services Research and Development.

Wensing M, Weijden van der T and Grol R (1998). Implementing guidelines and innovations in general practice: Which interventions are effective? *Br J Gen Pract.* **48**:991–997.

Woerkom C van (1990). *Voorlichting als Beleidsinstrument. Inaugurale Rede [Education as a policy instrument. Inaugural address].* Wageningen: Wageningen University.

Chapter 9

Dissemination of innovations

Richard Grol and Michel Wensing

KEY MESSAGES

- Effective dissemination of innovations, guidelines and best practices is a necessary but insufficient measure to ensure their use in practice.
- The aim of dissemination is to advise and inform the target group about the required practice, and to stimulate them to use the innovation for education, local arrangements, audit of care practices or improving the quality of care.
- Distinctions can be drawn between mass media or non-personalised methods and personal methods of dissemination. Probably, a combination of the two is the most effective, particularly if the target group is kept informed via several channels.

Box 9.1 Dissemination of guidelines among physicians (Grol 2001; Grol et al. 1998)

To speed up the introduction of national guidelines for primary care, a special package was put together that contained 10 national guidelines for general practice and various materials to enable self-evaluation with these guidelines. In a controlled study, two methods for disseminating the package were compared:

▨ Sending it by post to all local co-ordinators of continuous medical education and to representatives of local general practitioner (GP) groups (one district);

▨ Sending it by post (as above), with the additional support of two colleague–physician outreach visitors, who sought contact with key figures, enquired whether they required any form of assistance with using the materials and if necessary offered support at group meetings (one comparable district).

▨ The rest of the country served as control group – people were informed about the existence of the materials by publications in journals. If they were interested, they could request them.

All doctors in the two districts (527 and 504, respectively) and 500 from the rest of the country were asked to complete a questionnaire before and after the intervention period (1.5 years). A total of 762 physicians filled in questionnaires. The results are given below.

Situation after intervention	By post and outreach visitor, $n = 269$ (%)	Only by post, $n = 244$ (%)	Control group, $n = 249$ (%)
Were aware of the existence of the package	66	25	20
In possession of the materials	49	14	6
Have read the materials	35	9	6
Made use of the materials	25	4	2

There was clearly more effect in the district that received the combined intervention (i.e. with the input of so-called outreach visitors) than in the district that received post only or where advertisements had been placed in the media. However, the actual use of the materials was limited, even in the district where the target group had been reached most effectively.

INTRODUCTION

To adapt new insights or procedures to existing routines, it is a pre-requisite that the target group be aware of their existence, take notice of them, understand what they are about, be prepared to study them carefully and actually does something with them (read them or discuss them with colleagues). It is therefore necessary to present people with the new information, preferably in a stimulating manner. In itself, dissemination of an innovation does not necessarily lead to its actual application. However, implementation often fails if effective dissemination among the target group fails. The importance of systematic and well-planned dissemination is often underestimated. There are many examples of beautifully designed printed guidelines, prevention programmes and improvement schemes that did not leave the shelf. In a dissemination plan, consideration must be given to, for example (NHMRC 2000):

- Definition of the target group – Lomas (1997) distinguished five target groups, namely policy makers and politicians, managers and administrators, care providers and healthcare policy-makers, patient or consumer (groups), and researchers (including developers of support materials or instruments);
- The most suitable media or channels for distribution must be established;
- A budget must be available for the development, production and distribution of the various forms of presentation of the innovation (for some forms of presentation, such as video recordings and CD Roms, the price can be fairly high);
- The development, production and distribution of the various presentation forms for the different subgroups must be set up and conducted as a distinct project, with adequate measurements (of the aims being achieved and financial cost) and feedback.

To disseminate the innovation, distinction can be made between *mass media* or *non-personalised* and *personal communication* channels:

- Mass media:
  - Publication in scientific journals;
  - Publication in professional journals;
  - Direct mailing of texts, books, folders, diskettes;
  - Dissemination of CD Roms;
  - Audiovisual communication;
  - Computerised databases (Medline, Cochrane Library, etc.);
  - Communication by internet, e-mail.
- Personal:
  - Continuous medical education courses or congresses;
  - Local group meetings, network meetings;
  - Bringing in key figures and opinion leaders;
  - Individual approaches by trained outreach visitors;
  - Inter-collegial contact;
  - Advice by telephone.

The literature supports the hypothesis that usually a range of approaches (mass media and personal) best reaches the target group. A one-off presentation in a journal, on the television or in another way is seldom sufficient to reach the whole target group (*Box 9.2*). Dissemination activities usually have to be repeated and continued for a considerable period of time. The target group must have the information repeatedly placed right under their noses, as it were, via the same channel or different channels, for them to become aware of it.

As well as the channel along which the 'message' is relayed, the source and form of the message are very important during dissemination. Chapter 4 gives a

---

Box 9.2 Influence of published research on patient management (Mead *et al.* 1999)

Between 1989 and 1992 several leading medical journals (including the *Lancet* and *New England Journal of Medicine*) published seven large investigations, which involved thousands of patients. They reported that anticoagulation therapy in patients with atrial fibrillation (cardiac dysrhythmia) reduced the risk of stroke. Mead's study investigated patients from 180 British primary care practices who had been admitted to hospital because of a stroke in the period from 1990–1997. The study group included 161 patients with cardiac dysrhythmia who did not have any contraindications for anticoagulation therapy. Only 22% had been using the medication. The conclusion was that publications in medical journals led to insufficient change in prescription behaviour. This gives rise to questions about the value of publication, both as a means of effective dissemination of scientific insights (do people know about them, have they been discussed in the work setting and do people support them?) and as a method of implementation (if people know about them, are they being applied?).

Box 9.3 Credibility of the source of dissemination (Marriot *et al.* 2000)

In 1951, American doctors were asked to estimate how correct a series of statements about antihistamines were. The same information was presented in an article in the *New England Journal of Medicine* and in an article in a popular magazine. The target group was far more convinced by the information in the medical journal than by that in the popular magazine, even though the information was exactly the same.

detailed description of the form in which guidelines, new procedures or proposals for changes should be presented. The credibility of the source or the medium of information about a guideline or proposal for change is another important factor in the success of implementation. Care providers are more readily convinced by information from reputable journals (*Box 9.3*, but also see *Box 9.4*), by guidelines from their own professional society (see *Box 9.6*) and by professional opinion leaders from their own social network.

A combined approach is not necessary in every case. New insights or working methods that can be incorporated easily into existing routines and do not require too much knowledge and expertise can sometimes be introduced perfectly adequately via an intensive media campaign (Gatignon and Robertson 1985). An example is a finding published in the *Nederlands Tijdschrift voor Geneeskunde* that syringotomy for acute otitis media in children does not produce better results than a watchful waiting policy and medication therapy (Van Buchem *et al.* 1985). As mentioned before, for the majority of doctors this publication was sufficient for them to abandon the intervention. Another example is that

of cot death in infants. In 1987, paediatricians in the Netherlands gave the advice, supported by scientific research, not to put babies to sleep lying on their stomach. This recommendation was adopted quickly by all the home-nursing services and communicated to all infant care bureaux. Subsequently, use of the prone position decreased rapidly (60% in 1987 to 15% in 1990) and, simultaneously, the incidence of cot death decreased sharply (from 1.01 per 1000 in 1985–1987 to 0.64 in 1998–1999; De Jonge 1992).

Before we elaborate further on the possible effects of using mass media and personal channels to inform care providers and others about innovations, it is worth saying that rigorous research in this area, in which measures such as familiarity, interest, 'the-use-of' and such like are routinely used as measures of effect, is still fairly scarce.

MASS MEDIA APPROACH

The majority of new clinical innovations or new procedures and techniques are reported in scientific and specialist journals. Target groups are also often

Box 9.4 Diffusion of magnetic resonance imaging (Ramsey *et al.* 1993)

Sometimes implementation is rapid and independent of publications about its value. An example is magnetic resonance imaging (MRI). The authors conducted a literature study over the period from a few years prior to the clinical introduction of MRI to the first 5 years afterwards. In about 1700 citations in the literature, MRI was the central theme, but it had been compared to other technologies in only 28%. A considerable number of MRI units were purchased before adequate studies had been performed and before MRI had been compared to alternative diagnostic approaches. The conclusion was that among radiologists, non-scientific and non-objective information sources were more important than scientific sources. Publications in scientific journals apparently have little influence on the implementation of such new technologies.

Box 9.5 US national guideline clearing-house

In co-operation with the American Medical Association (AMA) and the American Association of Health Plans (AAHP), the US Agency for Healthcare Research and Quality (AHRQ) took the initiative to start placing evidenced-based guidelines on the web in 1998. In-coming guidelines are screened on their quality (criteria include systematic literature search and not older than 5 years), then a structured summary is made of every guideline. At present, over 1000 guidelines have been entered, including more than 120 from outside the USA.

informed about new research findings or new products and procedures via mail. In addition, increasing use is being made of the internet and computerised databases, such as the Cochrane Library or US guideline clearing house (*Box 9.5*).

The problem with a written approach is that many care providers from target groups do not read the information at all, or do not read it properly or only choose items that are in line with their preferences or interests. When the first guidelines appeared from the National Institute of Health in the 1980s, a study was performed to investigate the extent to which these guidelines reached the target group after dissemination via medical journals, the lay press, press conferences and mailing to key figures. The results showed that only 40% of the intended target group knew that a guideline had been developed and only 20% knew the recommendations (Kosecoff *et al.* 1987). A study from Sweden (Troein *et al.* 1991) evaluated the extent to which doctors were aware of existing guidelines for the treatment of hypercholesterolaemia. The majority had received information about it, either via the guideline documents or in another way. However, only a small minority knew the recommended values for starting treatment. Salem-Schatz *et al.* (1990) investigat-ed the level of knowledge of surgeons and anaesthetists regarding published guidelines on blood transfusion policy. Less than 50% were aware of the risks, and only 30% knew the correct indications for blood transfusion. The physicians with the most faith in their own judge-ment in this field were also the ones with the poorest awareness of the guidelines. A study by Lomas *et al.* (1989) on the dissemination of a guideline on caesarean section among obstetricians showed that 90% were aware of the existence of the guideline. However, only 3% could correctly repeat all eight central recommendations. After the guideline had been published for 2 years, 33% said that they had adapted their obstetric practice; however, in reality, the number of caesarean sections had increased by between 15 and 49%, whereas the aim of the guideline was to reduce them.

The situation in some countries may now be slight-ly more favourable, in view of the relatively transpar-ent procedures adopted by scientific societies of medical specialists and other organisations in the development of clinical guidelines.

The way in which primary care physicians obtain information about guidelines is fairly well-document-ed (*Box 9.7*). Less is known about other professional

---

Box 9.6 Dissemination of guidelines among medical specialists in the Netherlands (van Everdingen *et al.* 2003)

Via a written survey among six groups of medical specialists (cardiologists, paediatricians, anaesthetists, chest physicians, neurologists and urologists) information was obtained about both their knowledge of four nationally developed guidelines in their own field and the sources they had used to acquaint themselves with that knowledge. The percentages of physicians who were aware of the guidelines ranged from 23% for the urologists to 73% for the chest physicians. Major sources are given below.

Type of source (%)	Cardiologists	Paediatricians	Anaesthetists	Chest physicians	Neurologists	Urologists
Journal from own society	33	10	16	7	3	6
General professional journal	13	11	14	16	25	6
CME courses	22	14	11	25	25	7
Scientific meeting	17	9	10	26	16	9
Mailing from own society	10	9	15	12	21	6

The results of this study showed that an average of about half of medical specialists were informed about the existence of specific national guidelines in their own field; also, various sources had been used, both written and personal, to become informed. Rates varied between specialists, depending on the existence of adequate scientific journals in their own field or continuing medical education (CME) courses.

groups, partly because systematic guideline development by central organisations is still relatively new.

The results of existing studies show that care providers use various sources and channels to obtain information about guidelines and new procedures, and that different subgroups use different sources (*Boxes 9.8* and *9.9*). This means that it is a good idea to disseminate innovations via multiple channels.

Box 9.7 How do primary care physicians find out about guidelines? (Grol *et al*. 1998)

A written survey among over 1000 doctors in the Netherlands (response rate 67%) was conducted to explore the sources they used to obtain information about new guidelines. Major sources were the scientific journals (85%), local group (53%), contact with colleagues (43%), CME courses (33%) and via medical representatives or drugs sales persons (12%). Various subgroups or segments of the target group used the different sources in different ways, for example:

- Information from scientific journals – mostly used by members of the professional society, younger physicians and doctors involved in the training of practitioners;
- Information via discussion of the guidelines in the local group – mostly used by physicians actively involved in local quality improvement;
- Information via contact with colleagues – mostly used by physicians who were participating in local CME courses, working in group practices and who were not a member of the professional society;
- Information via drugs sales persons (pharmaceutical companies) – mostly used by physicians who were not a member of the society and by solo practitioners.

In addition, a specific question was asked about the extent of their knowledge of eight specific nationally developed guidelines. The physicians had greater knowledge when they:

- Had used the scientific journal as an information source;
- Were a member of the professional society;
- Were in the younger age group;
- Were involved in the training of physicians;
- Had not drawn on information from pharmaceutical companies.

Box 9.8 Which information sources do medical specialists use to obtain information about new developments and insights? (van Everdingen *et al*. 2003)

Via written surveys among random samples of six groups of medical specialists in the Netherlands, data were obtained about the use of guidelines and the different sources used to keep informed about new developments. Percentages of specialists who use the guidelines from different sources are presented below.

Use (always or often) of guidelines from	Cardiologists	Paediatricians	Chest physicians	Neurologists	Urologists
Own society	93	70	78	83	81
Independent national institute	41	52	70	52	8
College of family doctors	3	10	27	7	9
Foreign organisations	55	40	50	35	16

Specialists used guidelines from their own society most often. In comparison with the other specialists, the chest physicians used guidelines from other sources more often. Guidelines for family physicians were not very popular among the majority of specialists. Foreign guidelines were consulted regularly.

Box 9.9 Which information sources do specialists use to stay informed about new developments in their field? (Van Everdingen *et al*. 2003)

From the same sources as in *Box 9.8*, specialists were informed about the new developments through different sources.

Source	Cardiologists	Paediatricians	Chest physicians	Neurologists	Urologists
Own society journal (%)	96	83	37	44	77
CME (%)	95	88	92	94	89
Scientific meetings (%)	89	77	91	84	95
Local partnership meetings (%)	76	58	68	68	71
Foreign congress (%)	91	65	87	68	93
Mailing from own society (%)	71	71	66	74	78
Internet (%)	31	39	32	32	34
Industry meeting (%)	60	37	47	37	59
Representatives from pharmaceutical companies (%)	43	31	39	36	55
National scientific journal (%)	56	77	68	78	61

CME, scientific meetings, partnership meetings and foreign congresses were used, as well as written media, to keep up-to-date about new developments. A great deal of information was also obtained via industry, particularly by the urologists and cardiologists. About one-third of the specialists used the internet.

Many people have high expectations of electronic databases that summarise information about the most effective interventions, such as the Cochrane Library. In 1996, Prescott *et al*. (1997) found that practising physicians made hardly any use of these types of databases. At that time, far more use was made of familiar (scientific) journals. A study by Wyatt *et al*. (1998), which involved gynaecologists, to stimulate the use of the Cochrane Library also showed that the consultation of such databases remained limited. This may change as increasing use is made of the internet, both within healthcare and also among the general population.

In general, the mere availability of databases, the opportunity to read journals or the mailing of information material cannot be expected to adequately attract the attention of the target group to new insights and working methods in healthcare. When things are read, this is usually by subgroups who are open to new ideas or who are searching for new information themselves. Some segments of the target group read, while others obtain information chiefly via personal channels.

To increase the chance that a mass media approach will achieve its goal, the following measures can be considered:

- The essence of the new information should be summarised into a concise, easy-to-grasp text with an attractive presentation. For example, guidelines might be summarised on a plastic card that can be kept in a folder. Reading the core recommendations from such a guideline should not take more than 10 minutes, particularly when it contains practical flow charts for diagnostics and treatment that can be consulted rapidly and easily.
- A summary of a proposed procedure of care process can also be presented in one or more concise, attractive brochures adapted to the various target groups and distributed on a large scale. This information should ideally be based on pre-existing questions from the relevant target groups. As well as recommendations on practical management, the brochure should also contain scientific background information. The design could therefore be as follows:

- Presentation of a relevant question or problem in practice;
- Confrontation of the reader with their own routines (what are people used to doing at present?);
- Summary of the new insights, the most crucial recommendations;
- Explanation of why old routines are less desirable and arguments in favour of new routines (how good is the evidence?)
- Information about possible problems with changing the present management practices and how they can be solved;
- Where people can find out more.

▦ The summary can also be published simultaneously on the internet (e.g. on the site of the professional society) and in diverse professional journals read by the target group. This can also be accomplished in the form of an interview with a key figure who explains the proposed change and its performance. On a local or institute level, the proposed routines can be sent by e-mail to the people involved and further distributed through internal newsletters.

▦ In addition, attempts can be made to publish popularised versions of an innovation in regional or national daily newspapers or weekly (news) magazines and in magazines read by large groups of patients. Special versions for patients and policy makers are very useful. Over the past few years, many of the guidelines for GPs in the Netherlands have, for example, been published in an easily accessible form in a Dutch consumer magazine. Attention from radio or television can obviously also give an extra impetus, so that patients can consult their care provider with the correct expectations (see Chapter 13).

In general it is a good idea to use multiple channels and to repeat the 'message' many times. The target group should be exposed to the information continuously for a period of time (Tierney *et al.* 1990). However, this is not straightforward as, at a certain stage, its effect may be lost and it may even lead to irritation.

PERSONAL APPROACH

A mass media approach may fail to bring an innovation to the attention of the target group, particularly if it involves complex or sensitive information. Personal approaches can then offer additional support (Rogers 1995; Jacoby and Rose 1986). Informing the target group and motivating them so that they wish to study the

innovation can be achieved by, for example:
▦ CME courses and conferences;
▦ Social networks of care providers;
▦ Key figures and opinion leaders;
▦ Personal introduction by advisers and facilitators.
Chapter 10 elaborates more fully on educational innovations, particularly where they concern the effects on actual performance. Below, we discuss the possible role of educational approaches in the dissemination of innovations.

CME courses and conferences

Congresses, courses and national and local CME programmes can make an important contribution to effective information transfer with regard to new developments. This is certainly the most popular manner and generally is reasonably well appreciated.

A problem with courses and conferences as a method of information transfer is that people often choose subjects they already find interesting and consequently, keep up-to-date with them better than with other subjects (Sibley *et al.* 1982). People's skill in assessing their own competence and performance proves to be limited (Norman 1999). In addition, much of such education is fairly passive and requires little input from the participants. A systematic literature review of methods used to introduce guidelines (Grimshaw and Russell 1993) showed that interactive methods of education, in which participants were actively (as opposed to passively) involved in the course, seemed to be more effective in persuading the target group to change their behaviour in line with the guidelines. This finding was later confirmed many times in systematic literature analyses of various forms of education (e.g. Davis *et al.* 1999). Indeed, much of the present professional development in many countries is gradually adopting this interactive character, partly inspired by educational developments in the field of problem-based learning.

To achieve a successful dissemination of innovations, it appears to be important to:
▦ Design educational programmes for the innovation that are based on concrete, recognisable problems, questions or cases from everyday practice (Spencer and Jordan 1999);
▦ Allow room for discussions between participants and the exchange of existing working methods – people then realise that colleagues have different opinions and use different routines, which stimulates their interest to find out more about the innovation;

■ Present data on existing routines, variations in such routines and deviations from the proposed (new) working method – the basis for attracting interest often lies in confrontation with deviations from existing norms and the feeling that something actually ought to change (Grol and Lawrence 1995).

Networks

The dissemination of innovations and changes can occur through local networks of care providers and key figures and opinion leaders within these groups. Relationships with colleagues and other important persons in the direct vicinity strongly help to determine the decisions that are made (McLeroy *et al.* 1988; Bandura 1986). Social–psychological research into, for example, voting behaviour showed that people were more led by individuals in their social network than by the media, particularly when these individuals were considered to be competent, popular and open (Marriot *et al.* 2000). The social network provides new information, access to new sources of information and support for adequately fulfilling one's own tasks. These networks differ considerably between professional groups (*Box 9.10*).

An analysis of the networks within the target group might therefore be of importance to establish the precise flow path of information and the key figures in this (Rogers 1983, 1995). However, Grimshaw *et al.* (2000) were unable to identify social networks for primary care physicians in two districts in Scotland, although they could be identified for doctors in secondary care. Therefore, the presence of social networks cannot always be assumed in all settings.

Many care providers are not prepared to accept new rules of behaviour until a local consensus has been reached. Consensus arises, in the first instance, by local communication about the advantages and risks of the

recommended performance and by the availability of local education programmes and demonstrations of the method (Greer 1988). At two large health centres in Sweden, a study was performed in which observations were made for 3 months to evaluate how new information about the treatment for elevated cholesterol levels was transferred (Diwan *et al.* 1997). Observations showed that much of the transfer of information took place in implicit interactions between care providers (who knew the procedure) and 'newcomers'. A large part of the learning process occurred via continuous discussions and exchanges of information and experiences within the team. Within this process, factors such as hierarchy between care providers and gender also played a role.

Optimal involvement of the social network in dissemination and implementation might therefore mean:
■ Actively involving the social network and its representatives in the development and execution of a dissemination strategy;
■ Adapting dissemination interventions to the ideas, needs and capacities of the network;
■ Making use of prearranged meetings of the networks to plan the interventions.

Key figures and opinion leaders

The person who presents or introduces the innovation is judged by the target group on his or her level of trustworthiness, expertise and acceptability (Kok 1987). In the case of healthcare professionals, the authority and prestige of the presenter is of particular importance. For some people this applies to the scientific status of the presenter, while for others this is not important. If the presenter is regarded as being someone who is too far removed from practice or as someone with revolutionary ideas, then this makes it more difficult to

---

Box 9.10 Dissemination of AIDS education programmes among teachers (Paulussen *et al.* 1995)

A study was performed of 698 teachers at secondary schools to find out whether they were aware of the existence of various acquired immune deficiency syndrome (AIDS) education programmes and whether they had been using them. Dissemination took place by advertisements in magazines and newspapers, and by mailing. About two-thirds of the respondents were aware of the existence of one or more curricula. A large proportion of these teachers mentioned colleagues as the information source – they had talked about it (34%) or knew of colleagues who had applied such a curriculum (63%). Knowledge of the curricula seemed to be particularly dependent on norms and values and on the frequency of inter-collegial contact. The conclusion was that both the presence of colleagues who were considered to be setting an example and contact between colleagues played a very important role in acquiring knowledge of the programmes.

increase acceptance than if the presenter is regarded as being 'one of us'. Many practising care providers are sceptical about scientists. They know that scientific findings are often at odds with each other and that the scientific literature is sometimes more a channel for communication between experts than a way to reach practising care providers (Greer 1988). Therefore, the question is, "Who has the most power of expression in a specific target group or subgroup to inform them about, and involve them in, changes in care?"

During the introduction of new working methods, a special role is reserved for the *key figures* within local networks (Lomas 1993; Rogers 1983, 1995). They form both the first target group for the introduction and the channel along which the introduction will be the most effective, "The heart of the diffusion process consists of interpersonal network exchanges and social modelling between individuals who had already adopted and those who then would be influenced to do so" (Rogers 1983). The term *key figures* implies respected and well-informed professionals within a target group, who filter incoming information and pass it on to the people around them. They are not usually the 'innovators' within a group, but the persons who best personify the group norms and group culture. They judge new developments in the light of existing group norms.

An example of using key figures was reported in a study for which specially selected hospital physicians enrolled in a course that dealt with medication for rheumatoid arthritis (Stross *et al*. 1983). These physicians had, subsequently, to transfer the information to other physicians. Comparison with a control group showed an improvement in the prescription behaviour of these physicians. One of the conclusions was that during the dissemination and introduction of new insights it was very effective to aim at a group of care providers who become rapidly interested in the subject and also have authority in the target group. Another well-known example is the study by Lomas *et al*. (1991), in which guidelines for the application of caesarean section were introduced by key figures and opinion leaders at 16 hospitals. One group received the guidelines only, a second group participated in staff meetings with feedback over a period of 3 months and in a third group the opinion leaders were identified and subsequently recommended the guidelines. A letter from an authoritative colleague was also circulated. In addition, regular enquiries were made about guideline application. A (small) effect on management was seen only in the third group.

The literature, however, does not always show a positive attitude to all issues concerned with the use of key figures and opinion leaders:

- Firstly, it is sometimes difficult to establish precisely who the key figures are – it is not always clear precisely what are the important characteristics of key figures, so they are difficult to identify;
- Effects on management vary, as shown in the reviews by Davis *et al*. (1995), Oxman *et al*. (1995) and Thomson *et al*. (1998) – Chapter 10 deals more fully with this issue.

In summary, by investing a great deal of time in the key figures, by visiting them, contacting them by telephone, showing interest in the specific local situation and involving them in the proposed change and in the planning of the introduction to their network, the dissemination of an innovation may be facilitated (Box *9.11*).

Personal introduction by advisors

Another method to bring innovations to the attention of a target group is to approach them personally and

---

Box 9.11 Using the services of key figures in the introduction of professional collaboratives in primary care (Grol 1987)

The introduction of an innovative method for quality improvement in primary care in the Netherlands (i.e. quality circles or professional collaboratives) was started at the beginning of the 1980s in a group of highly motivated physicians. After they had gained experience for a while, other groups were recruited, both by mail and by telephone. Potential participants were invited to a group meeting, in which the members of the pioneer group related their experience and answered questions. In this way, hundreds of doctors became motivated to participate in this new method (Grol 1987). In a later phase of the introduction, key figures from local groups were trained to chair and supervise quality circles specially aimed at the use of national guidelines. After a short training period of 4–6 days, the participants made a start on their own groups. Evaluation showed that participants were reasonably successful in initiating this form of quality improvement. It is estimated that, presently, more than 60% of all family doctor groups are using this method regularly.

give them information and tuition (*Boxes 9.12* and *9.13*). This can be carried out by a trained colleague or an expert in a particular field who visits the target group in their own working environment and – depending on personal needs or questions – offers them support in understanding the innovation. The influence of such a consultation (in the literature, referred to as outreach visits or academic detailing) on actual implementation is described further in Chapter 10.

However, there is evidence that personal tuition, tailored to the questions of the persons involved and given by a respected outreach visitor, can contribute to arousing interest and creating a positive attitude towards innovations (see *Box 9.1*).

Box 9.12 Outreach visits to improve smoking cessation (Cockburn *et al.* 1992)

A package with materials that advised patients to stop smoking was delivered to physicians in Australia in three different ways:

- Personally by a trained nurse or physiotherapist, who demonstrated the materials and encouraged the physician to use the materials;
- By a courier;
- By mail.

The study showed that physicians in the first group remembered more often that they had received the materials and used more often at least one component of the package. There were no differences with respect to actual use of the minimal intervention strategy for smoking cessation or the overall attitude regarding the materials among physicians. The effects have to be assessed in the light of the costs – personal delivery by a trained person was 12 times more expensive than the courier and 24 times more expensive than mailing.

Box 9.13 Development of a dissemination plan for a national guideline on stroke (van der Weijden *et al.* 2004; Dautzenberg *et al.* 2003a,b)

A broad multidisciplinary Dutch working group analysed the scientific literature on the subject of stroke and subsequently formulated recommendations for medical practice. The recommendations were divided into four sections – care organisation, acute phase, secondary prevention, and recovery and rehabilitation. Recommendations for GPs, neurologists, rehabilitation specialists, neuropsychologists, nurses, ward orderlies, speech therapists, physiotherapists, home care organisations, etc., formed part of this guideline, which was therefore meant to be applied at all levels. The guideline served as a basis for locally developed protocols and agreements about the organisation of care. Effective dissemination among all the relevant care providers was therefore desirable. To promote dissemination, core recommendations were selected from the guideline to receive particular focus during implementation:

- There is evidence that improving and intensifying the organisation of care (a regional stroke service) leads to greater effectiveness and consequently to better functional health outcomes;
- Patients without atrial fibrillation but with amaurosis fugax or a transient ischaemic attach should receive 30–300 mg acetylsalicylic acid (aspirin) per day as secondary prevention;
- There is evidence that rehabilitation should be started as soon as possible in the acute phase.

In addition, factors that inhibited or promoted implementation were established for each recommendation. This was accomplished by brainstorming within the working group and by consulting external experts in the field. Bottlenecks with regard to a 'stroke service' were, for example:

- Vague definitions of a stroke unit or service;
- Co-ordination, transfer, communication and tuning of care between the disciplines involved;
- Shortage of specific expertise to set up a stroke service;
- Patients sometimes have other preferences concerning the care they receive.

Thus, in particular, bottlenecks in the domains of organisation and structuring of the care process and co-operation between disciplines were matters for consideration. In view of the large group of disciplines involved and that regional solutions had to be found for the restructuring of care for patients with stroke, it was decided to focus firstly on a dissemination plan. To achieve regional working agreements, people need to know about the guideline and not only develop the motivation to meet at the conference table with their own discipline, but also with other parties. Thus, the dissemination plan had to aim particularly at promoting local and regional discussion or communication about the new guidelines. Two major regions were compared in a pilot project – in one region nursing home and rehabilitation physicians were directly approached by a personal letter from their scientific society, while in a comparable region outreach visitors were called in to speak to key figures personally. Knowledge of and use of the guideline for local discussion was good in both regions after the dissemination, but did not differ between the two methods.

CONCLUSION

Literature on the dissemination of innovations shows that such dissemination may be best accomplished via various, closely linked channels:

- The target group must be presented with the innovations regularly and over a prolonged period of time via different mass media methods – magazines, journals, newsletters, internet, the lay press, summaries in an attractive form or personal e-mail;
- In addition to this, use must be made of personal channels – interactive education via existing educational programmes and local networks, with the assistance of key figures and opinion leaders. It is best to focus firstly on a group of relative frontrunners in the target group. Calling in the services of outreach visitors seems to be an appropriate method to accelerate the dissemination process in some cases.

It is important to realise, however, that different subgroups within the target group use different sources of information or have different preferences for sources. Some prefer scientific journals, others look to colleagues, while others might best be approached by outreach visitors or via the lay press.

A further concern is that effective dissemination does not guarantee implementation. Cameron and Naylor (1999) performed a study on the dissemination of the 'Ottawa Ankle Rules' at 63 hospitals. The guidelines were received with great enthusiasm. Subsequently, the effect of a 1 hour education session given by a trained expert at five hospitals was evaluated. The evaluation showed that, in comparison with a control group of five hospitals, there was no reduction in the number of radiographs taken of the ankle, and possibly even an increase. The conclusion drawn by the authors was that, even though the dissemination strategy may have been successful and the guideline broadly accepted, the influence on management still remained limited.

Effective dissemination and broad awareness and acceptance of an innovation are thus a necessary, but insufficient, step towards effective implementation. It is therefore – ultimately – of great importance to develop a 'dissemination plan' in close connection with the implementation plan and to involve the target group and key figures within the target group in the development of this plan and its enactment.

Recommended literature

Davis D, Thomson M, Freemantle N, *et al*. (1999). Do conferences, workshops, rounds and other traditional continuing education activities change physician behavior or health care outcomes. *JAMA* **282**:867–874.

Rogers E (1995). *Diffusion of Innovations*. New York: Free Press.

References

Bandura A (1986). *Social Foundations of Thought and Action*. Englewood Cliffs: Prentice Hall.

Buchem FL van, Peeters MF and Hof MA van't (1985). Acute otitis media: A new treatment strategy. *BMJ* **290**:1033–1037.

Cameron C and Naylor C (1999). No impact from active dissemination of the Ottawa Ankle Rules: Further evidence of the need for local implementation of practice guidelines. *Can Med Assoc J*. **160**(8):1165–1168.

Cockburn J, Ruth D, Silagy C, *et al*. (1992). Randomized trial of three approaches for marketing smoking cessation programmes to Australian general practitioners. *BMJ* **304**:691–694.

Dautzenberg M, van der Weijden T and Grol R (2003a). *Disseminatie van Richtlijnen Beroerte onder Verpleeghuisartsen en Revalidatieartsen. Een Interventiestudie [Dissemination of Stroke Guidelines among Nursing, Home and Revalidation Physicians. An Intervention Study]*. Maastricht/Nijmegen: WOK.

Dautzenberg M, van der Weijden T and Grol R (2003b). *Disseminatie van Richtlijnen Beroerte onder Verpleeghuisartsen en Revalidatieartsen. Een Cross-sectionele Studie [Dissemination of Stroke Guidelines among Nursing, Home and Revalidation Physicians. A Cross-Section Study]*. Maastricht/Nijmegen: WOK.

Davis DA, Thomson MA, Oxman AD, *et al*. (1995). Changing physician performance. A systematic review of the effect of continuing medical education strategies. *JAMA* **274**:700–705.

Davis D, Thomson M, Freemantle N, *et al*. (1999). Do conferences, workshops, rounds and other traditional continuing education activities change physician behavior or health care outcomes? *JAMA* **282**:867–874.

Diwan V, Sachs L and Wahlström R (1997). Practice–knowledge–attitudes–practice: An explorative study of information in primary care. *Soc Sci Med*. **44**:1221–1228.

Everdingen JJ van, Mokkink HGA, Klazinga NS, Grol R and Koekenbier GJS (2003). De bekendheid en verspreiding van CBO-richtlijnen onder medisch specialisten [The knowledge and distribution of CBO guidelines among medical specialists]. *TSG* **81**(8):468–472.

Gatignon H and Robertson T (1985). A propositional inventory for new diffusion research. *J Consum Res*. **57**:752–761.

Greer A (1988). The state of the arts versus the state of science. The diffusion of new medical technologies into practice. *Int J Technol Assess Health Care* **4**:5–26.

Grimshaw J and Russell I (1993). Effects of guidelines on medical practice. A systematic review of rigorous evaluations. *Lancet* **342**:1317–1322.

Grimshaw JM, Greener J, Ibbotson T, *et al*. (2000). *Is the Involvement of Opinion Leaders in the Implementation of Research Findings a Feasible Strategy?* Mimeo. Aberdeen: Health Services Research Unit.

Grol R (1987). *Kwaliteitsbewaking in de Huisartsgeneeskunde [Quality Improvement in General Practice]*. Proefschrift [Thesis]. Nijmegen: KUN.

Grol R (2001). Successes and failures in the implementation of evidence-based guidelines for clinical practice. *Med Care* **39**(S2):II46–II54.

Grol R and Lawrence M (1995). *Quality Improvement by Peer Review*. Oxford: Oxford University Press.

Grol R, Zwaard A, Mokkink H, *et al*. (1998). Dissemination of guidelines: Which sources do physicians use in order to be informed? *Int J Qual Health Care* **10**:135–140.

Jacoby J and Rose M (1986). Transfer of information and its impact on medical practice: The US experience. *Int J Technol Assess Health Care* **1**:107–115.

Jonge G de (1992). Wiegedood in Nederland 1985–1990 [Cot death in the Netherlands]. *Med Contact* **47**:215–218.

Kok G (1987). Theorieën over gedragsbeïnvloeding. In: Damoiseaux V and Visser A. *Gezondheidsvoorlichting en -opvoeding [Health Information and Education]*. Assen/Maastricht: Van Gorcum.

Kosecoff J, Kanouse D and Rogers W (1987). Effects of the National Institutes of Health Consensus Development Program on physician practice. *JAMA* **258**:2708–2713.

Lomas J (1993). *Teaching Old (and not so Old) Docs New Tricks: Effective Ways to Implement Research Findings*. CHEPA Working Paper 93–4. Hamilton: Centre for Health Economics and Policy Analysis.

Lomas J (1997). *Beyond the Sound of Hand Clapping: A Discussion Document on Improving Health Research Dissemination and Uptake*. Sydney: University of Sydney.

Lomas J, Anderson G, Domnick-Pierre K, *et al*. (1989). Do practice guidelines guide practice? The effect of a consensus statement on the practice of physicians. *N Engl J Med*. **321**:1306–1311.

Lomas J, Enkin M, Anderson G, *et al*. (1991). Opinion leaders versus audit and feedback to implement practice guidelines. *JAMA* **265**:2202–2207.

Marriot S, Palmer C and Lelliott P (2000). Disseminating health care information: Getting the message across. *Qual Health Care* **9**:58–62.

McLeroy K, Bibeau D, Steckle A, *et al*. (1988). An ecological perspective on health promotion programs. *Health Educ Q*. **15**:351–377.

Mead G, Wardlaw J, Lewis S, *et al*. (1999). The influence of randomised trials on the use of anticoagulants for atrial fibrillation. *Age Ageing* **28**:441–446.

NHMRC (2000). *How to Put the Evidence into Practice: Implementation and Dissemination Strategies*. Canberra: NHMRC.

Norman G (1999). The adult learner: A mythical species. *Acad Med*. **74**:886–889.

Oxman AD, Thomson MA, Davis DA, *et al*. (1995). No magic bullets: A systematic review of 102 trials of interventions to improve professional practice *Can Med Assoc J*. **153**:1423–1431.

Paulussen T, Kok G, Schaalma H, *et al*. (1995). Diffusion of AIDS curricula among Dutch school teachers. *Health Educ Q*. **22**:227–243.

Prescott K, Lloyd M, Douglas HR, *et al*. (1997). Promoting clinically effective practice: General practitioners' awareness of sources of research evidence. *Fam Pract*. **14**:320–323.

Ramsey S, Hillman A, Renshaw L, *et al*. (1993). How important is the scientific literature in guiding clinical decisions? *Int J Technol Assess Health Care* **9**:253–262.

Rogers E (1983). *Diffusion of Innovations*. New York: Free Press.

Rogers E (1995). *Diffusion of Innovations*, Fourth Edition. New York: Free Press.

Salem-Schatz S, Avorn J and Soumerai S (1990). Influence of clinical knowledge, organizational context and practice style on transfusion decision making. *JAMA* **264**:476–483.

Sibley J, Sackett D, Neufeld V, *et al*. (1982). A randomized trial of continuing medical education. *N Engl J Med*. **306**:511–515.

Spencer J and Jordan R (1999). Learner centred approaches in medical education. *BMJ* **318**:1280–1283.

Stross JK, Hiss R, Watts C, *et al*. (1983). Continuing education in pulmonary disease for primary care physicians. *Am Rev Respir Dis*. **127**:739–746.

Thomson MA, Oxman AD, Haynes RB, *et al*. (1998). *Local Opinion Leaders to Improve Health Professional Practice and Health Care Outcomes*. The Cochrane Library, Issue 3. Oxford: Update Software.

Tierney W, Miller M and McDonald C (1990). The effect on test ordering of informing physicians of the changes for outpatient diagnostic tests. *N Engl J Med*. **322**:1499–1504.

Troein M, Rastam L and Selander S (1991). Dissemination and implementation of guidelines for lipid lowering. *Fam Pract*. **8**:223–228.

Weijden T van der, Hooi JD, Grol R and Limburg M (2004). A multidisciplinary guideline for the acute phase of stroke. Barriers perceived by Dutch neurologists. *J Eval Clin Pract*. In press.

Wyatt J, Paterson-Brown S, Johanson R, *et al*. (1998). Randomised trial of educational visits to enhance use of systematic reviews in 25 obstetric units. *BMJ* **317**:1041–1046.

Chapter 10

Educational interventions

Michel Wensing and Richard Grol

KEY MESSAGES

- The effects on professional behaviour and health outcomes of reading educational materials or attending courses are often limited. Small-scale and interactive education may be more effective, but still little research evidence supports this.
- Factors that may increase the effectiveness of education include longer time period, an appropriate group composition, needs assessment before the activity, active participation, individualisation and the use of local opinion leaders.
- Although the effects of education on behaviour may be limited, it is often a necessary first step in a process of implementation of innovations. Education is particularly valuable if it is part of a broader implementation strategy that includes other interventions as well.

Box 10.1 Shortening the learning curve for a new surgical procedure (Hasan *et al.* 2000)

When a new surgical procedure is introduced, there is a learning curve – a period during which rates of mortality and complications gradually reduce to the lowest possible. It is important that this period is as short as possible.

When they introduced a new procedure to replace heart valves, surgeons from two British hospitals applied the following strategies. Each surgeon took a course on the procedure and practised on artificial material. The first operation on a patient was carried out with an expert. Subsequently, operations were carried out by two surgeons, but one was always responsible for the patient. Of the 20 patients who were operated on, one died within a few weeks of the operation (5%), and most of the others had only minimal or mild complications. Previously, in the first year after the introduction of this operation procedure, about 20% of the patients operated on had died.

INTRODUCTION

This chapter focuses on 'educational interventions' for (teams of) healthcare professionals, the aim of which is to implement evidence, clinical guidelines, new procedures or best practices. These interventions comprise different types of activities intended to increase the knowledge and skills of the target group in relation to the innovation, with the expectation that this will result in actual use of the innovation. Traditionally, education is the approach most often used to stimulate change and improvement in healthcare. The continuing education of healthcare professionals takes much time and money, so some understanding of the cost effectiveness

of different types of education and improvement of patient care is crucial (Hutchinson 1999). As with medical care for patients, education of care providers should be as 'evidence based' as possible (Petersen 1999). This chapter provides an overview of different types of continuing education, the effects of education on the process and outcomes of care provision, and the factors that may improve the effectiveness.

A number of educational theories are described in Chapter 2. The basic and continuing education of healthcare professionals has been studied for several decades. The medical knowledge of physicians increases during their basic training, but gradually decreases over subsequent years (Van Leeuwen *et al.* 1995); this is probably similar in other healthcare professionals. Knowledge and skills are associated only weakly with actual performance (Ram *et al.* 1999), so actual performance has increasingly become the yardstick in education. Both in basic and continuing education, large-scale, passive methods of education have been replaced by small-scale, motivational types of education (see also Chapter 2, subsection on educational theories). This means, for instance, that students work together in small groups on a variety of real problems, to allow for students' different learning needs and styles. Continuing education has gradually developed into 'continuing professional development', with the focus on the learning needs of the individual care provider.

Motivational education is mostly based on theories of 'adult learning' (*Box 10.2*). These theories assume that adults are intrinsically motivated to learn and that they can guide the learning process themselves (Kaufman 2003; Newman and Peile 2002). Adults prefer to learn new insights by means of specific problems that they have experienced in their daily work ('problem-based learning'; Irby 1995; Albanese and Mitchell 1993). An important principle of problem-based learning is that individuals have different learning styles – some want to experience things first before they start to study to gain a better insight, while others want to understand fully before they start to act. Therefore, education should meet these differing learning styles. Chapter 2 provides more information about the theoretical background of educational theories.

The dissemination of a new product or insight through a target group is also often done by means of information or education (Chapter 9). This chapter considers education, however, as a strategy aimed at actual behaviour change. The chapter first describes different types of educational interventions and then provides an overview of their effectiveness. Next, the possible determinants of effectiveness that potentially can be used to improve the effectiveness of education are described.

TYPES OF EDUCATIONAL INTERVENTIONS

The different types of educational interventions vary from educational materials to individual instruction. The Cochrane Effective Practice and Organisation of Care Group (EPOC) distinguishes the following:

■ *Educational materials* – publication or mailing of written recommendations for clinical care, including guidelines, audiovisual material, electronic publications (through the internet) and educational computer programmes;

■ *Large-scale educational meetings* – participation of care providers in conferences and lectures that are large scale, so that participation is usually of a passive character;

■ *Small-scale educational meetings* – participation of care providers in workshops, skills training, educational groups, local consensus groups and quality circles or peer-review groups outside the practice setting, so meetings are of a small-scale nature in which participation is usually active;

■ *Outreach visits* – contact in the practice setting of care providers with a trained individual who provides information, instruction and support, and sometimes also feedback, on current practice;

■ *Use of opinion leaders* – educational activities provided by 'opinion leaders', individuals who are seen as influential in a specific clinical area, a strategy treated as a determinant of the effectiveness of education in this chapter (see later).

The distribution of educational materials can achieved in different ways. For instance, the publication of new insights in journals, mailing leaflets to healthcare professionals, distributing messages to email mailing lists or broadcasting educational programmes on radio or television (where a larger audience can be reached). Interactive internet websites and distant learning programme are in this category, although they are more interactive than are most other methods in it. Educational computer programmes can also be cate-

---

Box 10.2 Portfolio learning (Mathers *et al.* 1999)

Individualisation of an educational programme by means of a 'portfolio' is a method based on the principles of adult learning. This method helps the care provider to choose an individual programme for continuing education that is based on individual needs and objectives, and individual gaps in knowledge and skills. It is assumed that this approach promotes the learning process and the motivation to learn. A qualitative study among physicians showed that they used the portfolio approach quite differently. The approach was evaluated positively by most users, although the physicians did not like the paper work that had to be done.

gorised here, although computerised 'decision-support systems' are seen as reminders (see Chapter 11). The distribution of educational material with the intention not only to inform care providers (dissemination), but also to change their behaviour assumes that they are prepared to be guided by such information and that barriers to change are minimal or absent.

In large-scale educational meetings (more than 25 people) the focus is on the presentation of information in an oral and/or visual format. This category includes lectures, seminars, presentations, courses and conferences. Practical limitations mean this type of education is usually teacher-orientated and passive. As with written educational materials, once the format of the meeting has developed it is relatively easy to reach a large group of individuals. There is, again, the assumption that care providers are prepared to use the information to change behaviour.

Small-scale educational meetings have a range of functions, formats and purposes, such as skills training to learn technical or communication skills, local consensus development and continuing education courses in which participants work in small groups. Quality circles and supervision groups can also be seen as small-scale educational meetings, although they may use additional educational strategies, such as feedback on practice routines (Beyer *et al.* 2003). One classic example is the 'grand round', the visit to patients in hospital by a small group of resident or trainee doctors, who are taught by an experienced physician. The format of small-scale educational meetings can be similar to that of large-scale meetings, but they are usually more orientated towards individual needs and motivations.

Outreach visits are a specific type of education, based on the techniques used by the pharmaceutical industry to influence the prescribing patterns of physicians. The visit comprises individual explanation, instruction and support in the practice of the care provider by a specially trained person. The visitor may be a physician, nurse, pharmacist or other. This type of education has been applied mainly to rationalise physician-prescribing behaviour, but has been used for other purposes, such as to promote prevention in primary medical care (Hulscher *et al.* 1997). This approach is particularly suited to tailor a programme to the individual needs of the care provider. Specific techniques of outreach visits (sometimes labelled as 'academic detailing') include, among others, interviews to investigate baseline knowledge and motivations for current patterns, defining clear educational and behavioural objectives, stimulating active physician participation in educational interactions and providing positive reinforcement of improved practices in follow-up visits (Soumerai and Avorn 1990).

EFFECTIVENESS OF EDUCATION

When compared to most other implementation strategies, there is a relatively large body of research evidence on the effectiveness of educational interventions. These evaluative studies are summarised in different reviews, but these draw on the same studies to a greater or lesser extent. *Table 10.1* describes 39 reviews that report on

Table 10.1 Overview of reviews of controlled trials on educational strategies

Study	Conclusions
Educational material	
Cohen and Dacanay (1992)	Review of 37 studies of computerised learning programmes for care providers. The effectiveness, reported as the difference of mean scores in intervention group and control group divided by the standard deviation in the control group, varied between −1.02 and 2.64; the mean value was 0.41.
Davis *et al.* (1995)	Review with 11 studies of educational materials. Four studies showed a positive effect, the remaining seven showed no effect.
Freemantle *et al.* (1998)	Review with nine studies of educational materials. Estimation of the effectiveness varied between +3% and +243% (never significant), but the practical relevance of the changes was limited.
Gill *et al.* (1999)	Review of seven studies of educational materials about prescribing medication. This was effective in three studies.
Grimshaw *et al.* (2004)	Review with 18 studies on the dissemination of educational materials compared to no intervention, which showed modest improvements that may be short lived. The effects varied between +3.6 and +17% absolute change in four randomised trials. *(cont.)*

Table 10.1 (*cont.*) Overview of reviews of controlled trials on educational strategies

Study	Conclusions
Educational material	
Hulscher *et al.* (1999)	Review with three studies of educational materials about prevention in general practice and family medicine. The effects varied.
Oxman *et al.* (1995)	Review with 12 studies of educational materials. Most studies did not show any differences in practice routines or patient outcomes between intervention group and control group.
Pippalla *et al.* (1995)	Review with four studies on the effect of educational material on medication prescribing. The mean effect was 0.51.
Soumerai *et al.* (1989)	Review with eight studies of educational material about prescribing medication. This was effective in three studies, but not effective in the remaining five studies.
Van der Weijden *et al.* (2000)	Review with four studies of dissemination of educational material to improve test ordering. A reduction of 4–20% was found in three studies. The fourth study showed an increase of 2%.
Large-scale educational meetings	
Davis *et al.* (1995)	Review with seven studies of formal continuing education. One study showed a positive effect, the remaining six studies showed no or negative effects.
Davis *et al.* (1999)	Review with four studies of formal continuing education. None of the studies showed positive effect.
Grimshaw *et al.* (2004)	Review with three studies on educational meetings against no intervention. The results suggested that the effects, if any, were small to modest.
Oxman *et al.* (1995)	Review with 17 studies on educational conferences. These were not effective if no effort was made to facilitate the change process. The comprehensive strategies (e.g. including the opportunity to practice) were effective.
Small-scale educational meetings	
Hulscher *et al.* (1999)	Review of four studies of group continuing education about prevention in general practice and family medicine. Changes in preventive care varied between –4% and +31%.
Davis *et al.* (1999)	Review of six studies of interactive continuing education, of which four showed an effect on physicians' routines. Five out of seven combinations of formal and interactive continuing education showed positive effects.
Lancaster *et al.* (1998)	Review of an uncertain number of studies of training on smoking cessation in primary care. There was clear improvement in the process of care (advice, arrangements, etc.). One out of 50 patients who received advice actually stopped smoking.
Pippalla *et al.* (1995)	Review of three studies of group meetings to discuss prescribing medication. The mean effect size was 0.31 (compared to 0.56 on average, see above).
Smits *et al.* (2002)	Review of six trials of problem-based learning in continuing education. These studies provided little evidence that problem-based learning increased participants' performance and patients' health.
Soumerai *et al.* (1989)	Review of two studies on small-scale group education (conferences, lectures, seminars, etc.). Both were effective.
Thomson O'Brien *et al.* (2001)	Review of 32 studies (36 comparisons) of continuing education meetings and workshops. For 10 comparisons of interactive workshops, moderate or large effects occurred in six studies and small effects in four studies. For 19 comparisons that combined workshops and didactic presentations, there were moderate or large effects in 12 comparisons and small effects in seven comparisons. In seven comparisons of didactic presentations, only one showed some significant results.
Outreach visits	
Davis *et al.* (1995)	Review of two studies of outreach visits by an external person. Both studies showed positive results.
Gurwitz *et al.* (1990)	Review of two studies of the effects of outreach visits by an external person on the prescribing of medication in nursing homes. One study showed a positive effect on prescribing behaviour (reduction of 18%), the second study did not show an effect.

Table 10.1 (*cont.*) Overview of reviews of controlled trials on educational strategies	
Study	**Conclusions**
Outreach visits	
Hulscher *et al.* (1999)	Review of two studies of individual instruction regarding prevention in general practice and family medicine. The changes in preventive care varied between 5 and 44%.
Oxman *et al.* (1995)	Review of eight studies of outreach visits by an external person. The strategy improved prescribing behaviour and, to a lesser extent, increased preventive activities.
Pippalla *et al.* (1995)	Review of eight studies of one-on-one meetings about prescribing behaviour. The mean effect size was 0.64 (compared to 0.56 on average, see above).
Qureshi *et al.* (2002)	Review of seven studies of educational outreach visits for non-prescribing interventions in general practice. All of the studies reported that the visits had a positive effect, though the impact varied greatly between the studies. The impact was mainly on the process of care.
Soumerai *et al.* (1989)	Review of six studies of face-to-face education about prescribing behaviour. This was effective in five studies, and in one study not effective.
Thomson *et al.* (1998a)	Review of three studies of practice visits by an external person compared to a control group without intervention. This was (partly) effective in two studies; the relative improvements varied between 24 and 50%.
Van der Weijden *et al.* (2000)	Review of two studies of educational visits that resulted in an absolute reduction of 8–12% in test ordering.
Education, other or not specified	
Bower *et al.* (2001)	Review of three comparative studies (and five before-and-after studies) of educational interventions to improve child and adolescent mental services in primary care teams. One comparative study showed some differences, while the other two showed few differences.
Brown *et al.* (2002)	Review of nine studies of continuing professional development, which included an economic evaluation. The studies did not allow empirical conclusions to be drawn about the economic value of continuing professional development.
Davis *et al.* (1992)	Review of 15 studies of education (individual instruction, computerised information, presentations, knowledge tests, printed materials, workshops, etc.). 11 studies reported on the effects on process of care, of which seven showed positive effects. Six studies reported on patient outcomes, of which one study showed positive effects.
Greenhalgh *et al.* (2003)	Review of trials on online education, which found one small randomised trial (results not reported).
Harvey *et al.* (2001)	Review of three studies on educational interventions to improve obesity management. These studies showed some positive effects, but suffered from substantial methodological limitations.
Solomon *et al.* (1998)	Review of five studies of education on test ordering. Three out of five studies showed positive effects.
Thomas *et al.* (1998)	Review of nine studies on the instruction on the use of guidelines, sometimes combined with education. Positive effects were found in four out of five studies for process measurements. Six out of eight studies with patient outcome measurements showed positive effects.
Waddell (1991)	Review of 34 studies of continuing education for nurses (lectures, discussions, written exercises, clinical training, use of audiovisual materials, demonstrations, etc.). Cohen's *d* was 0.73, which implies that about three-quarters of the participants experienced a positive effect.
Wensing *et al.* (1998)	Review of (a) seven studies of individual instruction, peer review groups or patient reports, and (b) 17 studies of written material, group education and patient education. In group (a), two of seven studies showed positive effects, three showed partly positive effects and two had no effect. In group (b) two of 17 studies showed positive effects, six showed partly positive effects and nine had no effect.
Worrall *et al.* (1997)	Review of six studies of education in primary care. This was effective in three out of six studies.
Zwarenstein *et al.* (2000)	Review on interprofessional education (education of members of different disciplines), which did not identify any studies that met the inclusion criteria.

controlled trials of educational strategies. The following general picture emerges:

- The effectiveness of educational materials is at best modest, although according to several reviews they are clearly ineffective;
- The effectiveness of large-scale educational meetings is variable and, in some reviews, these appear to be ineffective;
- The number of studies on small-scale education is more limited, but this strategy seems promising as most studies suggest that it is effective;
- The effects of outreach visits are mainly positive, but a positive effect was not always found and the number of available studies is limited;

The effectiveness of educational strategies combined with other strategies, such as audit and feedback, is discussed in Chapter 14.

Educational material

Freemantle et al. (1998) found nine studies on the effects of dissemination of educational material on healthcare providers' behaviour and patient outcomes. None of the studies met the methodological criteria set. The studies focused, among others, on the effect of written material on medication prescribing (the effectiveness in these studies varied between –3 and +12%) and on the use of radiology guidelines in primary care (31–34% change). Although some of the relative differences were large, none were statistically significant and the practical relevance was uncertain.

A review of 58 studies of the implementation of prevention in primary medical care contained three studies on the effectiveness of educational material (Hulscher et al. 1999). Providing general practitioners with materials for smoking cessation had a small but significant effect on physicians' routines (Kottke et al. 1989). Two

other studies (one on hypertension, the other on different types of prevention) did not show any effects.

A more recent review found 18 studies that showed, overall, modest effects of dissemination of educational material (Grimshaw et al. 2004). It may be helpful to distinguish between dissemination of reading materials (such as guideline text), on the one hand, and educational packages for active self-study (such as distant learning programmes) on the other. Active self-study can actually change professional behaviour, while it is unlikely that reading materials have such an effect. The costs of educational materials are relatively limited, so that the strategy may be cost-effective despite moderate effectiveness (Box 10.3).

Large-scale educational meetings

A literature overview of different types of education contained four studies on formal educational interventions (Davis et al. 1999). These studies focused on cholesterol screening, general practice care, mammography and cervical screening. None of the interventions changed physicians' routines (Box 10.4). Wensing et al. (1998) found 17 studies on providing educational material and formal group education, sometimes supplemented with patient-education materials. Two of these studies showed positive effects and six studies showed partly positive effects. The remaining nine studies did not show any positive effects.

Small-scale educational meetings

Thomson et al. (2001) found 10 comparisons of interactive workshops, with moderate or large effects in six and small effects in four of the studies. For 19 comparisons that combined workshops and didactic presentations, there were moderate or moderately large effects

---

Box 10.3 Guidelines for head injuries (Thomson *et al.* 1994)

Patients with head injuries have a risk for damage by a cerebral haematoma. If they attend the emergency department, this risk should be assessed adequately. In day-to-day practice a high number of inappropriate radiographs are ordered, so guidelines were developed for the appropriate management of these patients. The guidelines provided recommendations for the use of radiographs, such as loss of consciousness or amnesia, neurological symptoms, clear fluid or blood from the nose or throat, etc. The guidelines were printed on posters and charts and disseminated among all emergency departments in the north of England. An evaluation showed no consistent differences from the pre-intervention measurement. For example, there was an improvement in the number of radiographs ordered in one particular department, but a deterioration was seen in another department. The percentage of head-injury patients that were appropriately managed was 69% before the intervention and 64% after the intervention (no significant difference). The dissemination of educational materials was insufficient to change practice routines – a more intensive implementation strategy was thought to be needed.

Box 10.4 Guideline implementation in community pharmacies (Watson *et al.* 2002)

A randomised trial assessed the effects of educational strategies to implement evidence-based guidelines for the sale of over-the-counter (OTC) anti-fungals in community pharmacies. The study with 60 pharmacies compared postal dissemination of the guideline (control) with attendance at a continuing professional education session (intervention 1) and an educational outreach visit (intervention 2). Attendance of the educational session provided 2.5 hours of accreditation (locum costs and travel expenses were reimbursed). Pre- and post-intervention simulated patient visits were made to participating pharmacies to measure the effects (the simulated patients completed assessment forms after each visit). The primary outcome was the appropriateness of sale or no sale of OTC anti-fungals. There were no significant differences in the proportion of appropriate outcomes for any of the interventions.

in 12 comparisons and small effects in seven comparisons. So, interactive small-scale educational meetings seem to be at least moderately effective (*Box 10.5*). Davis *et al.* (1999) also found seven studies on mixed types of interactive and non-interactive education, five of which showed positive effects on physicians. Three of these seven studies also assessed the effects on patient outcomes – two showed positive results. Interestingly, there is little evidence that problem-based learning in continuing education is effective (Smits *et al.* 2002).

Educational outreach visits

Thomson *et al.* (1998a) found three studies in which educational outreach visits were compared with a group that did not receive an intervention – one study focused on the prescribing of NSAIDs (50% relative improvement after the intervention), a second focused on the prescribing of benzodiazepines (4% relative improvement compared to a group that only received written material) and a third group focused on the prescribing of cholesterol-lowering medication (27–50% relative improvement). Hulscher *et al.* (1999) found two further studies on educational outreach visits that aimed to improve prevention in primary care. The effects varied between the two studies, with one showing significant differences. *Box 10.6* illustrates a study of outreach visits in gynaecology departments.

DETERMINANTS OF THE EFFECTIVENESS OF EDUCATION

A range of factors may influence the effectiveness of educational strategies to implement innovations in clinical

Box 10.5 Pharmacological quality circles (von Ferber *et al.* 1999)

In a German project, 79 physicians participated in small-scale group meetings that took place eight times over a period of 18 months. These physicians were selected because of their relatively expensive prescribing patterns. In each meeting a specific clinical problem was discussed and written information on medication was provided, as was feedback on their prescribing behaviour. After this programme the physicians prescribed less medication that was not evidence-based, such as specific anti-rheumatic medication. Furthermore, there was less inappropriately long prescribing of medications, such as benzodiazepines and non-steroidal anti-inflammatory drugs (NSAIDs). Relatively new medications, such as proton-pump inhibitors, were not prescribed significantly more often. The study concluded that this method was appropriate to improve the quality of prescribing and reduced the costs of healthcare.

Box 10.6 Outreach visits in gynaecology departments (Wyatt *et al.* 1998)

In a randomised experiment, 25 gynaecology departments were allocated to an intervention group or a control group. The 12 practices in the intervention group were visited by a respected gynaecologist, who discussed the effectiveness and use of several procedures and introduced a copy of the Cochrane database, along with other materials. The control group did not receive an intervention. Outcome measures in this study included the number of clinical procedures, such as antibiotics prophylaxis before Caesarean sections and the prescribing of corticosteroids for premature deliveries. Data from medical records were collected, at baseline and after 9 months, for 30 patients whose care covered 10–14 days of clinical practice. The study showed that both the intervention and control groups adhered well to the scientific evidence and the outreach visit added nothing.

practice. A number of factors described by educational theories are presented in Chapter 2. This chapter focuses on five factors, described by reviews of empirical studies on educational interventions:

- Duration of the education;
- Group composition;
- Needs assessment;
- Active participation;
- Use of opinion leaders.

It is plausible that an educational programme may be more effective if more time is invested in it. The participants thus have more exposure to what is being taught and more repetition can be integrated into the programme. One review showed that continuing education that lasted 1 day is less effective than education of several days, but there was hardly any difference between education of 2 days and education of more than 12 months (Beaudry 1989).

Another possible factor is the composition of the group of care providers who participate in the programme. There was no difference between the education of nurses compared with a multidisciplinary group that included nurses along with other healthcare professionals (Beaudry 1989). However, educational programmes were more effective if all the participants were from one organisation compared to groups of care providers from different organisations (Beaudry 1989).

A third factor is the assessment of the learning needs of care providers prior to an educational activity (*Box 10.7*). This fits within the model for implementation, described in this book, in which an analysis of the target group and setting precedes the choice of an implementation strategy. This assessment may focus both on the content (which topics) and/or on the format of the educational programme (which format fits with the preferences and learning styles). The programme can be built to the needs of the target group, or a range of programmes can be delivered to meet individual needs ('tailoring').

One review showed that formal needs assessment did not result in better effects (Beaudry 1989), but other reviews suggested that the identification of care providers with poor performance or of barriers to change clearly improved the effectiveness of continuing education (Davis *et al.* 1995, 1999). A simple reference to deficiencies in care provision was not related to the effectiveness of education (Davis *et al.* 1995). The actual effect of needs assessment on educational interventions remains unclear (*Box 10.8*).

Active participation of professionals in the educational programme, and control over the learning process, is also expected to improve the effectiveness of education. This was confirmed in a review of studies on computerised learning (Cohen and Dacanay 1992). Active participation may increase motivation and

---

Box 10.7 Why do care providers participate in continuing education?

The literature suggests a range of motivations:

- Education is seen as part of their profession – they are interested in the subject, they think that continuing education can confirm or change behaviour that they have learned, they have specific objectives (knowledge or behaviour) and they feel it is an escape from routines and an opportunity to meet colleagues (Richards and Cohen 1980);
- An educational programme is more likely to be chosen if it contributes to accreditation, if the subject is important, if presenters have a good reputation, if there are no conflicting social and/or family obligations and if the travelling distance is not too large (Slotnick *et al.* 1994);
- Professionals participate in continuing education because they like to learn new things, want to develop as a professional, experience external pressure, expect social interaction and want to escape from routine and boredom (Tassone and Heck 1997).

Box 10.8 Effectiveness of two educational strategies (Borgiel *et al.* 1999)

In a controlled trial of 56 physicians, practice routines were assessed and a 'Practice Assessment Report' provided, along with targeted support from tutors. The effects were measured in almost 2400 patients, with respect to quality of routines, registration, prevention, prescribing and patient satisfaction with care. There were no differences between the intervention group and the control group after the intervention. Adding targeted education based on the assessment of performance measurements did not contribute to the effectiveness of care.

provide the opportunity to focus the programme on personal learning needs. Another review suggested that the effectiveness is largest if the incidental participation of the learner is integrated into the educational programme. The effects of programmes with incidental participation were better than those of programmes without participation or programmes with frequent, systematic participation (Beaudry 1989).

Finally the use of opinion leaders in educational activities may influence effectiveness (*Table 10.2*).

Opinion leaders are individuals whom others see as authorities in a specific area. There are structured methods to identify these persons by interviewing healthcare professionals in a specific setting or discipline. The opinion leaders may have different roles, varying from signing a letter that accompanies educational material to delivering lectures during educational meetings, chairing a local group session or visiting care providers in their practice (*Box 10.9*). The literature shows that the use of opinion leaders has overall small positive effects, although there are also examples of studies in which no effects were found.

DISCUSSION AND CONCLUSIONS

Education of care providers can lead to changes of professional behaviour, but the effects of most types of education are small (less than 10% absolute change). Health professionals learn in many ways other than by formal education, particularly through contacts with colleagues, patients and others (Owen *et al.* 1989). The small changes may, nevertheless, be clinically relevant. For instance, an increase from 60 to 70% adherence to a recommendation or new procedure is similar to an odds ratio of 1.55, which may be regarded as clinically relevant if it was related to pharmacological treatment. In addition, the consequences of continuing education for reducing the costs and improving effectiveness and efficiency of healthcare provision may be substantial, if small effects can be achieved on a large scale in the healthcare system. The literature also suggests that the effectiveness of education can be improved if the programme has specific characteristics, such as a longer duration, a needs assessment prior to the programme, the opportunity

Table 10.2 Reviews of studies on use of opinion leaders in education

Study	Conclusions
Davis *et al.* (1995)	Review of three studies – all the studies showed positive effects for at least some of the outcome measures.
Oxman *et al.* (1995)	Review of five studies – the effectiveness varied from not significant to substantially effective.
Thomson *et al.* (1998b)	Review of six studies – five of the six studies showed some effect on at least one outcome measure. The absolute risk on inappropriate routines (for instance, corticosteroids instead of aspirin for rheumatoid arthritis patients) was reduced; the reduction varied between −0.08 and 0.31.

Box 10.9 Implementation of dementia guidelines by neurologists using opinion leaders (Gifford *et al.* 1999)

A written survey was performed among a sample of neurologists in six areas in the USA to identify 12 local opinion leaders, who were then used in an educational programme on guidelines for dementia from the American Academy of Neurology. The educational strategy was a mailed self-learning package, materials (such as a questionnaire for depression in dementia patients), a chart with factual information for patients and carers and several reminders of the messages. In addition, neurologists in the intervention group were invited to a seminar of 3 hours, during which opinion leaders gave lectures. The evaluation showed that neurologists in the intervention group adhered better to about half of the recommendations compared to neurologists in the control group (measured with paper-based scenarios). This effect was stronger in those neurologists who actually attended the seminar (about half of the total number invited).

for active participation, a voluntary character and the use of opinion leaders in the education. Developers of educational programmes should integrate these characteristics as much as possible.

There are indications that education that is interactive and personal (small-scale educational meetings and educational outreach visits) is more effective than passive education (written material and large-scale educational meetings). The social interaction element may strongly motivate specific health professionals and facilitate learning processes that could not be achieved through self-study. However, written material is not necessarily ineffective, particularly if it requires active self-study by using knowledge tests, needs assessment and practical exercises. Most important may be that education be related to individual motivations of participants – social interaction integrated into the education programme is one method to achieve this. Education of health professionals is probably a necessary component of any implementation strategy, but it is likely that additional interventions are needed most of the time to change behaviour and maintain the changes.

Recommended literature

Davis D, O'Brien MA, Freemantle N, *et al*. (1999). Impact of formal continuing medical education: Do conferences, workshops, rounds, and other traditional continuing education activities change physician behavior or health care outcomes? *JAMA* **282**:867–874.

Grimshaw JM, Shirran L, Thomas R, *et al*. (2001). Changing provider behavior. An overview of systematic reviews of interventions. *Med Care* **39**:S2–45.

References

Albanese MA and Mitchell S (1993). Problem-based learning: A review of literature on its outcomes and implementation issues. *Acad Med*. **68**(1):52–81.

Beaudry JS (1989). The effectiveness of continuing medical education: A quantitative synthesis. *J Cont Educ Health Prof*. **9**:285–307.

Beyer M, Gerlach FM, Flies U, *et al*. (2003). The development of quality circles/peer review groups as a tool for quality improvement in Europe. Results of a survey in 26 European countries. *Fam Pract*. **20**:443–451.

Borgiel A, Williams J, Davis D, *et al*. (1999). Evaluating the effectiveness of two educational interventions in family practice. *Can Med Assoc J*. **161**:965–970.

Bower P, Garralda E, Kramer T, Harrington R and Sibbald B (2001). The treatment of child and adolescent mental health problems in primary care: A systematic review. *Fam Pract*. **17**:373–382.

Brown CA, Belfield CR and Field SJ (2002). Cost effectiveness of continuing professional development in health care: A critical review of the evidence. *BMJ* **324**:652–655.

Cohen PA and Dacanay LS (1992). Computer-based instruction and health professions education. A meta-analysis of outcomes. *Eval Health Prof*. **15**:259–281.

Davis DA, Thomson MA, Oxman AD, *et al*. (1992). Evidence for the effectiveness of CME. A review of 50 randomized controlled trials. *JAMA* **268**(9):1111–1117.

Davis DA, Thomson MA, Oxman AD, *et al*. (1995). Changing physician performance. A systematic review of the effect of continuing medical education strategies. *JAMA* **274**:700–705.

Davis D, O'Brien MA, Freemantle N, *et al*. (1999). Impact of formal continuing medical education: Do conferences, workshops, rounds, and other traditional continuing education activities change physician behavior or health care outcomes? *JAMA* **282**:867–874.

Ferber L von, Bausch J, Köster I, *et al*. (1999). Pharmacotherapeutic circles. Results of an 18-month peer-review prescribing-improvement programme for general practitioners. *Pharmacoeconomics* **16**:273–283.

Freemantle N, Harvey EL, Wolf F, *et al*. (1998). Printed educational materials to improve the behaviour of health care professionals and patient outcomes. The Cochrane Library, Issue 3. Oxford: Update Software.

Gifford DR, Holloway RG, Frankel MR, *et al*. (1999). Improving adherence to dementia guidelines through education and opinion leaders. A randomized controlled trial. *Ann Intern Med*. **131**:237–246.

Gill PS, Mäkelä M, Vermeulen KM, *et al*. (1999). Changing doctor prescribing behaviour: A review. *Pharm World Sci*. **21**(4):158–167.

Greenhalgh T, Toon P, Russell J, Wong G, Plumb G and Macfarlane F (2003). Transferability of principles of evidence based medicine to improve educational quality: Systematic review and case study of an online course in primary care. *BMJ* **326**:142–145.

Grimshaw J, Thomas RE, Maclennan G, *et al*. (2004). Effectiveness and efficiency of guideline dissemination and implementation strategies. *Health Technol Assess*. **8**(6):1–84.

Gurwitz JH, Soumerai SB and Avorn J (1990). Improving medication prescribing and utilization in the nursing home. *J Am Geriatr Soc*. **38**(5):542–552.

Harvey EL, Glenny AM, Kirk SFL and Summerbell CD (2001). Improving health professionals' management and the organisation of care for overweight and obese people. The Cochrane Library, Issue 2. Oxford: Update Software.

Hasan A, Pozzi M and Hamilton JRL (2000). New surgical procedures: Can we minimise the learning curve? *BMJ* **320**:171–173.

Hulscher MEJL, Drenth BB van, Wouden JC van der, *et al*. (1997). Changing preventive practice: A controlled trial on the effects of outreach visits to organize prevention of cardiovascular disease. *Qual Health Care* **6**:19–24.

Hulscher MEJL, Wensing M, Grol RPTM, *et al*. (1999). Interventions to improve the delivery of preventive services in primary care. *Am J Public Health* **89**(5):737–746.

Hutchinson L (1999). Evaluating and researching the effectiveness of educational interventions. *BMJ* **318**:1267–1269.

Irby DM (1995). Teaching and learning in ambulatory care settings: A thematic review of the literature. *Acad Med*. **70**:898–931.

Kaufman DM (2003). Applying educational theory in practice. *BMJ* **326**:213–216.

Kottke T, Brekke ML, Solberg LL, *et al*. (1989). A randomized trial to increase smoking intervention by physicians. Doctors helping smokers, round I. *JAMA* **261**:2101–2106.

Lancaster T, Silagy C, Fowler G, *et al*. (1998). Training health professionals in smoking cessation. The Cochrane Library, Issue 4. Oxford: Update Software.

Leeuwen YD van, Mol SSM, Pollemans MC, *et al*. (1995). Change in knowledge of general practitioners during their professional careers. *Fam Pract*. **12**:313–317.

Mathers NJ, Challis MC, Howe AC, *et al*. (1999). Portfolios in continuing medical education – effective and efficient? *Med Educ*. **33**:521–530.

Newman P and Peile E (2002). Valuing learner's experience and supporting further growth: Educational models to help experienced adult learners in medicine. *BMJ* **325**:200–202.

Owen PA, Allerly LA, Harding KG, *et al*. (1989). General practitioners' continuing medical education within and outside their practice. *BMJ* **299**:238–240.

Oxman AD, Thomson MA, Davis DA, *et al*. (1995). No magic bullets. A systematic review of 102 trials of interventions to help health care professionals deliver services more effectively or efficiently. *Can Med Assoc J*. **153**:1423–1431.

Petersen S (1999). Time for evidence based medical education. Tomorrow's doctors need informed educators and not amateur tutors. *BMJ* **318**:1233–1234.

Pippalla RS, Riley DA and Chinburapa V (1995). Influencing the prescribing behaviour of physicians: A meta evaluation. *J Clin Pharm Ther*. **20**:189–198.

Qureshi N, Allen J and Hapgood R (2002). A systematic review of educational outreach visits for non-prescribing interventions in general practice. *Eur J Gen Pract*. **8**:31–36.

Ram P, Grol R, Rethans JJ, *et al*. (1999). Assessment of general practitioners by video observation of communicative and medical performance in daily practice: Issues of validity, reliability and feasibility. *Med Educ*. **33**:447–454.

Richards RK and Cohen RM (1980). Why physicians attend traditional CME programs. *J Med Educ*. **55**:479–485.

Slotnick HB, Raszokowski RR, Jensen CE, *et al*. (1994). Physician preferences in CME including insights into education versus promotion. *J Cont Educ Health Prof*. **14**:173–186.

Smits PBA, Verbeek HAM and De Buisonjé CD (2002). Problem based learning in continuing education: A review of controlled evaluation studies. *BMJ* **324**:153–156.

Solomon DH, Hashimoto H, Daltroy L, *et al*. (1998). Techniques to improve physicians' use of diagnostic tests. *JAMA* **280**:2020–2027.

Soumerai SB and Avorn J (1990). Principles of educational outreach ('academic detailing') to improve clinical decision making. *JAMA* **263**:549–556.

Soumerai SB, McLaughin TJ and Avorn J (1989). Improving drug prescribing in primary care: A critical analysis of the experimental literature. *Milbank Q*. **67**:268–317.

Tassone MR and Heck CS (1997). Motivational orientations of allied health care professionals participating in continuing education. *J Cont Educ Health Prof*. **17**:97–105.

Thomas LH, McColl E, Cullum N, *et al*. (1998). Effect of clinical guidelines in nursing, midwifery, and the therapies: A systematic review of evaluations. *Qual Health Care* **7**:183–191.

Thomson R, Gray J, Madhok R, *et al*. (1994). Effect of guidelines on management of head injury on record keeping and decision making in accident and emergency departments. *Qual Health Care* **3**:86–91.

Thomson MA, Oxman AD, Davis DA, *et al*. (1998a). Outreach visits to improve health professionals' practice and health care outcomes. The Cochrane Library, Issue 3. Oxford: Update Software.

Thomson MA, Oxman AD, Haynes RB, *et al*. (1998b). Local opinion leaders to improve health professionals' practice and health care outcomes. The Cochrane Library, Issue 3. Oxford: Update Software.

Thomson O'Brien MA, Freemantle N, Oxman AD, Wolf F, Davis DA and Herrin J (2001). Continuing education meetings and workshops: Effects on professional practice and health care outcomes. The Cochrane Library, Issue 2. Oxford: Update Software.

Waddell D (1991). The effects of continuing education on nursing practice: A meta-analysis. *J Cont Educ Nurs*. **22**(3):113–118.

Watson MC, Bond CM, Grimshaw JM, Mollison J, Ludbrook A and Walker AE (2002). Educational strategies to promote evidence-based community pharmacy practice: A cluster randomized controlled trial. *Fam Pract*. **19**:529–536.

Wensing M, Weijden T van der and Grol R (1998). Implementing guidelines and innovations in general practice: Which interventions are effective? *Br J Gen Pract*. **48**:991–997.

Weijden T van der, Wensing M, Giffel M, *et al*. (2000). *Interventions Aimed at Influencing the Use of Diagnostic Tests*. Report. Maastricht: WOK.

Worrall G, Chaulk P and Freake D (1997). The effects of clinical practice guidelines on patient outcomes in primary care: a systematic review. *Can Med Assoc J*. **156**(12):1705–1712.

Wyatt JC, Paterson-Brown S, Johanson R, *et al*. (1998). Randomised trial of educational visits to enhance use of systematic reviews in 25 obstetric units. *BMJ* **317**:1041–1046.

Zwarenstein M, Reeves S, Barr H, Hammick M, Koppel I and Atkins J (2000). Interprofessional education: Effects on professional practice and health care outcomes. The Cochrane Library, Issue 3. Oxford: Update Software.

Chapter 11

Feedback and reminders

Trudy van der Weijden and Richard Grol

KEY MESSAGES

- Feedback and reminders can change behaviour effectively, but their effect is dependent on the underlying evidence, the degree of understanding of the barriers to adherence to the new system and the level to which the content and format of the reminders is tailored to the barriers to change.
- The effectiveness of feedback and reminders may be influenced by the motivation of the recipient, the timing and frequency of feedback and reminders, and the type of data on which feedback or reminders are given (source, validity, volume, format, active or passive).
- Feedback can be comparative – data from peers are given for comparison. This may engage the recipients, which makes it more likely that they will study the feedback data. In addition, meeting in small groups, with interprofessional differences as the focus for discussion, may increase the effect.
- Feedback and reminders seem to work well for implementing guidelines on test ordering, prescription and primary prevention.

Box 11.1 Feedback regarding preventive action (Szczepura *et al.* 1994)

The effect of various forms of feedback were evaluated in an experiment that involved almost 200 physicians. Focus group meetings were organised beforehand to determine the content for the feedback. The doctors were asked what information would help them set priorities for improving quality of care. They wanted feedback about the extent to which a range of risk factors were recorded in their patients' records. The final content of the feedback reports was:

- Number and quality of cervical swabs;
- Proportion of children immunised;
- Proportion of children undergoing developmental screening;
- Proportion of children with a low birth weight;
- Proportion of children whose mothers smoked;
- Proportion of children breastfed at the age of 1 month;
- Number of laboratory tests requested per 1000 patients annually;
- Number of other risk factors (weight, smoking, alcohol consumption, blood pressure, etc.).

The investigators audited the patient records.

The feedback was returned in schematic and standardised forms so that the physicians could compare their own data with those of colleagues. A second group of doctors received this feedback and an outreach visit to their practices 4–6 weeks later. The visitor used a protocol for discussing the figures with the physicians. However, the choice to initiate improvements was left to the practitioners themselves. Feedback about the same items was given again 12 and 24 months after the first feedback report.

A range of organisational changes were in place at the practice level after both 1 and 2 years. Apart from these there were no significant changes. The doctors reported having no problems with the validity of the feedback data. The degree of acceptance of the schematic feedback itself was very high, although 30% of those who had received the feedback followed by a visit judged this negatively.

INTRODUCTION

One of the most common methods for implementing innovations or changes in clinical practice is to give feedback on the care that has been delivered and possible departures from optimal practice. In addition, one can also give information or a signal (reminder) at the moment a decision has to be made and certain actions should, or should not, be performed.

In this chapter, 'feedback' refers to returning information about their actions to professionals, practices or institutions to increase their insight into these actions. The information covers a specified time period, and is collected from data on actual practice, often referred to as an 'audit' or 'clinical audit' in the literature. It is not clear exactly how feedback works to change behaviour. However, it is reasonable to assume that it increases awareness of any discrepancy that exists between what people think they are doing or want to do, and what they are really doing. Such a discrepancy is not acceptable for many people and therefore encourages change.

In this chapter, the term 'reminder' refers to information (whether verbal, on paper or on a computer screen) that has been designed to remind a professional of a certain recommendation for good care and to let him or her take action at a certain moment. This appears to be effective in some instances, but not in others.

The purpose of this chapter is to provide some insight into the range of options when developing feedback or reminder strategies to help implement innovations or changes in patient care. We suggest that the effectiveness may be increased in a number of ways:

- Taking into account existing barriers to improving care;
- Acquiring insight into the target group;
- Adjusting the content, form, frequency and timing of the feedback or the reminder to the needs of the target group;
- Choosing the right person or organisation to distribute the feedback or reminders.

Feedback and reminders have been used as interventions to change healthcare for many years (Box 11.2). Sometimes, the purpose is to decrease redundant medical actions (e.g. unnecessary diagnostic tests or prescriptions) and the costs of the care at the same time. Sometimes, the aim is to improve the quality of care and increase actions in line with existing guidelines or scientific insights. Feedback and reminders are potentially effective interventions, but in literature reviews their effectiveness varies from study to study (Grimshaw *et al.* 2001, 2004; Walton *et al.* 1999; Hunt *et al.* 1998; Thomson *et al.* 1997; Balas *et al.* 1996; Buntinx *et al.* 1993, Mugford *et al.* 1991). The difference in effectiveness among the various studies is partly because they differ widely in the form and content of the feedback or reminders, in the target groups, in the clinical subjects or the type of care to be improved, and in the methods used to study the effect of the feedback or reminders. This means that it is not possible to design an optimum intervention solely on the basis of the published evidence.

The various theories about effective implementation (see Chapter 2) suggest that feedback and reminders are likely to be appropriate interventions to change clinical practice. Communication theories, for instance, emphasise effective communication with specific attention to the characteristics of the recipient. This could be achieved by giving individualised comparative feedback that shows how an individual's behaviour compares to that

Box 11.2 Reminders regarding internists' test requests (Tierney *et al.* 1988)

Decision-making theory assumes that a doctor makes better decisions regarding test ordering if the disease probability of the individual patient has been estimated correctly. This estimation seems to be difficult for doctors. Therefore, investigators at the Indiana University School of Medicine developed computer software to estimate, on the basis of clinical patient information, disease probabilities for individual patients. The aim was to reduce the costs of the tests requested by internists. For eight selected tests [including urine tests, chest radiography and electrocardiograms (ECG)], 112 participating internists were asked for a small number of items of clinical patient data (seriousness of the complaints or symptoms), the reason for testing and an estimation of the chance for an abnormal test result. Data that had already been entered in the computerised patient file, such as previous laboratory results, diagnoses and prescribed therapies, were also used. An automatic reminder showing the chance of an abnormal test appeared when one of the eight tests was requested. The doctor then had to choose 'cancel' or 'continue'. During the 6 month experiment, the costs of the eight tests dropped by 9% compared with those in the control group.

of peers. Education theory emphasises intrinsic motivation and learning on the basis of experience. Feedback on behaviour can heighten awareness of one's own way of working and its problems. Economic theories emphasise management via financial incentives and budgets. Feedback about the costs that a professional incurs in comparison with those of colleagues may be used, or reminders about costs of investigations given at the time of the ordering could be considered.

Providing professionals with *new* clinical information about patients that does not directly reflect the clinical practice of the professional, such as quality of life scores from an instrument for measuring depression, are not addressed here. They are discussed in Chapter 13, on patient-oriented interventions. Giving performance information to policy makers or to the community instead of to teams, groups of professionals or individual professionals also does not fall within the scope of this chapter (Domenighetti *et al.* 1988).

Here, we first elaborate the definitions of feedback and reminders, then the current state of knowledge about the effectiveness of feedback and reminders are described and some practical examples are presented to illustrate the literature. Finally, we give some suggestions as to how feedback and reminders may be built into an effective implementation plan.

DEFINITIONS OF FEEDBACK AND REMINDER

The various characteristics of feedback and reminders are described below (for a summary, see *Table 11.2*).

Feedback

Feedback is concerned with sending information back to an individual professional, practice, team or institution. This information can be collected on the basis of an internal audit, in which the professionals actively participate in the data collection, or it can be based on an assessment of care conducted by others (external audit). The information concerns a given period and is usually about a patient population, although it may also be given on individual patients. It may be about aspects of clinical performance, about costs or about outcomes of care, and it can be oral or written and with or without supporting materials. It can be non-comparative or it can contain a comparison with colleagues, or a judgement with reference to guidelines, criteria, best practices or recommendations for optimal care. Feedback is generally given *after* the actual care described has ended and thus is a retro-

spective approach, although the area of activity, such as test ordering, is usually ongoing.

There are multiple possible variations in the configuration of the content and delivery of feedback. The messenger (who gives the feedback?), the method (how?), the content of feedback, the frequency of feedback (how often?) and the intensity (how much?) can all vary.

We can distinguish between two types of origin of feedback data. The information can be based on direct observation of care provision (by audio- or videotapes of consultations, by physically being present at patient contacts or by the use of and report by simulated patients). Alternatively, the information can be based on indirect observation, such as self-monitoring (computerised or not), patient record audit, structured interviews or enquiries among professionals (*Box 11.3*). It can also be based on data provided by third parties (population morbidity and mortality data, error or critical incidence registers, performance figures from the healthcare insurer, prescription data from pharmacies, request data from laboratories or patients' opinions about the care provided).

Providing comparable information about the clinical practice of colleagues is a potentially powerful addition to the feedback information.

Reminders

A reminder is a piece of patient- or consultation-specific information or information on groups of patients that is intended to remind a professional to perform or to avoid a specific clinical action. The reminder is usually given *before* or *during* the patient contact and thus can be seen as a prospective approach.

The following taxonomy of reminders (adapted from Thorsen and Mäkelä 1999) details both the content of reminders and their timing (the degree to which the reminder is linked to the moment of clinical decision making).

Content
Implicit reminders
Implicit reminders, for example, give the predictive value of a test result together with the test result itself (without giving an explicit recommendation for action) or they give information about the costs of specific tests requested.

Administrative support
Administrative support, for example, involves stickers on patient files as a system for follow-up appointments

Box 11.3 A feedback report (Verstappen *et al.* 2003)

The number of tests related to heart disease and/or hypertension requested by a primary care physician in 6 months, standardised to a Dutch norm practice of 2350 patients, are presented in this report. The clinical chemical tests involved are cholesterol (chol), high-density lipoprotein (HDL), potassium (K), creatinine (creat), low-density lipoprotein (LDL), sodium (Na), triglycerides (TG) and urea. The function tests involved are the ECG and the exercise ECG (E-ECG).

For serum cholesterol tests, the first column shows 34 cholesterol tests ordered per 6 months (for this particular physician, left column). The column in the centre shows the average number of requests made by physicians in the local group (*n* = 69 cholesterol tests per 6 months). The column on the right shows the average regional figure (*n* = 56 tests ordered). The doctor illustrated here requests relatively few cholesterol tests (too few?) and a relatively high number (too many?) of exercise ECGs and urea tests. The white (lowest) parts of the columns show the proportion of the tests with abnormal results, the so-called 'diagnostic yield' of the test. A diagnostic yield that deviates from the regional figures can be an indication of underuse or overuse of diagnostic test ordering.

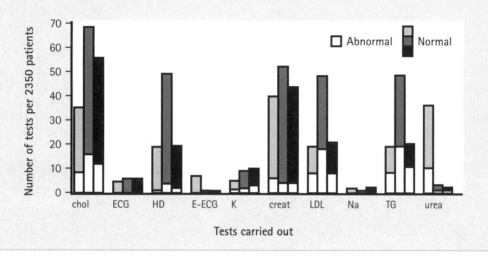

(to remind a professional of specific guideline recommendations) or posters in the work place with a reminder message that is not patient specific.

Comprehensive medical report

Comprehensive medical report are reports sent direct to the professional from, for example, the laboratory, diagnostic centre or chemist after an abnormal result has been noticed or a medication with interaction risks has been prescribed. Such a report contains additional information with specific recommendations for action, such as providing a signal that a certain preventive check is necessary.

Computerised, decision-making support

Computerised, decision-making support is an active 'knowledge system' in which patient data are used to generate patient-specific advice. For example, when a medicine is prescribed, the computer may suggest alternative medication. This reminder method has two forms – proactive and reactive computerised reminders. The professional can deliberately consult the proactive reminder in specific cases by using a decision-making support system. An example of a proactive reminder is when the doctor clicks the reminder function to check whether he or she should prescribe a flu vaccination for this particular patient (*Box 11.4*). The reactive reminder, unasked, sends a signal to the professional if the knowledge system runs into clinical actions that do not satisfy the medical indications, or if specific clinical actions have not been performed. An example of a reactive reminder is when, during office hours, and after the electronic patient files have been updated, a doctor receives a message that the diabetes patient concerned has not yet had a vaccination.

Timing

Simultaneous, concurrent reminders

Information is directed to the professional at the moment of a contact, to remind him or her of (un)desired actions for individual patients. An example is to show the professional a reminder of the correct medication dose in the patient file.

Reminders between two contacts with the same patient (intervisit reminders)

Information is directed to a professional or team after a patient contact, just before a following contact, when it has become clear that care for this patient is suboptimal, for example when a notice of the correct follow-up after an abnormal test result does not appear in the patient's file.

RESEARCH ON THE EFFECTS OF FEEDBACK AND REMINDERS

Over the past ten years there has been a marked increase in the number of published studies reporting the effects of implementation strategies, and particularly of feedback and reminders. These have been accompanied by several literature overviews that summarise the results of these studies. Grimshaw and Russell (1993), for example, summarised the effects of strategies to implement clinical guidelines. They described 59 controlled studies – feedback was evaluated in 11 of these and the effect of reminders in 22. Wensing *et al.* (1998) described 143 stud-

Box 11.4 An electronic reminder (Bindels *et al.* 2000)

An example of a reactive electronic reminder for test-ordering behaviour is illustrated below (vraagstelling, question; chemisch bloed, chemical blood; overige, rest; beeldvorming, imaging; cervix, cervical). The doctor has to give the knowledge system certain patient-specific data, such as the intended test(s) to be ordered, the working hypothesis, the reason for request, etc. The system then prompts the doctor with a reminder if the ordering is not in line with the guideline recommendations. This example focuses on the unnecessary use of diagnostic tests.

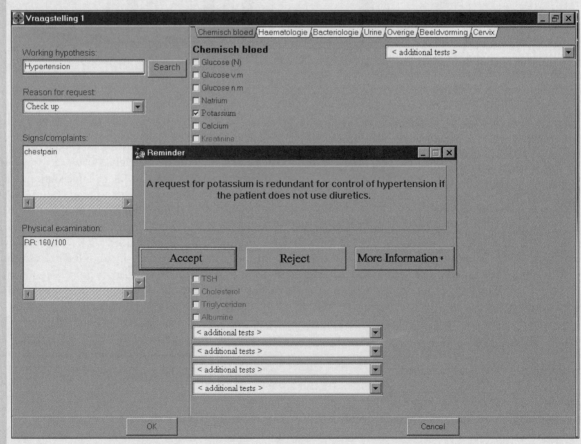

ies (of which 61 were controlled studies) on the effect of implementing guidelines on the performance of professionals in general practice. At least 32% of these studies investigated the effect of feedback, and 27% that of reminders. In a recent review by Grimshaw *et al.* (2004), again looking at strategies to implement clinical guidelines, 235 controlled studies were included, of which 28% evaluated the effect of feedback (4% as single interventions and 24% as part of multifaceted interventions), and 44% the effect of reminders (13% as single intervention and 31% as part of multifaceted interventions).

As well as these general reviews, there are specific literature overviews of the effects of feedback and reminders (examples are given in *Table 11.1*). There are also reviews of a range of implementation strategies, but within specific clinical domains, such as preventive care and test ordering, in which feedback and reminders play an important part (again, examples are given in *Table*

11.1). Feedback or reminders were used in about half the studies on the improvement of test ordering (van der Weijden *et al.* 2000; Solomon *et al.* 1998). Often, feedback was used to reduce the overuse of laboratory tests; reminders, however, were often used to improve adherence to guidelines on appropriate test ordering.

The effectiveness of feedback and reminders appears to be variable (*Table 11.1*). This can be explained partly by the heterogeneity of the studies. The content of the feedback and the reminders differed considerably between studies. Even if the interventions were comparable with respect to content, they often differed in terms of intensity or format – some studies looked at intensive feedback or reminders and others at minimal forms. Other sources of variation were the differences between the types of professionals or the patient populations. In addition, there were shortcomings in the research meth-

Table 11.1 Literature reviews of studies of the effects of feedback and reminders

Review	Domain	Total studies	Intervention	Results, author's summary
Literature reviews specific to the effect of feedback and/or reminders				
Mugford *et al.* (1991)	Preventive care, diagnostic tests, prescription behaviour, certain surgical procedures	36 CT[a]	36 Feedback	Varying effects: the closer to the moment of care giving, the more the effect of the feedback. Especially effective for motivated professionals.
Buntinx *et al.* (1993)	Preventive care and diagnostic tests in primary care	26 CT	19 Feedback 9 Reminders	Varying effects: 5–50% improvement in volume measures. Reminders seem to have a little more effect than feedback on adherence to guidelines.
Austin *et al.* (1994)	Preventive care	10 CT	10 Reminders	Reminders may increase provision of preventive care services. Significant odds ratios for cervical screening (1.18) and for tetanus vaccination (2.82).
Balas *et al.* (1996)	Diagnostic tests, prescriptions and total costs of care	16 CT	16 Feedback[b]	No effect in two studies, varying effects in the others. Pooled odds ratio of 1.1, statistically significant, but clinically irrelevant.
Shea *et al.* (1996)	Preventive care	16 CT	16 Reminders	Computer reminders increased six groups of preventive practices; combined odds ratio 1.77 (95% confidence interval, range 1.38–2.27)
Beilby and Silagy (1997)	Diagnostic tests, prescriptions, referrals to specialists	6 CT	6 Feedback on costs	Feedback on costs may change behaviour in all areas. Sustainability of the changes was not studied.
Thomson *et al.* (1997)	Preventive care, diagnostic tests, general management of medical problems	37 CT	37 Feedback	The relative difference between intervention and control group varied from −16% to +152%. (cont.)

Table 11.1 (*cont.*) Literature reviews of studies of the effects of feedback and reminders

Review	Domain	Total studies	Intervention	Results, author's summary
Literature reviews specific to the effect of feedback and/or reminders (cont.)				
Hunt *et al.* (1998)	Preventive care, differential diagnosis, test ordering and prescribing behaviour, general management of medical problems, procedures for hospital admission and discharge	68 CT	68 Reminders, computerised decision-support systems	In 65 studies the effects were described at the doctor's level with a positive effect in 43. In 14 studies the effects were described at the patient's level with a positive effect in six.
Walton *et al.* (1999)	Determining the optimum drug dose	18 CT	18 Reminders, computerised decision-support systems	Computer support helps doctors in hospitals to tailor drug doses more closely to the needs of individual patients. Further research is necessary to evaluate the benefits of general use.
Literature reviews of the effect of implementation strategies in specific clinical areas				
Solomon *et al.* (1998)	Use of diagnostic tests	49 PP[c] and CT	24 Feedback 5 Reminders	13 of 21 studies with single interventions were successful. 24 of 28 studies with combined interventions were successful.
Hulscher *et al.* (1999)	Preventive primary care: cervical screening, occult blood faeces, alcohol, smoking, dietary counselling, vaccination programmes	58 CT	22 Feedback 28 Reminders	Feedback only: some studies showed no effect, others 4–26% improvement. Reminders only: 6–24% improvement. Combinations with feedback: some studies showed no effect, others 4–57% improvement. Combinations with reminders: 7–35% improvement.
Gill *et al.* (1999)	Prescribing behaviour	79 CT	33 Feedback or Reminders	In about half of these studies positive findings were found.
van der Weijden *et al.* (2000)	Use of diagnostic tests to reduce over use of tests or improve adherence to guidelines	80 CT	25 Feedback 18 Reminders	Varying effects: feedback can be effective in reducing unnecessary use of tests and in improving following clinical guidelines; reminders (particularly computerised decision support) seem more suitable for improving adherence to guidelines.

[a]CT, controlled trials, controlled studies.
[b]Feedback with comparisons with colleagues (profiling reports).
[c]PP, pre- and poststudies, uncontrolled studies.

ods used. Methods of randomisation were often poor or not done at all. This may have resulted in incomparable test groups – for example, in non-randomised designs, professionals more motivated to improve quality may be more likely to volunteer for a study and thus have a greater chance of being allocated to the intervention group. This may have introduced bias into the study with the possible overestimation of any effects of the intervention.

DETERMINANTS OF EFFECTIVENESS OF FEEDBACK AND REMINDERS

No clear general conclusions can be drawn from the literature reviews above about any consistent effects of feedback and reminders, nor the attributes that might influence such effects. However, they do give insight into some of the possible determinants of successful feedback and reminder strategies, discussed further in this section (*Table 11.2*).

Two examples that show the variable effect of feedback and the impact of specific determinants are given in *Boxes 11.5* and *11.6*. O'Connell *et al.* (1999; *Box 11.5*) showed that impersonal written feedback on data derived from a central database was not effective, despite comparisons with colleagues. However, Winkens *et al.* (1992, 1995, 1996; *Box 11.6*) showed that personal feedback with general and patient-specific characteristics, given by a respected colleague, can be effective. This feedback was maintained for a long time and was integrated into a regional approach of continuing medical education and distribution of clinical guidelines on test ordering.

The *source* and the *messenger* for the feedback or reminder information may be important. The initiator or provider of the information should ideally be a respected institute, a respected colleague or a person more highly placed in the work hierarchy. In the studies described, the feedback information is sometimes personally given to an individual or group. The person who is directly responsible for clinical decision making should receive the information directly and, preferably, so should the superiors or policy makers who exercise control over the organisation's quality-improvement activities.

Table 11.2 Feedback and reminder characteristics

Timing in the care process	Characteristics of the strategy	To be combined with
Feedback		
Afterwards	The data source: validity of the data dependent on the professional's direct or indirect observation	Educational materials or meetings
	The messenger: colleague (opinion leader), academic investigator, insurer or financier, authority	
	The method: written or electronic, orally given to professional, reported descriptively or schematically, timing of the feedback	Reminders
	The content: information without judgement (passive feedback) or assessment of quality, using criteria or benchmarks (active feedback), formative or summative purposes, patient-specific or general, with or without peer data for comparison	Peer review groups or quality circles
	The intensity: the frequency or duration of feedback	Outreach visits
Reminders		
Before or during	The initiator of the reminder: colleague (opinion leader), academic investigator, medical computing expert, insurer or financier, healthcare organisation	Educational materials (e.g. guidelines) or educational meetings
	The method: written or electronic, timing of the reminder before or during the care process, proactive or reactive	
	The content: implicit (reminder for additional information) or explicit (recommendation to do or to avoid a clinical action), patient-specific or general	Feedback
	The intensity: the frequency and/or duration of the reminders	

Box 11.5 Feedback about prescription behaviour (O'Connell *et al.* 1999)

In a large study involving 2440 physicians in Australia, the effect of feedback on prescription routines was evaluated. The purpose of the study was to rationalise prescription behaviour and reduce medication costs. The null hypothesis was that a simple, unifactorial and relatively cheap intervention, such as sending feedback reports, would have an effect that, although small, would be relevant on a large scale. Feedback reports with a graphical reproduction of their standardised prescription behaviour over a period of 2 years were posted to the practitioners. The reports dealt with five often-prescribed medicines – angiotensin-converting enzyme (ACE) inhibitors, statins, stomach acid inhibitors, non-steroidal anti-inflammatory drugs (NSAIDs), and oral antibiotics. Schematic comparisons with colleagues were enclosed, as were educational newsletters. A second feedback report followed 6 months after the first.

The average prescription behaviour with respect to these medicines did not change after the intervention. There were no indications that the variation in the prescription behaviour diminished, or that the outliers, both above and below (individual practitioners prescribing much or little compared to their peers), changed.

Box 11.6 Feedback about requests for diagnostic tests (Winkens *et al.* 1992, 1995, 1996)

The Maastricht Diagnostic Centre was established in 1979 and co-ordinates all diagnostic requests from the approximately 90 practitioners in Maastricht and the surrounding area. The distribution of individual feedback, to improve the quality of test-ordering behaviour, was started in 1985. Twice a year the physicians received a personal report from a well-known respected internist that critiqued the volume and quality of their test requests in a random but recent month. The feedback was based on the test-ordering forms, on which the practitioners had noted clinical data from the history taking and physical examination, as well as on the possible diagnosis for the patient. Requests in general, as well as requests that related to individual patients, were discussed, and suggestions for a more rational test use made. The feedback was valued as positive – more than 85% of the practitioners indicated that they appreciated it. The beginning of the feedback process was accompanied by a considerable change in the number of requests. The total number of tests diminished by 24% after 2 years of feedback. Reductions of more than 90% were seen for specific tests. The number of requests remained smaller than that of doctors using a control laboratory during the further course of the feedback process. The cost reduction for the year 1990 on the basis of this feedback was estimated at 450,000 euros for the 90 GPs.

The studies conducted so far tell us little about the ideal *quantity of data* and the ideal *form* in which the feedback or reminder should be cast. The feedback was provided in a written form mostly, as a printout of a computer file. Consequently, some questions arise as far as the design of the feedback or reminder is concerned. Do we want the information about behaviours on the computer screen or on paper? Should it be a narrative report, an overview of figures or a schematic reproduction? What quantity of data must be worked into the feedback report? How will the signal function of the reminder be designed? Careful preparation and piloting of the chosen form is desirable before a strategy is implemented on a larger scale.

The feedback information can be provided in the 'active' or 'passive' form. *Passive feedback* gives only quantitative information without comment about performance, for example the total number of prescriptions, requested diagnostic tests or referrals in the previous 6 months, or the costs of certain procedures. Feedback about the costs of practices is given in some studies, with varying effects. The sustainability of the effects has not been investigated in most studies. In the hospital setting, passive feedback about the costs of tests did not bring about a change, but it had some effect in primary care. Passive feedback can become more interesting for professionals if it encourages peer review within small groups and therefore is combined with this (*Box 11.7*). If *comparisons* with colleagues' data are added to feedback data on individual professionals, the feedback seems to gain effect (Balas *et al.* 1996).

Active feedback or *reminders* contain an implicit or explicit judgement of the practice observed, and sometimes also advice about the preferred clinical practice.

An interpretation, educational information or a guideline for optimal care may accompany the information in active feedback or reminders. This enables professionals to react to differences between their current and the desired performance. In a randomised controlled trial by Kiefe *et al.* (2001) the use of achievable benchmarks significantly enhanced the effectiveness of physician performance feedback. It is important that the professional can recognise himself or herself in the guidelines or benchmarks presented (*Boxes 11.8* and *11.9*).

The *timing* of the feedback or reminder information is another important consideration. Larger effects appear to occur if the information is linked directly to the moment of decision making (Grimshaw and Russell 1993). Overhage *et al.* (1996) and Safran *et al.* (1995) give examples of this (*Boxes 11.10* and *11.11*, respectively). The information can best be given in direct connection to everyday work and tailored as much as possible to the decisions that are subject to intervention.

The various studies in the reviews showed large differences in the *frequency* with which the feedback or reminders were given. Sometimes there was one occurrence only, while in other studies they were given with a fixed regularity, such as weekly. While it is reasonable to suggest that repeated feedback or reminders should have more effect, this needs to be explored further.

The *duration* of the period in which feedback and reminders were provided also varied in the studies. It is unclear how long the feedback and reminders must continue after a change has been achieved. Often, professionals relapse to the old level of functioning after an intervention ends (*Box 11.12*). To consolidate the desired performance, it appears necessary to maintain the feedback or reminder process for a long time or to

Box 11.7 Feedback with peer comparisons and small-group education and peer review (Verstappen *et al.* 2003)

An intervention to improve test-ordering behaviour in a project that involved 200 practitioners in the south of the Netherlands was evaluated. The participating physicians received written feedback about their own practice regarding the usual tests in three clinical domains. The feedback report consisted of a schematic reflection of the individual data, which was contrasted with the average test-ordering data of the local practitioners' group and the regional data (see *Box 11.3*). The doctors received the report, together with national clinical guidelines for the tests. The local practitioner groups discussed differences in each others' feedback data during a meeting held about 2 weeks after they received the feedback report.

The local medical co-ordinator, who had been trained for the purpose, chaired this peer-review session. In addition to discussing the reports, they exchanged knowledge about the clinical guidelines for test ordering during the meeting. They practised communication techniques used to reassure patients that a test was not needed. Those present at the meeting were also encouraged to make individual and group plans for change. The results of the process evaluation showed that the participants highly valued such feedback reports and the small group activities. The combination of feedback and peer review in small groups proved to reduce test ordering significantly, by about 20%.

accompany the process with other interventions. Ideally, the feedback or reminders are built into a system for continuous monitoring and improvement of the quality of care. This system can be used to deter-mine whether improvements are still necessary and what progress has been made.

Considering the knowledge available at this moment, reminders, even more than feedback, seem to

Box 11.8 Active, patient-specific feedback (Smeele *et al.* 1999)

Smeele's quasi-experimental study evaluated the effects of introducing a monitoring system by which individual data regarding asthma or chronic obstructive pulmonary disease (COPD) patients were fed back to the primary care physicians. 24 practitioners registered data about lung function [forced expiratory volume 1 (FEV1)], smoking habits, medication and compliance with follow-up of 299 asthma and COPD patients and sent the information to the research centre. The centre processed this information as patient-specific feedback on the basis of the data provided. The practitioners also received feedback about their performance compared with the average

of their colleagues. The report also gave an opinion about the performance based on indicators for optimal quality of care. The written feedback was sent to the practitioners and then discussed in three small-group meetings spread over 1 year. The results of this group were compared with those of a reference group of 17 physicians with 223 asthma and COPD patients without intervention. The feedback group showed significant improvements after a year. The improvements were related to knowledge, skills, equipment in the practice, influenza vaccination and medication prescription according to national clinical guidelines.

Box 11.9 Improving feedback using achievable benchmarks (Kiefe *et al.* 2001)

A group of 70 physicians were randomly assigned to receive either physician-specific feedback on their performance regarding the management of diabetes mellitus patients, or the identical intervention plus achievable benchmark feedback. The benchmarks were calculated from the performance of all members of a peer group and represented a standard attained by the top 10% in that group. The benchmark was calculated for each specific indicator (e.g. as the percentage of eligible patients receiving an influenza vaccination). Adjustments were made to account for differences in the number of patients per physician. An adjusted performance fraction (APF) was calculated for each physician by dividing the

number of patients who received the vaccination plus 1 by the number eligible for vaccination plus 2. The clinicians were then ranked from highest to lowest according this APF. The achievable benchmark for influenza vaccination turned out to be 82%. To be eligible each physician was required to have a minimum of 25 eligible diabetic patients. For baseline and follow-up measurements an average of 20 records per physician were selected randomly and reviewed. The intervention period was 18 months. The proportion of patients who received influenza vaccine improved from 40 to 58% in the experimental group, versus from 40 to 46% in the comparison group ($p < 0.001$).

Box 11.10 Computerised reminders in a hospital (Overhage *et al.* 1996)

All the departments in a hospital in Indianapolis used the same electronic patient-recording system. A patient's file contained the data about admissions and outpatient contacts. The doctors working in the hospital also ordered all requests for laboratory tests and prescriptions electronically. 22 recommendations regarding preventive care were selected from American guidelines and translated into decision-making rules that were incorporated as reminders in the patient-registration system. Analyses of all the files of patients admitted by the general internists were run every night. The internists received a reminder in one of two ways. Firstly, the reminders appeared in a summary at the top of the patient report that the attending doctor printed out daily. Secondly, one-line reminders appeared on the computer screen with suggestions for screening at the point that the doctor wanted to order tests. This combined form of reminders was evaluated in a randomised, controlled study that involved 78 general internists. No significant differences were found among the internists who had been exposed to the reminders and those who had not. The authors of the study attributed the absence of an effect to the fact that the internists were too busy with curative care and, unlike primary care doctors, received no remuneration for providing preventive care during hospitalisation.

Box 11.11 Reminders for the treatment of HIV-infected patients (Safran *et al.* 1995)

Safran *et al.* observed the practices of 126 doctors who provided the outpatient care for 349 patients infected by human immune deficiency virus (HIV). The doctors had access to a computer network, for example to consult laboratory data and supporting decision trees. The patient's medical data (problem lists, medication lists, journals, etc.) were available online during every consultation. Recommendations for the care of HIV-infected patients were developed in 1990. These guidelines were delivered to the intervention group by means of patient-specific reminders via the computer network, but not to the doctors in the control group. The doctors in the intervention group received reminders onscreen with the suggested action to be taken within the framework of the recommendations, such as:

■ Requests for total blood count, toxoplasmosis titre or cervical swab;
■ Prescribing influenza or pneumococcus vaccination;
■ Adjusting the dosage of a zidovudine prescription.

The study included all HIV-infected patients who visited the outpatient department during 18 months. One of the effect measures was the number of days between the patient presenting and the point at which the recommendations for optimal care were met. The median response to the recommendations was 114 days in the intervention group and more than 500 days in the control group. In other words, the doctors in the intervention group provided their patients with the necessary diagnostics and prescriptions on average three times faster than the doctors in the control group.

Box 11.12 Reminders for the management of venous thromboembolism prevention (Durieux *et al.* 2000)

Using a time-series design and based in an orthopaedic surgery department of a teaching hospital in Paris, France, the investigators studied whether presentation of venous thromboembolism prophylaxis guidelines using a clinical decision-support system (CDSS) increases the proportion of appropriate clinical practice decisions made. A CDSS designed to provide immediate information on venous thromboembolism prevention among surgical patients was integrated into daily medical practice during three 10 week intervention periods, alternated with four 10 week control periods, with a 4 week washout between each period. Physicians complied with guidelines in 82.8% [95% confidence interval (CI), 77.6–87.1%)] of cases during control periods and in 94.9% (95% CI, 92.5–96.6%) of cases during intervention periods. During each intervention period, the appropriateness of prescription increased significantly ($p < 0.001$). Each time the CDSS was removed, physician practice reverted to that observed before initiation of the intervention. The relative risk of inappropriate practice decisions during control periods versus intervention periods was 3.8 (95% CI, 2.7–5.4).

be especially suitable for encouraging the adherence to clinical guidelines (*Box 11.13*). Reminders may also play a role in processing complex information more easily (Buntinx *et al.* 1993). Computerised decision support seems to be particularly effective in improving preventive care and prescription behaviour (Hunt *et al.* 1998), and in following guidelines for test ordering (van der Weijden *et al.* 2000).

Box 11.13   Effect of feedback versus reminders on primary care radiology (Ramsay *et al.* 2003; Eccles *et al.* 2001)

In this study the aim was to assess the effect of feedback versus educational reminder messages on reducing redundant requests for radiological tests in general practice. The design was a cluster randomised trial with a 2 × 2 factorial design in 244 general practices. A random subset of the patient records per practitioner was examined for adherence to clinical guidelines. The main outcome measure was the number of radiograph requests per 1000 patients per year. Each practice was randomised twice. Firstly, for allocation to the feedback or control, and secondly to the educational reminder messages or control. Thus, four groups (feedback, reminder, feedback-plus-reminder and control) could be compared. The intervention period was 12 months. All practitioners were sent the clinical guidelines by post. The research team prepared the feedback report using routine data of the previous 6 months provided by hospital radiology departments. It was sent twice to the physicians – at the start of intervention and 6 months later. Educational messages were attached to the reports of radiographs requested during the 12 month intervention, to remind the doctors of the indications for requesting radiographs. The relative reduction caused by the feedback reports was not significant, at about 1%, and the relative reduction of the educational reminder messages was significant, at about 20%. The authors also demonstrated that the significant effect of the educational reminder messages began at the start of the intervention period and was maintained at this level throughout the 12 month intervention period.

DISCUSSION OF EFFECTIVENESS OF FEEDBACK AND REMINDERS

Although the effectiveness of feedback and reminders has been much investigated, many questions remain unanswered and many hypotheses need further investigation. One example is the hypothesis that feedback and reminders are especially effective in situations in which the desired behaviour is complex, as in complex technical actions, or in situations in which there is little spontaneous peer feedback regarding the clinical actions, such as in prevention. Feedback and reminders are probably more effective for professionals in training than for well-established professionals, because those in training are more open to self-reflection. Individualised feedback is probably more effective than group feedback or feedback posted in the professionals' meeting-room. It may make a difference whether feedback with data about the functioning of a team is sent to every professional separately or whether it is presented in general during a team meeting. It is unknown whether it makes a difference if professionals themselves carry out the audit of their own activities or are shown the results of an external audit in a feedback report. Perhaps it is crucial to the professionals' motivation to change that they be provided with a useful alternative when confronted with the feedback or reminder.

Characteristics of the clinical context may also determine the success of feedback and reminders. Professionals may, for instance, be less sensitive to feedback if they have no control over the facilities or resources necessary for change. The feedback and reminders must also be attuned to the clinical context in which the individual professional must take decisions. Feedback in the context of home care by a district nurse looks different to feedback about postoperative infections in a department of surgery or feedback about individual internist's decisions to order blood tests. How the characteristics of the feedback and reminders and the characteristics of the professional precisely determine the effect of these strategies is unclear and must be studied further.

Feedback can lead to various reactions in the target group (Grol and Lawrence 1995). One's own practice performance may appear to be more or less in agreement with the current or new insights. Some professionals experience this as a matter of course and do not give it much thought. It gives others an awareness of the strengths in their own approach and management. This can lead to greater self-confidence and an incentive to strive for improvement on other points.

A different situation is created when an individual's routines appear not to be in agreement with the current guidelines or new insights. This can create tension between self-image and external reality (cognitive dissonance). This usually results in one of the following reactions. There may be *acceptance* of the discrepancy, whereby the new insights are weighed critically, as is the divergence from it. This can be called 'active acceptance'. There may also be 'passive acceptance', that is, the necessity of the change is seen, but this does not result in motivation for any real change. The new practice may be viewed as unwelcome, as hardly attainable or as something that interrupts normal routines. Supplementing the performance data with that of colleagues for comparison can influence the motivation favourably at such a moment, especially if the data can also be discussed with colleagues under expert guidance. Then the social influence of the group is potentially an important mechanism – group values and colleagues' opinions can be crucial in adjusting one's own behaviour.

Finally, one can also *reject* the discrepancy. Professionals who are confronted with a gap between the desired practice and actual care provision can set up defence mechanisms. This can be done in a number of ways, such as not trusting the feedback data and putting it down to clerical or analytical mistakes, or by emphasising the exceptional nature of one's own work setting or one's patient population. One can also reject the advocated clinical guideline, new procedure or benchmark as unrealistic, too ambitious, not in line with the practice or not well-enough evidence based. In the case of negative feedback, it is also possible that the professional feels hurt. Receiving unwelcome feedback can cause confusion, uncertainty or anxiety. There may be a threat of losing stability or there may be uncertainty about what will replace the current practice routines. This means that care must be taken in creating feedback and reminders, and they must be well prepared with involvement of the target group. More research into the impact of feedback on professionals is required to be able to design the optimal procedures.

The proposed mechanism of feedback, namely, an increasing awareness of the discrepancy that exists between what one thinks he or she is doing and the actual provision of care does not unconditionally encourage a change in behaviour. Providing information alone, apparently, does not automatically lead to change. We have seen in various reviews that the effect of reminders is somewhat greater than that of feedback. The prospective character of reminders, whereby the professional can immediately react to the information, partly explains this. Such is not the case with feedback because of its retrospective nature (Greco and Eisenberg 1993).

Many professionals do not apply the new procedures or practices, or do not apply them well, because they forget what, exactly, is expected of them. Under the pressure of daily work, they relapse into habitual activity. The reminder method is particularly intended to support busy professionals. Most professionals' work is becoming more and more complicated. It is impossible for the individual to know constantly and in every area what the desired action is, precisely what a new procedure entails or when a certain action is desirable.

Long ago Samuel Johnson wrote, "Men more frequently need to be reminded than informed."

CONCLUSIONS

Feedback and reminders can be an effective way to improve the quality of care, but success is not guaranteed. As single interventions, the effects of feedback and reminders are variable. If there are effects, then they are usually limited. Good insight into the target group, setting and existing barriers to change and linking the strategies to these insights can optimise the effect. "Success may require an understanding of the motivations underlying current practice" (Greco and Eisenberg 1993).

Although scientific knowledge about the effects of various forms of feedback and reminders is still limited, the literature nonetheless offers stepping stones for their application in implementation plans and projects.

It appears sensible to aim feedback at concrete, carefully selected aspects of care provision for which the professional is unaware of a deviation from a guideline or best practice. Further, the recipient target group's acceptance of the source of the feedback or the reminder seems to be an important influence on the effect. Feedback or reminders in the form of recognisable messages, possibly delivered via a personal approach from an experienced colleague or expert, linked to accepted guidelines, can be helpful. Obviously, the data on which the feedback or reminders are based must be valid and reliable. The quantity of data to be transmitted and the form into which the feedback or the reminder is shaped must be well prepared and tested beforehand, and correspond to the target group's experience and possibilities.

Delivering information in an active rather than a passive form also appears to be important. It is likely to be more effective if the recommendations clearly describe actions in specific conditions for specific patient populations. Implementation strategies in which the professional first receives an educational refresher course pointing him or her in the right direction and then receives patient-specific information appear intuitively promising. Finally, the timing (as close as possible to the patient contact), the frequency and duration (as continuous as possible, or part of a continuous system of monitoring) of the feedback and reminders are probably important. Clearly, good development and practical piloting are recommended for feedback or reminder strategies before the definite form and content is determined.

Recommended literature

Jamtvedt G, Young JM, Kristoffersen DT, Thomson O'Brien MA and Oxman AD (2003). Audit and feedback: Effects on professional practice and health care outcomes (Cochrane Review). The Cochrane Library, Issue 3. Oxford: Update Software.

References

Austin SM, Balas EA, Mitchell JA and Ewigman GB (1994). Effect of physician reminders on preventive care: Meta-analysis of randomized clinical trials. *Proc Ann Symp Comput Appl Med Care* **1994**:121–124.

Balas EA, Boren SA, Brown GD, *et al.* (1996). Effect of physician profiling on utilization. Meta-analysis of randomized clinical trials. *J Gen Intern Med*. **11**:584–590.

Beilby J and Silagy CA (1997). Trials of providing costing information to general practitioners: A systematic review. *MJA* **167**:89–92.

Bindels R, Clercq PA de, Winkens RAG and Hasman A (2000). A test ordering system with automated reminders for primary care based on practice guidelines. *Int J Med Inform*. **58–59**:219–233.

Buntinx F, Winkens R, Grol R and Knottnerus JA (1993). Influencing diagnostic and preventive performance in ambulatory care by feedback and reminders. A review. *Fam Pract*. **10**:219–228.

Domenighetti G, Luraschi P, Casabianca A, *et al.* (1988). Effect of information campaign by the mass media on hysterectomy rates. *Lancet* **ii**:1470–1473.

Durieux P, Nizard R, Ravaud P, Mounier N and Lepage E (2000). A clinical decision support system for prevention of venous thromboembolism: Effect on physician behavior. *JAMA* **283**:2816–2821.

Eccles M, Steen N, Grimshaw J, *et al.* (2001). Effect of audit and feedback, and reminder messages on primary-care radiology referrals: A randomised trial. *Lancet* **357**:1406–1409.

Gill PS, Mäkelä M, Vermeulen KM, *et al.* (1999). Changing doctor prescribing behaviour: A review. *Pharm World Sci*. **21**(4):158–167.

Greco PJ and Eisenberg JM (1993). Changing physician's practices. *N Engl J Med*. **329**:1271–1273.

Grimshaw JM and Russell IT (1993). Achieving effect of clinical guidelines on medical practice: A systematic review of rigorous evaluations. *Lancet* **342**:1317–1322.

Grimshaw JM, Shirran L, Thomas R, *et al.* (2001). Changing provider behavior. An overview of systematic reviews of interventions. *Med Care* **39**:S2–S45.

Grimshaw J, Thomas RE, Maclennan G, *et al.* (2004). Effectiveness and efficiency of guideline dissemination and implementation strategies. *Health Technol Assess*. **8**(6):1–84.

Grol R and Lawrence M (1995). *Quality Improvement by Peer Review*. Oxford: Oxford University Press.

Hunt DL, Haynes RB, Hanna SE and Smith K (1998). Effects of computer-based clinical decision support systems on physician performance and patient outcomes. A systematic review. *JAMA* **280**:1339–1346.

Hulscher MEJL, Wensing M, Grol RPTM, van der Weijden T and van Weel C (1999). Interventions to improve the delivery of preventive services in primary care. *Am J Public Health* **89**:737–746.

Kiefe CI, Allison JJ, Williams OD, Person SD, Weaver MT and Weissman NW (2001). Improving quality improvement using achievable benchmarks for physician feedback. A randomized controlled trial. *JAMA* **285**:2871–2879.

Mugford M, Barfield P and O'Hanlon M (1991). Effects of feedback of information on clinical practice: A review. *BMJ* **303**:398–402.

O'Connell D, Henry D and Tomlins R (1999). Randomised controlled trial of effect of feedback on general practitioners prescribing in Australia. *BMJ* **318**:507–511.

Overhage JM, Tierney WM and McDonald CJ (1996). Computer reminders to implement preventive care guidelines for hospitalized patients. *Arch Intern Med*. **156**:1551–1556.

Ramsay CR, Eccles M, Grimshaw JM and Steen N (2003). Assessing the long term effect of educational reminder messages on primary care radiology referrals. *Clin Radiol*. **58**:319–321.

Safran C, Rind DM, Davis RB, *et al.* (1995). Guidelines for management of HIV infection with computer-based patient's record. *Lancet* **346**:341–345.

Shea S, DuMouchel W and Bahamonde L (1996). A meta-analysis of 16 randomized controlled trials to evaluate computer-based clinical reminder systems for preventive care in the ambulatory setting. *J Am Med Inform Assoc*. **3**(6):399–409.

Smeele IJM, Schayck CP van, Grol RPTM, *et al.* (1999). Implementing national guidelines on asthma/COPD in general practice; the effects of continuous monitoring and feedback at patient level. In: Smeele IJM. *Improving Care for Patients with Asthma and COPD in General Practice*. Thesis. Nijmegen: Catholic University of Nijmegen.

Szczepura A, Wilmot J, Davies C, *et al.* (1994). Effectiveness and cost of different strategies for information feedback in general practice. *Br J Gen Pract*. **43**:19–24.

Solomon DH, Hashimoto H, Daltroy L, *et al.* (1998). Techniques to improve physicians' use of diagnostic tests. A new conceptual framework. *JAMA* **280**:2020–2027.

Thomson MA, Oxman AD, Davis DA, *et al.* (1997). Audits and feedback improve health professional practice and health care outcomes. (Part I + II). The Cochrane Library. Oxford: Update Software.

Thorsen T and Mäkelä M (1999). *Changing Professional Practice. Theory and Practice of Clinical Guidelines Implementation*. DSI Report 99.05. Copenhagen: Danish Institute for Health Services Research and Development.

Tierney WM, McDonald CJ, Hui SL, *et al.* (1988). Computer predictions of abnormal test results. Effects on outpatient testing. *JAMA* **259**:1194–1198.

Verstappen W, Weijden T van der, Sijbrandij J, *et al.* (2003). Effect of a practice-based strategy on test ordering performance of primary care physicians. A randomized trial. *JAMA* **289**:2407–2412.

Walton R, Dovey S, Harvey E and Freemantle N (1999). Computer support for determining drug dose: Systematic review and meta-analysis. *BMJ* **318**:984–990.

Weijden T van der, Wensing M, Giffel M, *et al.* (2000). *Interventions Aimed at Influencing the Use of Diagnostic Tests.* Report. University of Maastricht: Centre for Quality of Care Research (WOK).

Winkens RAG, Pop P, Grol RPTM, *et al.* (1992). Effect of feedback on test ordering behaviour of general practitioners. *BMJ* **304**:1093–1096.

Winkens RA, Pop P, Bugter-Maessen AM, *et al.* (1995). Randomised controlled trial of routine individual feedback to improve rationality and reduce numbers of test requests. *Lancet* **345**:498–502.

Winkens RA, Pop P, Grol R, *et al.* (1996). Effects of routine individual feedback over nine years on general practitioners' requests for tests. *BMJ* **312**:490.

Chapter 12

Organisational and financial interventions

Michel Wensing, Niek Klazinga, Hub Wollersheim and Richard Grol

---

KEY MESSAGES

- Organisational and financial interventions include changes at the microlevel (change of professional tasks, multiprofessional collaboration, leadership), mesolevel (disease management, knowledge management, quality management) and macrolevel (reimbursement and co-payments).
- The research literature suggests that organisational interventions can effectively change processes of care delivery. As with other types of intervention, there is no magic bullet.
- The effectiveness of specific organisational and financial interventions is influenced by the context in which these are applied, which can reduce the generalisability of individual studies.

Box 12.1 Impact of total quality management and organisational culture on outcomes of care for patients with bypass surgery (Shortell *et al.* 2000)

A prospective cohort study assessed the outcomes of 3045 coronary artery bypass graft (CABG) patients from 16 hospitals. Outcomes measured were clinical, functional health status, costs and satisfaction with care, the organisational culture of the hospitals and the level of implementation of quality management in the hospitals. Healthcare outcomes varied between the hospitals by a factor of two to four. However, only a very small amount of the variation could be attributed to either the use of total quality management (TQM) or the organisational culture of the hospital. Patients who had surgery in a hospital with a high TQM score were more satisfied with the nursing care, but had a higher likelihood of staying more than 10 days in hospital. A supportive group culture was associated with shorter post-surgical intubation, but a longer stay in the surgical theatre. A supportive group culture was also associated with better physical and mental health status 6 months after surgery. The authors concluded that TQM and organisational culture had little measurable effect on healthcare outcomes of coronary bypass patients. They highlighted the need for a more detailed study at the level of the primary process to discover how, in the microsystem, clinical care can be improved.

INTRODUCTION

This chapter focuses on the effectiveness of various organisational and financial interventions to change the behaviour of patients and (teams of) healthcare professionals. Organisation is a complex concept and definitions often use the word 'organising'. The meaning of this verb is 'arranging that different components make up a systematic whole, collaborate well'. An organisational intervention implies 'arranging something'. The 'systematic whole' refers to the variety of care providers, technology, communication structures, managers and funders organised around the primary process of patient care. In this chapter a healthcare organisation is defined as a local system the members of which (such as physicians, nurses and other health professionals) have a shared healthcare goal, which they achieve by performing professional labour within a fixed set of regulations and collaborations (Klazinga 2000).

One of the first efforts to develop a scientific basis for the management of organisations was by Taylor (1856–1915), who developed an organisational theory which is now known as Scientific Management. This theory is based on the following principles:

- Specification of tasks as part of the production process;
- Specialisation of labour between individuals;

- Selection and training of workers;
- Task performance according to plan;
- Incentives based on clear criteria.

These ideas from the end of the nineteenth century are still relevant when considering specific types of quality assurance within which production processes are disentangled into different components and the assumption is made that patient care can be planned. Taylor's ideas have led to a descriptive and control-oriented management approach, which is consistent with the first phases of quality management in the 1950s and 1960s (*quality assessment* and *quality control*). The most important critique of Taylor's work was that it alienated the worker from the work and payed insufficient attention to human motivation. The rise of organisation sociology and psychology led to other organisational theories that took these into account. In 1930 Mayo developed an organisational theory that emphasised interpersonal relationships. His studies in the Hawthorne factory of Western Electric Company showed the relevance of motivation and relations between workers. McGregor (1960) elaborated this theory (called Human Resource Theory) and emphasised the capacity of each worker to develop themselves.

Over the past three decades system theory and contingency theory have strongly influenced thinking about organisations. In these approaches, organisations are seen as social systems in which individuals continuously learn about their tasks. The dynamics in the organisation are determined by both the mutual relationships and the interaction between organisation and environment (Lawrence and Lorsch 1967). Important aspects of the systems approach are:

- Principle of self-organisation and group autonomy;
- Enhancement of learning capacities of individuals and groups;
- Recognition that there is not only a formal technical system but also other systems – such as the (informal) social system – and that objectives can be achieved by different approaches.

In these approaches organisations are seen as open systems. Formal and informal regulations mainly aim to reduce uncertainty regarding future events.

In the past 20 years many examples of decentralisation of responsibilities, self-guided teams and continuous adaptation of the organisational structure have developed. The management literature has focused not only on the dynamics of organisational structures (Mintzberg 1983), but also increasingly on the organisational culture (Morgan 1986). In the 1990s the focus for attention on the 'soft' side of organisations was on 'knowledge management' and 'learning organisations' (Garvin 1993; Argyris 1992).

To summarise the management literature, a broad conclusion is that two approaches can be distinguished. On the one hand, there is a 'technical' approach that sees the organisation as a system maintained by clear objectives, planning, explicit processes, tasks and responsibilities. On the other hand, there is a 'social science' approach that sees the organisation as a group of individuals with specific behavioural routines that fit together by means of a set of shared regulations that aim to achieve common goals. Each organisation has an area of tension between the regulations and planning, on the one hand, and the autonomy of each worker to design the job according to individual knowledge and preferences, on the other. In healthcare institutions this tension is particularly relevant, because many workers belong to well-developed professions, which are groups of workers with a recognised body of knowledge and skills.

This chapter presents an overview of the available scientific knowledge of the effectiveness of various organisational and financial interventions that can support and enhance the implementation of innovations. Specific interventions targeted at health professionals (such as written materials or feedback on their performance) or patients (such as telephone counselling or self-management education) are presented in previous chapters. This chapter focuses on broader strategies that aim to change the organisational and financial structures in which patients and providers operate. Usually, a distinction is made between the microlevel of care (primary process), the mesolevel (organisation, e.g. hospital or nursing home) and macrolevel (healthcare system, including reimbursement system). This chapter presents a range of organisational interventions at these different levels, the final aim of which is to impact at the microlevel of providing optimal patient care:

- Microlevel – change of professional tasks and multiprofessional collaboration;
- Mesolevel – disease management, knowledge management, quality management and leadership;
- Macrolevel – changes of reimbursement and co-payment.

CHANGE OF PROFESSIONAL ROLES

A range of interventions focus on changing the role, tasks and responsibilities of professionals, such as delegation of tasks to nurses (e.g. diabetes nurses in the hospital or practice nurses in general practice) or enlarging the tasks of pharmacists (e.g. in patient education or quality of prescribing). The rationale for changing professionals' roles varies from responding to previously unmet health needs (e.g. making home visits to elderly patients) and internal development in specific professions (e.g. nurses or pharmacists) to improving the effectiveness of healthcare services (e.g. through more appropriate prescribing) and increased efficiency (e.g. by delegation of tasks to nurses). Eight reviews focused on the effects of change of roles, tasks and responsibilities – five drew positive conclusions and three (Bower and Sibbald 2000; Thomas *et al.* 1998; Soumerai *et al.* 1989) drew negative or inconsistent conclusions. In addition, one review focused on case management, which was defined as 'the use of physician or non-physician providers to maintain continuous contact with patients via telephone or home visits in order to prevent disease exacerbation through intensive assessment and education techniques' (Ferguson and Weinberger 1998). It found that patient satisfaction, quality of life and functional status improved with case management programmes, but at an unknown cost.

It is difficult to draw general conclusions from these reviews because of the variety of organisational changes and outcome measures. The absence of a difference regarding outcome measures between study groups may sometimes be a desirable study result, for instance if the focus was on improving efficiency (where similar outcomes at lower costs would be desirable). The available studies provide evidence from various settings that the quality of care could be maintained or improved after changing professionals' roles or the involvement of a case manager (*Table 12.1*).

Table 12.1 Overview of reviews on change of professional roles	
Overview	**Conclusion**
Beney *et al.* (2000)	A review of 14 studies of the effects of enlarging the role of the public pharmacist in the areas of information delivery and collaboration with other care providers. Non-planned use of care was reduced, as was the number of visits to medical specialists and the costs of medication (six studies). Ten of 13 studies that reported patient outcomes showed positive effects. If the pharmacist focused on other care providers, rather than directly on patients, positive effects were achieved in all nine available studies.
Bower and Sibbald (2000)	A review of 40 trials of on-site mental-health professionals in primary care. Most studies focused on replacing the primary care physician with a mental-health worker in primary care, but a minority focused on consultation with a more specialised mental-health worker. There were inconsistent effects on consultation rates and prescriptions, with a tendency to reduced psychotropic prescribing. Prescribing and referring in the wider patient population was unchanged.
Ferguson and Weinberger (1998)	A review of nine trials of case management in specific clinical conditions. All of the six studies that examined patient-centred outcomes reported a positive impact and both studies that examined clinical parameters found a positive impact. Of the seven studies that investigated the impact on health-resource use, only two found a positive impact.
Gurwitz *et al.* (1990)	A review of two small controlled studies of the introduction of a pharmacist into medication prescription in the nursing home. This had the intended effects on prescribing in one study and increased blood pressure in another study (which was interpreted by the authors as a positive outcome).
Horrocks *et al.* (2002)	A review of 11 trials of nurse practitioners working in primary care. Patients were more satisfied with care by a nurse practitioner (standardised mean difference = 0.27). Health status was unchanged. Nurse practitioners had longer consultations (weighted mean difference = 3.67 minutes) and ordered more tests [odds ratio (OR) = 1.22], but no differences in other aspects of care were found.
Hulscher *et al.* (1999)	A review of four studies of the effectiveness of task delegation and arrangements of procedures on preventive care in general practice. The effects, which varied between 3 and 30% improvement, were significant in all four studies.
Pippalla *et al.* (1995)	A review of five studies of the effects of the introduction of a pharmacist on prescription behaviour. The average effect size in the five available studies was 0.53, a moderate effect.
Soumerai *et al.* (1989)	A review of two studies of the effectiveness of clinical pharmacy services. There was no effect in one study and the effect was unclear in the other.
Thomas *et al.* (1998)	A review of six studies of the effects of delegating tasks to nurses. None of the studies reported a significant effect.

MULTIPROFESSIONAL COLLABORATION

Improving collaboration between different professions and professionals has received much attention in the past decade (*Box 12.2*). Many current theories of organisational change highlight the relevance of working relations with respect to the creation of a shared vision and culture of collaboration (Berwick and Nolan 1998). Many clinical interventions require multiprofessional collaboration, but it is often difficult to determine the effects of multiprofessional collaboration as such, because other factors are usually involved. For instance, 'comprehensive geriatric assessment' implies a comprehensive assessment of the health problems, a focus on the functional problems and a co-ordinated delivery of services. It is the total package that achieves the effects. In addition, such specialised multiprofessional teams may be difficult to distinguish from disease management systems, both conceptually and practically.

Specialised teams in palliative care and geriatric care have tended to achieve intended patient outcomes (Hearn and Higginson 1998; Stuck *et al.* 1993). The number of controlled studies that focus on multiprofessional collaboration as such is limited (*Table 12.2*). A review of interventions to improve the collaboration between physicians and nurses (Zwarenstein and Bryant 2000) found only two relevant studies.

DISEASE MANAGEMENT

Disease management refers to the organisation of delivery systems and, usually, comprises a team of care providers, explicit task allocation and management of patient contacts (appointments, follow-up; Hunter and Fairfield 1997). A disease management system aims to provide effective and efficient healthcare to a well-defined category of patients, such as patients with diabetes or elderly patients. The system is designed to meet

---

Box 12.2 An organisational strategy, combined with education, that focused on collaboration between cardiologists and general practitioners (Vlek 2000)

In a study of the effects of shared consultations between a cardiologist and general practitioners (GPs), patients whom the GP was uncertain whether to refer or not were seen collaboratively. This randomised study involved 49 GPs in 16 groups and 13 cardiologists who had monthly sessions during 1.5 years. Patients were allocated at random to a shared consultation or usual care (148 patients in the intervention group, 158 patients in the control group). In the intervention group 34% of patients were referred, in the control group 55%. In the intervention group fewer diagnostic tests were ordered (7 versus 16%). The quality of care was similar in both groups.

Table 12.2 Overview of reviews on multiprofessional collaboration

Overview	Conclusion
Hearn and Higginson (1998)	This review comprised 18 studies, including five randomised trials, on specialised multiprofessional teams for patients with advanced cancer and their families. Four out of the five randomised studies reported similar or improved patient satisfaction and pain and symptom control, and reduced hospital stay.
Philbin (1999)	A review of comprehensive multidisciplinary programmes for the management of patients with congestive heart failure. Seven studies were found, including two trials. One trial showed improved quality of life and reduced hospital admissions. The other trial showed improved patient satisfaction, but not quality of life, and increased use of general medical and hospital care.
Stuck *et al.* (1993)	A review of 28 controlled trials of comprehensive geriatric assessment, which showed that this led to an increased likelihood of living at home, particularly for geriatric evaluation and management units (OR = 1.68) and hospital–home assessment services (OR = 1.49), and to a lesser extent for home-assessment services (OR = 1.20).
Zwarenstein and Bryant (2000)	A review of two studies of training, team development and other interventions to enhance working in teams of physicians and nurses. This resulted in a reduced hospital stay (6.06 versus 5.46 days on average). There was no difference in mortality.

patients' needs for healthcare. An underlying assumption is that resources can be used more effectively if the patient becomes the focus around which healthcare is organised (Hunter 2000). Systems differ in the extent to which responsibility for care of the patient remains in primary care and the degree to which specialised care providers, such as medical specialists or case managers, are involved (Wagner *et al.* 1996). In reality, most disease management systems comprise many different interventions, such as patient education, education of healthcare providers and feedback to care providers (Weingarten *et al.* 2002). An international comparison of integrated care for elderly patients suggested that common features of effective systems were a single entry point, case management, geriatric assessment, a multidisciplinary team and the use of financial incentives to promote downwards substitution (Johri *et al.* 2003). While the specific interventions can be studied separately, this section focuses on the evidence for disease management systems as a co-ordinated package of interventions.

Studies in this area have focused on specific diseases, such as diabetes, stroke, schizophrenia and total hip replacement. For instance, specialised stroke-unit interventions were defined as either a ward or team that managed stroke exclusively (dedicated stroke unit) or a ward or team that specialised in the management of disabling illnesses, which include stroke (mixed assessment and/or rehabilitation unit). One review showed that stroke units were associated with better patient outcomes and a shorter length of stay in hospital (Stroke Unit Trialist Collaboration 1997). A second review showed cost reductions, but no change of functional outcomes (Sulch and Kalra 2000), while a third reported potentially negative effects of in-hospital pathways (Kwan and Sandercock 2002). We conclude that the evidence of disease management in stroke is inconclusive (*Table 12.3*).

KNOWLEDGE MANAGEMENT (USE OF INFORMATION AND COMMUNICATION TECHNOLOGY)

Communication has a crucial role in care delivery, so information and communication systems are expected to facilitate changes of working processes. For instance, telephones facilitate the possibility of a telephone consultation hour and access to the internet facilitates answering questions from patients by email. The communication of test results, use of medication and patient transfer can be accelerated by information systems. Even less-advanced types of communication tools, such as the use of standard forms for medical records and to order tests, can influence professional behaviour. Not only can information systems and computer technology help to structure the information processes, but also they can provide direct decision support for the individual care provider (*Box 12.3*).

'Knowledge management' is the scientific approach of knowledge development and transfer in organisations. The boundaries between knowledge management and 'learning organisations' are unclear. A review of the organisational literature on both concepts showed that learning organisations are associated mostly with training, organisational development and human resources management, while knowledge management

Table 12.3 Overview of reviews on disease management in stroke	
Overview	Conclusion
Kwan and Sandercock (2002)	A review of ten controlled trials that compared in-hospital care pathways for stroke with standard medical care. No differences were found in death, dependency or discharge destination. Evidence from randomised trials suggested that patient satisfaction and quality of life may be lower in the care pathway group.
Stroke Unit Trialist Collaboration (1997)	A review of 19 randomised trials that compared organised in-patient stroke care with usual care. Stroke unit care was associated with a long-term reduction of death (OR = 0.83) and of other patient outcomes. Length of stay in hospital or institution reduced by 8%, but showed considerable heterogeneity.
Sulch and Kalra (2000)	A review of seven studies of the effects of disease management for stroke patients. It comprised protocol care delivery by, at least, medical and nursing care providers. The effects were 0.1–3.6 days reduction in hospital stay (six studies), 15–32% reduction of costs (four studies), reduced complications (one study) and no change in functional outcome (number of studies unclear).

Box 12.3 Computerised systematic surveillance of patients with diabetes in primary care (Griffin and Kinmonth 2000)

An analysis of five trials on the performance of systematic diabetes care in primary care showed that unstructured community care was associated with poorer follow-up, increased mortality and poorer control of blood sugar levels compared to care in hospital settings. A computerised central surveillance system, which reminds both the GP and the patient, can lead to a quality of diabetes care that is as good or even better than hospital care, at least in the short term. This analysis showed that the organisational conditions can be arranged for diabetes care to be provided adequately in primary care settings.

is associated mostly with information technology, intellectual capital and information systems (Scarbrough and Swan 2001). In knowledge management there is an emphasis on information and communication technology (ICT) that can support knowledge transfer within organisations (Garavelli et al. 2002).

Three reviews focused on the effects of introducing computerised medical records (*Table 12.4*). Balas et al. (1996) concluded that 13 of 19 studies had a positive result, while Sullivan and Mitchell (1995) calculated that in each of their 21 included studies there were improvements (of between 8% and 50%). A review on nursing record systems identified three trials of computerised nursing-care planning, which showed mixed results (Currell and Urquhart 1999). One study showed a negative effect on documented nursing-care planning, while two other studies demonstrated an increase in recording, but no change in patient outcomes. This review also examined client-held records and found no overall positive or negative effect for clients.

Table 12.4 Overview of reviews on information technology

Overview	Conclusion
Balas et al. (1996)	A review of 19 studies of the effects of the use of a computerised record system and access to information for patients. 14 studies (74%) reported positive effects.
Currell and Urquhart (1999)	A review of eight trials of nursing record systems. Three studies on computerised nursing-care planning showed mixed results. Three studies of client-held records showed no overall positive of negative effects. A study on paper-based systems showed improved documentation and a pain-management sheet showed a positive impact.
Currell et al. (2000)	A review of seven studies of the effects of telemedicine. While none of the studies showed clear disadvantages, the advantages were not clearly proved.
Hersch et al. (2001)	A review of 25 studies of telemedicine interventions, 21 of which were controlled. The strongest evidence for the efficacy of telemedicine in clinical outcomes came from home-based telemedicine in the areas of chronic disease management, hypertension and acquired immune deficiency syndrome (AIDS). The value for home glucose monitoring was unclear.
Mitchell and Sullivan (2001)	A review of 61 studies of primary-care computing systems that concluded these improve practitioner performance, particularly for health promotion interventions. Effects on patient outcomes are unclear.
Roine et al. (2001)	A review of studies on telemedicine, of which six were randomised trials. All but one trial showed unchanged patient outcomes; the exception was a study that showed improved compliance with medication. The only trial to include an economic analysis indicated that telemedicine was not cost-effective.
Sullivan and Mitchell (1995)	A review of 21 studies of the effects of the use of computers in general practice, particularly for prevention and prescribing. Each study showed improvements, varying between 8 and 50%. Three studies assessed patient outcomes, one showing positive effects.
Walton et al. (1999)	A review of 15 studies of computerised decision support on medication prescribing. A range of effects were found across the studies – a reduction of time to achieve therapeutic control (standardised mean difference, –0.44), decreased toxicity of medication (–0.12), decreased number of adverse events (–0.06) and reduced hospital stay (–0.32). These pooled effects were significant.

Telemedicine is the use of communication technology to capture and quickly transmit clinical data, such as patient information and test results, for consultation with a care provider who is geographically located elsewhere. The patient may be at home, in a primary care practice or in a remote hospital, for instance in a rural area. Three reviews have focused on telemedicine interventions (Hersch *et al.* 2001; Roine *et al.* 2001; Currell *et al.* 2000) and all concluded that the evidence to support the effectiveness of telemedicine is as yet limited (*Table 12.4*). Nevertheless, there are a number of successful examples, particularly in chronic disease management (Hersch *et al.* 2001).

Finally, computer technology has been used to provide support to clinical decisions or to provide reminders and feedback (*Table 12.4*). The effectiveness of feedback and reminders is described in Chapter 11. A broad review of primary-care computing showed that prescribing improved with computer support: prescribing of generic drugs increased and prescribing costs decreased (Mitchell and Sullivan 2001). This is consistent with another review on computer support for prescribing decisions, which showed a number of specific improvements (*Box 12.4*). Mitchell and Sullivans's review (2001) also concluded that disease management was improved by use of computers, for instance four studies on diabetes found improvements of 5–69% in the targets. The greatest improvement occurred when physicians used an electronic protocol.

There used to be considerable optimism about the use of computer technology to provide support to clinical decisions. Integrating the complexity of medical decisions, captured in computerised decision trees, together with scientific and professional knowledge, were expected to improve the quality of medical decision making. This optimism was reduced in the 1990s as it became clearer how complex the decision-making processes between doctor and patient actually are and how limited routine computer hardware was.

QUALITY MANAGEMENT

This section focuses on the effectiveness of strategies such as TQM and continuous quality improvement (CQI; Gustafson and Hundt 1995). These strategies cannot be seen as standardised interventions. Depending on which source is used, the focus of the intervention is more on standardisation and evaluation of care processes or on culture, leadership and motivation of health professionals. A review of 55 studies on the effects of TQM on care delivery reported that 42 studies concerned single-site projects (Shortell *et al.* 1995, 1998) and overall only three studies used a controlled design. Although a number of studies reported relevant improvements, the reviewers concluded that there was still insufficient evidence of hospital-wide positive effects on patient care (*Boxes 12.5 and 12.6*).

Another review brought together 21 studies of quality management in nursing homes, four of which used a controlled design (Wagner *et al.* 2001). The effects were inconsistent, but there was some evidence from the controlled studies that specific training and guidelines could influence the outcomes at the patient level. There is little evidence for the effectiveness of quality management models in primary care settings. It appears necessary to develop specific TQM models for small practices and to provide long-term, intense support to have any chance of implementing quality management successfully (Geboers *et al.* 1999; Solberg *et al.* 1998).

Box 12.4 Computerised decision support for medication dosages (Walton *et al.* 1999)

Walton *et al.* (1999) performed a meta-analysis of studies on the effectiveness of computer support for decisions on medication dosages. They analysed 18 comparative studies, published between 1966 and 1996, which had been identified by the Cochrane Effective Practice and Organisation of Care (EPOC) Group search strategy. The computer programs used individualised pharmacokinetic models to estimate the optimal dosage for medications such as theophylline, heparin, aminoglycosides, oxytocin and fentanyl. A meta-analysis of the data from 671 patients showed that higher serum concentrations of the medication (effect size 0.69, 95% reliability interval 0.36–1.02) and a reduced time period to achieve therapeutic control (0.44, 0.17–0.71) was achieved with computer support. The total medication use was unchanged, but the number of adverse events was lower in the intervention group. Five of six studies that assessed patient outcomes showed positive effects of computer support. The authors concluded that the use of computers to estimate the optimal dosage for an individual patient in a hospital setting could have positive effects. The computerised decision support appeared to support physicians in their choice for a higher dosage, if this seemed to be necessary for individual patients.

Box 12.5 Impact of CQI or TQM – concept versus implementation (Shortell *et al.* 1995)

A cross-sectional study examined the associations between organisational culture, quality improvement and selected hospital outcomes in 61 hospitals in the USA. Data were collected in participating hospitals for 7000 individuals. Operationalisation of quality improvement activities and the level of implementation of quality management was based on the Baldridge model [the American example of the European Framework for Quality Management (EFQM) model] and validated scales were used to measure organisational culture. The most important finding was that a participative, flexible, risk-taking organisational culture is associated with the implementation of quality management. Furthermore, a higher level of implementation of quality management was positively related to improved observed patient outcomes and improved human resource management. Larger hospitals showed lower clinical efficiency, mainly because additional bureaucratic layers appeared to inhibit the implementation of quality management. The authors concluded that an organisational culture that supports quality management and the possibility for flexible implementation seems to be important. Larger hospitals appear to have more difficulties with this.

Box 12.6 Use of CQI for the safe reduction of the number of Caesarian deliveries (Gregory *et al.* 1999)

A prospective observational study described how the Cedars Sinai Medical Center in Los Angeles participated in the 'breakthrough series' of the Institute for Healthcare Improvement in Boston. Over a period of 5 years (1994–1999) 17 interventions – partly clinical, partly administrative – reduced the percentages of Caesarian deliveries from 26.0% in 1993 to 20.5% in 1997, without an increase in complications. The researchers mentioned the limited validity of their study, but they claim it was plausible that CQI activities had an important role.

LEADERSHIP

The division of power among professions and healthcare institutions (hospital, nursing home and home care) may be problematic. Particularly in shared-care initiatives, there is a tendency to create new co-ordinating functions, in which new people (e.g. case managers, transfer nurses and circuit managers) are given new tasks, but do not necessarily have new competencies. One approach is to put physicians in a co-ordination role. Some studies in hospitals suggest that a model in which the physician is the co-ordinating care provider (physician-in-the-lead model) is most successful; the optimal management model in primary healthcare has not yet been found.

The general management literature on leadership needs to be read carefully in the context of healthcare because of both the type of organisations in which professionals work and their relative clinical autonomy. There is consensus that the leadership of professionals is crucial to implement change (*Box 12.7*). This idea is supported by both the idea of opinion leaders (Rogers 1995) and by the physician–leader concept (Berwick and Nolan 1998). The role of opinion leaders in educational interventions is discussed in Chapter 10. Apart from these studies on opinion leaders, we have not identified reviews of controlled studies in this area. The effectiveness of efforts to enhance leadership is largely unknown.

Box 12.7 Efficacy and effects of coaching on nursing managers, measured by satisfaction and absenteeism among workers (Weir *et al.* 1997)

In a Canadian hospital, nursing managers of seven departments received the option of external coaching for their leadership. A randomised controlled trial was performed to assess the effects on satisfaction of workers, absenteeism, the number of incidents in departments and patient satisfaction. The researchers concluded that coaching had a positive effect on the work atmosphere, but that absenteeism was equal in both groups. They point out that coaching was particularly effective in nursing managers who were open to it (a dose–response analysis supported this). Interventions to improve leadership capacities should focus on managers who are prepared to evaluate themselves and to work on their personal development.

CHANGES IN REIMBURSEMENT

Although macrolevel regulations may have an impact on the primary process of patient care, their impact is mainly indirect through supporting the microlevel and mesolevel organisational interventions described in the previous sections. For instance, national laws support the implementation of disease management systems for specific patient categories in the German healthcare system. Managed care seems to have reduced hospitalisation and use of high-cost discretionary services, increased preventive screening and be neutral in terms of patient outcomes (Steiner and Robinson 1998). While changes in the reimbursement system are usually arranged at the macrolevel, these can have a direct impact on patient care. This section focuses on financial interventions directly targeted at supporting or enhancing change in the performance of individual care providers and teams or in the behaviour of patients – this may include changed reimbursement for physicians or co-payments for patients.

Standard economic theory predicts that a higher fee for a service leads to a higher volume of that service, while prospective reimbursement systems (salary, capitation, budgets) put the financial risk on the side of the care provider and lead to lower volumes of the activities. A higher price should decrease demand for healthcare from citizens in a competitive market, but in most developed countries patients pay indirectly for healthcare through taxes or insurance premiums, so that this price mechanism is much weaker. Nevertheless, co-payments for patients have been used to decrease the demand for specific services. In this way changes in the reimbursement for professionals and payment by patients may support the implementation of innovations.

The number of studies of changes in reimbursement is limited (*Table 12.5*). Gosden and Torgerson (1997) and Gosden *et al.* (2000) concluded that fundholding in primary care reduced the costs of prescriptions and referrals and increased generic prescribing. Wensing *et al.* (1998) showed that the supply of resources, financial incentives to professionals, and financial regulations or incentives to patients were effective in one of three studies in primary care and partly effective in the remaining two studies. A comprehensive review by Chaix-Couturier *et al.* (2000) described the results of 89 studies. Different types of fundholding or fixed-payment systems reduced the volume of prescribing activities by up to 24% and the number of hospitalisations by 80% compared to fee-for-service systems. The authors claimed that financial interventions could contribute to a reduction in the use of resources in healthcare, better adherence to guidelines and achievement of

Table 12.5 Overview of reviews on financial interventions

Overview	Conclusion
Chaix-Couturier *et al.* (2000)	A review of 89 studies, including eight randomised experiments, of the effects of financial incentives. The provision of a fixed budget led to a reduction of up to 24% in the number of prescriptions and an 80% reduction in the number of days in hospital compared to fee per service. It is unclear which studies these figures were based on.
Giuffrida *et al.* (1999)	A review of 11 studies of the effects of targeted payments to patients in primary care. Six studies showed a significant effect. Two studies showed improvements in vaccination rates, but this was significant in one study only (*Box 12.8*).
Gosden and Torgerson (1997)	A review of nine studies of the effects of a fixed budget per general practice or group (fundholding). Eight of the studies showed effects on prescribing behaviour. Two studies showed a reduction of the number of referrals.
Gosden *et al.* (2000)	A review of four studies of the effects of different reimbursement systems on the behaviour of physicians in primary care. Payment per service, compared to fixed payments per period, led to increased numbers of patient contacts in primary care, more visits to medical specialists and more use of diagnostic and therapeutic services, but fewer referrals to the hospitals and fewer repeat prescriptions. Compared to a fixed salary payment, per service led to better continuity of care and better adherence to planned consultations, but to lower satisfaction with the accessibility of the physician.
Wensing *et al.* (1998)	A review of three studies of the effects of financial incentives in general practice. This was effective in one study and partly effective in the other two.

Box 12.8 Effect of financial sanctions on the vaccination level of children in families who receive social security (Kerpelman *et al.* 2000)

In the USA the low vaccination level among children in lower economic groups is an increasing problem. A randomised controlled trial was performed to assess the effects of financial sanctions. The study was performed between 1993 and 1996 among 2500 families with children under the age of 6 years who were dependant on a child social-security programme. In the experimental group payments were made only if there was proof of vaccination. The researchers concluded that this financial measure was an effective strategy to increase the vaccination level and apparently provided an incentive to keep the vaccination status of the children up to date.

healthcare targets. It could be an effective strategy to combine different interventions, depending on the specific aim of the healthcare programme. The review also showed the problems in organising the results of these studies, given the heterogeneity of the financial structures.

Although the majority of studies of financial interventions are targeted at changing professional behaviour, the use of financial incentives to influence patient behaviour has been receiving increasing attention. Giuffrida *et al.* (1999) published a review that assessed the impact of paying patients to comply with desired health behaviours. All 11 studies were from the USA and published between 1976 and 1996; ten studies showed that financial reimbursement to the patient led to better compliance than did alternative interventions (six of ten were significant). In only one study was the non-financial intervention more effective than the financial one. None of the studies compared the relative impact of differing levels of the payment. One study showed that the provision of free milk tickets to teenage mothers was more effective than the provision of presents.

CONCLUSIONS

A variety of interesting organisational and financial interventions are available, which have proved to be effective in specific settings. The research evidence is strongest for organisational interventions at the micro- and mesolevel – many interventions at these levels may be effective, although evidence for a generalised efficiency is limited. This is somewhat paradoxical in that it is a particular feature of organisational interventions that they may be targeted at improving efficiency rather than effectiveness.

The weaker evidence for macrolevel interventions partly reflects the difficulty of using a trial for such interventions. Overall, the generalisability of the studies is limited, not least because the effects are likely to be influenced by the organisational and financial system within which these have been conducted. Even more than with other implementation strategies, knowledge of the organisational and political setting is needed to select an intervention.

Recommended literature

Grol R (2001). Improving the quality of medical care. Building bridges among professional pride, payer profit, and patient satisfaction. *JAMA* **284**:2578–2585.

References

Argyris C (1992). *On Organizational Learning*. Cambridge MA: Blackwell Business.

Balas EA, Austin Boren S, Brown GD, *et al.* (1996). Effect of physician profiling on utilization. Meta-analysis of randomized clinical trials. *J Gen Intern Med*. **11**:584–590.

Beney J, Bero LA and Bond C (2000). Expanding the roles of outpatient pharmacists: Effects on health services utilisation, costs, and patient outcomes. The Cochrane Library. Oxford: Update Software.

Berwick DM and Nolan TW (1998). Physicians as leaders in improving health care. *Ann Intern Med*. **128**:289–292.

Bower P and Sibbald B (2000). Systematic review of the effect of on-side mental health professionals on the clinical behaviour of general practitioners. *BMJ* **320**:614–617.

Chaix-Couturier C, Durand-Zaleski I, Jolly D, *et al.* (2000). Effects of financial incentives on medical practice: Results from a systematic review of the literature and methodological costs? *Int J Qual Health Care* **12**:133–142.

Currell R and Urquhart C (1999). Nursing record systems: Effects on nursing practice and health care outcomes. The Cochrane Library. Oxford: Update Software.

Currell R, Urquhart C, Wainwright P, *et al.* (2000). Telemedicine versus face to face patient care: Effects on professional practice and health care outcomes. The Cochrane Library, Issue 2. Oxford: Update Software.

Ferguson JA and Weinberger M (1998). Case management programs in primary care. *J Gen Intern Med*. **13**:123–126.

Garavelli AC, Gorgoglione M and Scozzi B (2002). Managing knowledge transfer by knowledge technologies. *Technovation* **22**:269–279.

Garvin DA (1993). Building a learning organization. *Harv Bus Rev*. **71**:78–91.

Geboers H, Horst M van der, Mokkink H, *et al.* (1999). Setting up improvement projects in small scale primary care practices: Feasibility of a model for continuous quality improvement. *Qual Health Care* 8:36–42.

Giuffrida A, Gosden T, Forland F, *et al.* (1999). Target payments in primary care: Effects on professional practice and health care outcomes. The Cochrane Library. Oxford: Update Software.

Gosden T and Torgerson DJ (1997). The effect of fundholding on prescribing and referral costs: A review of the evidence. *Health Policy* 40:103–114.

Gosden T, Forland F, Kristiansen IS, *et al.* (2000). Capitation, salary, fee-for-service and mixed systems of payment: Effects on the behaviour of primary care physicians. The Cochrane Library. Oxford: Update Software.

Gregory K, Hackmeyer P, Gold L, *et al.* (1999). Using the CQI process to safely lower Cesarian section rate. *Jt Comm J Qual Improv.* 25:619–629.

Griffin S and Kinmonth A (2000). Diabetes care: The effectiveness of systems for routine surveillance for people with diabetes. The Cochrane Library. Oxford: Update Software.

Gurwitz JH, Soumerai SB and Avorn J (1990). Improving medication prescribing and utilization in the nursing home. *J Am Geriatr Soc.* 38(5):542–552.

Gustafson DH and Hundt AS (1995). Findings of innovation research applied to quality management principles for health care. *Health Care Manage Rev.* 20:16–33.

Hearn J and Higginson IJ (1998). Do specialist palliative care teams improve outcomes for cancer patients? A systematic literature review. *Palliative Med.* 12:317–332.

Hersch WR, Helfand M, Wallace J, *et al.* (2001). Clinical outcomes resulting from telemedicine interventions: A systematic review. *BMC Med Inform Decis Making* 1:9.

Horrocks S, Anderson E and Salisbury C (2002). Systematic review of whether nurse practitioners working in primary care provide equivalent care to doctors. *BMJ* 324:819–823.

Hulscher MEJL, Wensing M, Grol RPTM, *et al.* (1999). Interventions to improve the delivery of preventive services in primary care. *Am J Public Health* 89(5):737–746.

Hunter DJ (2000). Disease management: Has it a future? It has a compelling logic, but it needs to be tested in practice. *BMJ* 320:530.

Hunter DJ and Fairfield G (1997). Managed care: Disease management. *BMJ* 315:50–53.

Johri M, Beland F and Bergmann H (2003). International experiments in integrated care for the elderly: A synthesis of the evidence. *Int J Geriatr Psych.* 18:222–235.

Kerpelman LC, Connell DB and Gunn WJ (2000). Effect of a monetary sanction on immunization rates of recipients of aid to families with dependent children. *JAMA* 284:53–59.

Klazinga N (2000). *Sociale Geneeskunde: De Derde Weg*. Oratie. Amsterdam: Vossiuspers AUP.

Kwan I and Sandercock P (2002). In-hospital pathways for stroke. Cochrane Library. Oxford: Update Software.

Lawrence PR and Lorsch JW (1967). Organization and environment: Managing differentiation and integration. Boston: Harvard University Press.

McGregor D (1960). *The Human Side of Enterprise*. New York: McGraw-Hill.

Mintzberg H (198). *Structuring of Organizations*. Englewoods Cliffs: Prentice Hall Inc.

Mitchell E and Sullivan F (2001). A descriptive feast but an evaluative famine: Systematic review of published articles on primary care computing during 1980–97. *BMJ* 322:279–282.

Morgan G (1986). *Images of Organizations*. London: Sage Publishers.

Pippalla RS, Riley DA and Chinburapa V (1995). Influencing the prescribing behaviour of physicians: A meta evaluation. *J Clin Pharm Ther.* 20:89–98.

Philbin EF (1999). Comprehensive multidisciplinary programs for the management of patients with congestive heart failure. *J Gen Intern Med.* 14:130–135.

Rogers E (1995). *Diffusion of Innovations*, Fourth Edition. New York: Free Press.

Roine R, Ohinmaa A and Hailley D (2001). Assessing telemedicine: A systematic review of the literature. *Can Med Assoc J.* 165:765–771.

Scarbrough H and Swan J (2001). Explaining the diffusion of knowledge management: The role of fashion. *Br J Manage.* 12:3–12.

Shortell S, O'Brien J, Carman J, *et al.* (1995). Assessing the impact of CQI/TQM: Concept versus implementation. *Health Services Res.* 30:377–401.

Shortell SM, Bennett CL and Byck GR (1998). Assessing the impact of continuous quality improvement on clinical practice: What it will take to accelerate progress. *Milbank Q.* 76(4):593–624.

Shortell S, Jones R, Rademaker A, *et al.* (2000). Assessing the impact of total quality management and organizational culture on multiple outcomes of care for coronary artery bypass graft surgery patients. *Med Care* 38:207–217.

Solberg L, Brekke M, Kottke T, *et al.* (1998). Continuous Quality Improvement in primary care: What's happening? *Med Care* 36:625–635.

Soumerai SB, McLaughlin TJ and Avorn J (1989). Improving drug prescribing in primary care: A critical analysis of the experimental literature. *Milbank Q.* 67(2):268–317.

Steiner A and Robinson R (1998). Managed care: US research evidence and its lessons for the NHS. *J Health Serv Res Policy* 3:173–181.

Stroke Unit Trialist Collaboration (1997). Collaborative systematic review of the randomised trials of organised inpatient (stroke unit) care after stroke. *BMJ* 314:1151–1158.

Stuck AE, Siu AL, Wieland GD, Adams J and Rubenstein LZ (1993). Comprehensive geriatric assessment: A meta-analysis of controlled trials. *Lancet* 342:1032–1036.

Sulch D and Kalra L (2000). Integrated care pathways in stroke management. *Age Ageing* 29:349–352.

Sullivan F and Mitchell E (1995). Has general practitioner computing made a difference to patient care? A systematic review of published reports. *BMJ* 311:848–852.

Thomas LH, McColl E, Cullum N, *et al.* (1998). Effect of clinical guidelines in nursing, midwifery, and the therapies: A systematic review of evaluations. *Qual Health Care* 7:183–191.

Vlek H (2000). *Cardiologue. Joint Consultations of General Practitioners and Cardiologists in a Primary Care Setting.* Proefschrift. Maastricht: Universiteit Maastricht.

Wagner EH, Austin BT and Van Korff M (1996). Organizing care for patients with chronic illness. *Milbank Q.* 74(4):511–544.

Wagner C, Van der Wal G, Groenewegen PP and De Bakker DH (2001). The effectiveness of quality systems in nursing homes: A review. *Qual Health Care* **10**:211–217.

Walton R, Dovey S, Harvey E, *et al.* (1999). Computer support for determining drug dose: Systematic review and meta-analysis. *BMJ* **318**:984–990.

Weingarten SR, Henning JM, Badamgarav E, *et al.* (2002). Interventions used in disease management programmes for patients with chronic illness – which ones work? Meta-analysis of published reports. *BMJ* **325**:925–933.

Weir R, Stewart L, Browne G, *et al.* (1997). The efficacy and effectiveness of process consultation in improving staff morale and absenteeism. *Med Care* **35**:334–353.

Wensing M, Weijden van der T and Grol R (1998). Implementing guidelines and innovations in general practice: Which interventions are effective? *Br J Gen Pract.* **48**:991–997.

Zwarenstein M and Bryant W (2000). Interventions to promote collaboration between nurses and doctors. The Cochrane Library, Issue 4. Oxford: Update Software.

Chapter 13

Patient–mediated strategies

Michel Wensing, Glyn Elwyn and Richard Grol

KEY MESSAGES

- Patient involvement in the planning and delivery of healthcare services can serve several aims, including better implementation of innovations and quality improvement in clinical practice.
- Patient-mediated interventions can be targeted at the decision to seek professional care, at contacts with healthcare providers and at patients after they have received healthcare.
- Some strategies to implement innovations through patients are promising, but our understanding of the effects on professional behaviour and processes of care is, as yet, limited.

Box 13.1 Effect of a mass media campaign on the performance of a surgical operation (Domenighetti *et al.* 1988)

Between 1977 and 1983 the number of hysterectomies (surgical removal of the uterus) performed in Ticino, a district in Switzerland, increased from 323 to 472 per 100,000 women. Providing information on the wide variation in the number of operations between different areas had little effect on the clinical decisions of gynaecologists, even though, according to opinion leaders, a proportion of the operations were inappropriate. In 1984 a mass media campaign was conducted (newspaper, radio and television), in which the public were informed about the variation in the number of hysterectomies and it was suggested that the number of operations was too high. The rate of hysterectomies subsequently decreased to 349 per 100,000 women (26% lower than in 1983), while in another Swiss district, over the same period, the rate remained the same. The campaign probably influenced both patients and physicians, partly because physicians anticipated the knowledge and expectations of women.

INTRODUCTION

Most interventions to implement innovations in healthcare focus on (teams of) professionals or organisations. The patient is seldom directly involved in introducing change and improvement. Nevertheless, the needs and preferences of the patient can have a major impact on decisions about what healthcare is delivered (Sullivan and MacNaughton 1996). Increasingly, patients expect to be well-informed about treatment options and to be involved in making decisions. Effective implementation assumes that the patient appropriately uses any treatment or advice, so treatment compliance can be regarded as a component of the effective adoption of an innovation. A clinical guide-line or new procedure may provoke resistance if it contradicts expectations or preferences of patients. So, interventions targeted at patients may be used to enhance the implementation of innovations or improvements in clinical practice (Wensing and Grol 1998).

This chapter provides an overview of patient-mediated strategies in the context of the implementation of innovations in patient care – the patients' career in healthcare is used to categorise the strategies. An episode of care often starts with health problems that cause pain, limitations or concerns. In this phase information can be provided to help to make the decisions about whether or not to seek healthcare, and which care provider to attend, using evidence or guidelines to guide these decisions. In the next phase, in preparation for the contact with a care provider, practice or institution, patients' requirements for care can be documented and the patient can be prepared to play a specific role and ask for the appropriate type of care. During the contact with the care provider, the patient can be targeted by means of tailored patient education, shared decision-making strategies and explicit attention to compliance (or concordance) with treatment. Finally, after having received healthcare the patient can provide feedback as evaluations, complaints or comments. This feedback can influence the quality improvement activities of care providers, such as planned changes to service delivery or professional education.

This chapter describes the effectiveness of four types of patient strategies:

▪ Health education or advertising through the mass media;
▪ Preparation for contact with care providers;
▪ Communication during single contacts or within episodes of care;
▪ Feedback on healthcare received.

HEALTH EDUCATION THROUGH THE MASS MEDIA

The decision about whether or not to seek professional healthcare is influenced by many factors, such as the perceived seriousness of health problems, the extent of any limitations of daily activities, the expectation that self-management will not be effective and concerns of serious illness (Campbell and Roland 1996). The supply of information on health problems, on possible methods for self-management and on professional healthcare to people who are not yet a 'patient' may influence their illness behaviour and contribute to the implementation of a guideline or procedure. For instance,

bed rest is not effective for acute low back pain, advice that can be given by the physician or a physiotherapist, but also through the mass media. Information can be provided on a range of features of healthcare (e.g. quality, costs and outcomes) and may help patients make an informed choice between different care providers.

Different methods can be used to provide information, such as:

▪ Health information through the mass media – television commercials, articles in local newspapers, posters at bus stations, etc.;
▪ Books, leaflets, videos, etc., on specific health problems, targeted at specific groups;
▪ Internet websites that provide information on health problems.

Mass media programmes have been shown to influence the use of healthcare (*Table 13.1*). A systematic review found programmes that focused on a number of areas – vaccination and screening, reduction of delay in hospitalisation for suspected myocardial infarction and reduction in the number of hysterectomies (Grilli *et al.* 2001). In some of these examples the intention was to increase the use of the services, while in others the intention was to decrease their use. The effects of patient education via the internet have been studied increasingly in areas such as smoking cessation, education about nutrition, weight loss and pharmacy services. A review showed that internet information seemed to have positive effects on health outcomes, although the methodological quality of many studies was poor (Bessell *et al.* 2002). The effect on use of healthcare services was not specified in this review.

There is certainly no doubt in the commercial offices of pharmaceutical companies as to the impact of patient influences on health professionals and the services provided. In some countries, direct-to-consumer (DTC) advertising is allowed. As an example, the total DTC

Table 13.1 Effects of mass media interventions	
Overview	Conclusion
Bessell *et al.* (2002)	Review of ten comparative studies of internet interventions, which concluded that all the studies showed some positive effects on health outcomes.
Grilli *et al.* (2001)	Review of 20 studies of mass media interventions, of which 19 concluded that mass media effectively influenced the use of healthcare services. The effects were consistently in the expected direction, with a change in effect size that ranged from + 0.1 to –13.1.
Marshall *et al.* (2000)	Review of 21 articles, of which three examined the effect of public reports on outcomes of care (e.g. related to bypass surgery), some of which showed expected changes.

spend in the USA in 2000 was estimated to be 2.5 billion pounds (Mintzes 2002). A survey in the USA estimated that 20% of Americans said that DTC advertising prompted them to call or visit their doctor to discuss an advertised drug (Gottlieb 2002). Although rigorous evaluations on the effects of DTC were not identified, the available evidence suggests strongly that it is possible to influence healthcare practitioners by targeting patients.

There is little comparative research on the effects of the supply of information on the quality of care provided or adherence to guidelines by different care providers (*Box 13.2*). A review concluded that it is as yet unclear whether the supply of information about care providers can actually influence care provision and the implementation of innovations (Marshall *et al.* 2000). The most important conclusion was that consumers did not understand or trust the information and made little use of it in their choice of care provider. Physicians, too, are sceptical about these data, but hospitals may use them for internal quality improvement. The available information on care providers is not always relevant to patients' decisions (Hibbard and Jewtt 1997), and patients cannot reliably distinguish between appropriate and inappropriate healthcare – when faced with having to make co-payments, they reduce both (Newhouse 1993).

A sizeable body of research on the effects of health promotion programmes suggests a number of potential effect modifiers. The effectiveness of health education is greater if the theme is relevant for the target group, if the programme has been adapted to the individual's needs and if feedback, reinforcement and facilitation have been integrated into it (Kok *et al.* 1997). However, it is not always clear how health promotion programmes affected the use of healthcare services, so

the relevance of these potential effect modifiers in this context remains uncertain.

PREPARATION FOR CONTACTS WITH CARE PROVIDERS

In preparation for contacts with care providers, patients can document their health problems, quality of life, needs for care and then report this during the contact with the care provider. This strategy may help to identify issues that could otherwise go unnoticed or unmentioned and is particularly suited to situations in which underdetection is a problem that needs to be addressed. There is a range of possible methods for such problem or needs assessment prior to the contact between patient and care provider. Examples of such methods are:

■ Questionnaire on mental-health symptoms completed shortly before a contact by the patient and then attached to the medical records (Badger and Rand 1988);

■ Questionnaire on the need to discuss self-management (e.g. diet) completed by patients with diabetes shortly before a contact – the questionnaire comprised questions on motivation and problems of achieving adequate self-care (Osoba 1993);

■ Short session preceding a contact with a physician, in which the patient is helped to recognise relevant decisions and encouraged to discuss these with the physician (Greenfield and Kaplan 1985);

■ Written information alongside an exercise to clarify preferences for healthcare.

The routine use of condition-specific or general quality-of-life questionnaires has been studied in different settings and patients seem to accept the idea of completing questionnaires before a consultation (Buxton *et al.* 1998; *Table 13.2*; *Box 13.3*). Although, in some stud-

---

Box 13.2 Examples of public reports on performance data (Division of Research and Education 2000)

■ Ontario Hospital Association (voluntary): uses aggregate data, tabulates data by five numerically numbered and unidentified regions.

■ UK League tables (government legislation): ranks individual healthcare providers to identify 'good' and 'bad' performance; uses non-risk adjusted data.

■ UK high-level performance indicators and clinical indicators (government legislation): uses aggregate data, alphabetically orders and names NHS Hospital Trusts and Health Authorities by locality; indicators adjusted for age; similar Health Authorities combined graphically to enable social, economic and demographic information to be compared.

■ New York Cardiac Surgery Report System (required): the risk-adjusted mortality rates of high-volume surgeons who conduct over 200 coronary artery bypass graft (CABG) operations in a single hospital over 3 years are individually ranked and reported.

Box 13.3 Feedforwards of perceived quality of life (Jacobs *et al.* 2001)

Patients with asthma or chronic obstructive pulmonary disease (COPD) were seen periodically by their physician to monitor their condition and to change treatment as necessary – both clinical measures and quality of life were monitored. Patients completed a quality-of-life questionnaire shortly before a planned follow-up consultation and then brought the questionnaire to the consultation and the doctor looked at the scores. In one study the method was used by 14 physicians and 175 adult patients in a total of 537 consultations. In 57% of the consultations patients reported problems with their quality of life. This information was associated with interventions by the doctor. Physical symptoms were related to change of medication [odds ratio (OR) = 1.7] and patient education (OR = 1.9). Emotional symptoms were related to additional follow-up consultations (OR = 4.3) and counselling (OR = 7.3). Lower age was related to the provision of more patient education in most cases. Reports of physical or social disabilities or absence of work were not related to actions by the practitioner. Both patients and doctors were positive about the monitoring of quality of life as part of healthcare for asthma and COPD.

Table 13.2 Effects of questionnaires in routine practice

Overview	Conclusion
Centre for Reviews and Dissemination (2002)	Review of interventions to improve recognition and management of depression in primary care, summarising several other reviews, which comprised 16 studies on depression questionnaires and nine studies on health-related quality-of-life questionnaires. Most studies did not show effects of their use on process or outcomes of care.
Greenhalgh and Meadows (1999)	Review of 13 studies of patient-based measures of health in routine practice, which showed little evidence that their use substantially changed patient management or improved patient outcomes.

ies, it resulted in better recognition of health problems and higher satisfaction with healthcare, it did not influence clinical management or patient outcomes (Greenhalgh and Meadows 1999). A substantial number of studies have focused on recognition and management of symptoms of depression, and the results in this area are consistent with the general picture (Centre for Reviews and Dissemination 2002). It has been suggested that care providers should be better trained on how to use the information (Meadows *et al.* 1998).

Preparing the patient for an active role during the contact with a care provider is another intervention and can result in an improvement of clinical measures, as demonstrated in a classic study in which the blood glucose levels of patients with diabetes improved (Greenfield and Kaplan 1985). It is possible that patients feel more responsible if they are more involved and therefore comply better with any treatment. For instance, a leaflet to encourage uptake of pneumococcal vaccination led to a higher number of patients receiving the vaccination (Jacobson *et al.* 1999). *Table 13.3* describes the only review of studies that we identified.

COMMUNICATION WITH THE CARE PROVIDER

Patient education

Providing patients with information on their condition and treatment is, of course, an important component of care delivery, and an area for research and innovations

Table 13.3 Examples of strategies to prepare patients for a consultation

Overview	Conclusion
Harrington *et al.* (2004)	Review of 20 trials of interventions to increase patients' participation in medical consultations, that is, written or face-to-face encouragement to ask questions or raise concerns, provided pre-appointment. Half of the interventions resulted in increased patient participation, but few improvements in patient satisfaction with care were found. There were improvements in a range of other outcomes, such as in perceptions of control over health, preferences for an active role in healthcare, recall of information, adherence to recommendations, attendance and clinical outcomes.

in itself (Grol *et al.* 1999). Patient education may also contribute to the implementation of innovations in healthcare, because if patients know about the optimal treatment they may co-operate better with it, both during the consultation and later (patient adherence or concordance). Increasingly, attention is paid to the quality of patient information and its adequacy in reflecting current scientific insights, but unfortunately, many patient-education materials do not meet accepted standards (Coulter *et al.* 1999). Patient education in consultations can have different formats, including:

- Oral knowledge-transfer on the condition and its treatment (*Box 13.4*);
- Instruction regarding treatment, for instance the effective use of inhalers in asthma;
- Use of models, pictures, leaflets and (individualised) letters;
- Referral to external sources of information, such as internet websites;
- Tailored information – explicit recognition of patient needs and preferences in the information delivery.

Patient education tends to have small, but potentially relevant effects on patient outcomes, such as lifestyle change (Ashenden *et al.* 1997; *Table 13.4*). The effects of patient education on (other aspects of) the clinical management of patients are difficult to determine in the research literature, as this focuses mainly on patient outcomes rather than on the process of their care. 'Decision aids' are structured patient-education tools (e.g. leaflets) that aim to help patients participate in decisions on health treatment. Studies show that such decision aids had the intended effects on a number of psychological outcomes, such as having more realistic expectations and lower decision conflict (O'Connor *et al.* 2003). Personalised risk communication can increase the uptake of prevention and screening more than general risk communication (Edwards *et al.* 2002). Interestingly, patients may prefer more conservative

Box 13.4 Information on low back pain (Cherkin *et al.* 1996)

Many patients in primary care have non-specific low back pain. The treatment comprises patient education and advice – resume normal activities as quickly as possible, take physical exercise (walking, cycling, swimming) and increase the level of intensity of exercise. The objectives are to bring functional performance to a normal level and to prevent chronic back problems and dependence on care providers. A study compared two methods of delivering this information. The first method was a book given to patients with back pain who had visited their doctor. The second method was oral instruction by a trained nurse using the same book and delivered directly after a consultation with the doctor. Education by a nurse led to increased knowledge, higher satisfaction with care and better adherence to physical exercise. The book alone resulted in a limited increase in knowledge. However, these educational interventions had a limited effect, as there were no effects on the patients' limitations and use of care in the 12 months after the interventions.

Table 13.4 Effects of patient education interventions

Overview	Conclusion
Ashenden *et al.* (1997)	Review of 37 trials of patient life-style improving interventions in general practice. Many interventions showed small changes in patient behaviour; none appeared to produce substantial changes.
Balas *et al.* (1996)	Review of computerised interactive education and instruction, which led to positive effects in 14 of 19 comparisons (74%).
Edwards *et al.* (2002)	Review of 13 studies of personalised risk communication which showed that this was associated with an increased uptake of screening tests (OR = 1.5). The trend in the results was towards detailed personalised risk communication being associated with an increase in uptake of tests. Most of the included studies addressed mammography programmes.
O'Connor *et al.* (2003)	Review of 34 randomised trials of decision aids, which showed that decision aids had positive effects on psychological outcomes (realistic expectations, decisional conflict and active involvement in decision making), but no impact on satisfaction with decision making, anxiety and health outcomes. Decision aids had variable effect on which treatment was chosen.

treatments after being informed. For instance, a trial of an interactive multimedia decision aid on hormone replacement therapy (HRT) showed that more patients in the intervention group chose the option 'no therapy' after 3 months (46% versus 32% in the control group), although this difference had disappeared at 9 months (Murray *et al.* 2001).

Thus, it can be concluded that patient education can affect patient behaviour regarding healthcare services and that recent research has focused in more detail on different ways of presenting quantitative data to patients. Insights from cognitive psychology suggest that the way information is presented (focused on positive or negative consequences, using relative or absolute effects, etc.) can change its impact (Herrin 2002). However, it is as yet unclear how this affects clinical management and patient outcomes.

Active participation

Active participation during the contact implies that the care provider explicitly includes patients' needs and preferences within the contact and when making decisions. This can support the implementation of clinical guidelines, new procedures and other innovations. It is helpful to distinguish between:

■ Clarification of the patient's need for care – the care provider asks not only about a health problem, but also about the patients' needs and preferences (Mead and Bower 2000);

■ Shared decision making – the care provider informs the patient about the effects and risks of different treatments, identifies the patients' preferences and makes a decision together with the patient (Elwyn *et al.* 1999).

Insight into the effects of needs clarification and shared decision making is based mainly on observational studies, which tend to focus on subjective outcomes such as patient satisfaction (Mead and Bower 2000). The effects on patient management are largely unclear,

although a patient-oriented approach during contacts seems, in general, to be associated with better adherence by the patient to any advice given (Stewart 1984). *Box 13.5* describes a trial that showed general practitioners (GPs) involved patients at higher levels, which was positively evaluated by patients (Elwyn *et al.* 2004). However, if patients prefer a treatment that is not evidence based (such as tests for prostate cancer in lower urinary tract symptoms), patient participation may reduce adherence to clinical guidelines or best practice.

Interventions to enhance treatment uptake and compliance

Treatment compliance (also called adherence, concordance or persistence with treatment decisions) is crucial for effective treatment. Implementation can be successful only if the patient takes a prescribed treatment or adheres to the advice given, so compliance should be regarded as a crucial component of successful adoption. However, patients make independent evaluations with regard to a treatment (Foster and Hudson 1998). From the perspective of the patient it may be rational to not comply (partially or completely) with advice, perhaps because their perception of the expected health gains does not balance the burden, disadvantages or costs of treatment. Patient education, the provision of information, is often insufficient to influence patient behaviour. To improve compliance with treatment, different interventions can be used, such as:

■ A conversation technique that pays attention to patients' judgements of the quality of the advice and its perceived limitations (Lassen 1991);

■ Financial incentives to meet appointments;

■ Telephone reminders and counselling about the advice and instructions provided (*Box 13.6*).

The effects of different strategies to improve patients' treatment compliance are mixed and often limited (*Table 13.5*). A review of 158 studies on methods to increase treat-

Box 13.5 Shared decision making (Elwyn *et al.* 2004)

A cluster randomised trial was performed to evaluate the impact of skill development workshops and risk communication tools on the ability of clinicians to involve patients in decision-making processes. The study included 20 primary care physicians and 393 patients with menorrhagia, menopause and/or HRT therapy, lower urinary tract symptoms or atrial fibrillation. The clinicians were randomised to two interventions – interpersonal skill development and the use of risk communication tools – in a crossover design.

Independent raters assessed videotaped consultations using a validated scale (OPTION). As a result of the interventions, the clinicians ability to involve patients in decision making in consultations in clinical settings with real patients was increased. The level of involvement achieved by the risk communication tools was increased significantly by the subsequent introduction of skill-development workshops. The alternative sequence (skills followed by tools) did not achieve this effect.

Box 13.6 Increasing patient adherence in geriatric assessment (Reuben *et al.* 1999)

Many elderly adults living in the community have health problems that remain undetected and untreated. A brief, comprehensive geriatric assessment programme used validated questions to select adults 65 years of age or over who might have specific health problems, such as depression or urinary incontinence. These adults received (usually within 2 weeks) an in-depth, standardised, comprehensive geriatric assessment from a multidisciplinary team. The co-ordinating geriatrician telephoned the subject's primary care physician to convey the treatment recommendations. An adherence intervention targeted at patients was added – the patient received a written list of recommendations, a 'How to talk to your doctor booklet' and a telephone call approximately 2 weeks after the assessment. The aim was to ensure that the patient understood the recommendations, to assess their level of agreement with recommendations and to empower the patient to interact proactively with their physicians about the recommendations. A randomised trial showed that the geriatric assessment plus the adherence intervention led to improved physical functioning, fewer restrictions on activity and better self-reported functional status. During the 15 months after the geriatric assessment, patients adhered to 67% of all physician-initiated recommendations and 61% of all self-care recommendations.

Table 13.5 Effect of different interventions on treatment compliance

Overview	Conclusion
Balas *et al.* (1996)	Review of computerised reminders, which showed that 12 of 15 comparisons (80%) of patient reminders had the intended effects.
Giuffrida and Torgerson (1997)	Review of financial incentives to enhance patient compliance. Ten of 11 studies showed improvements in patient compliance with the use of financial incentives.
Gyorkos *et al.* (1994)	Review on interventions to enhance vaccination rates, which showed that patient reminders had a pooled effect size of 12% for influenza vaccination (14 studies) and mixed effects for other vaccinations (two studies).
Haynes *et al.* (2002)	Review of 33 randomised trials of interventions to enhance patient compliance with medication prescriptions, showed that 18 out of 36 interventions reported in 30 trials led to improved adherence, but only 16 led to improved clinical outcomes. Almost all of the interventions that were effective were complex and included combinations of strategies. Even the most effective interventions did not lead to large improvements in adherence and treatment outcomes.
Macharia *et al.* (1992)	Review of 23 studies of interventions to improve compliance with appointment keeping for medical services. The average rate of compliance with appointments was 58%. Mailed reminders and telephone prompts were consistently useful in reducing missed appointments (OR = 2.2 and OR = 2.9, respectively). An 'orientation statement' (OR = 2.9), 'contracting' with patients (OR = 1.9) and prompts from physicians (OR = 1.6) also showed positive effects.
Mandelblatt and Kantsky (1995)	Review of interventions to enhance mammography screening, which showed that patient reminders changed the proportion of women being screened by –6% to +7% (three studies) and the proportion of women undergoing physical examination by 23% and 24% (two studies).
McDonald *et al.* (2002)	Review of 33 unconfounded randomised trials of 39 interventions, which showed that 49% of the interventions were associated with significant increases in medication adherence, but only 17 reported significant improvements in treatment outcomes. Almost all the interventions that were effective for long-term care were complex, including combinations of more convenient care, information, counselling, reminders, self-monitoring, reinforcement, family therapy and other forms of additional supervision or attention.
Roter *et al.* (1998)	Review of 153 studies of interventions to improve patient compliance. Overall standardised effect sizes were 0.15 on health outcomes, 0.24 on direct measures of compliance, 0.46 on indirect measures of compliance, 0.17 on subjective reports and 0.11 on healthcare utilisation. The effectiveness of educational interventions, behavioural interventions, affective interventions and their combinations were not consistent and differed across the various outcome measures. The authors concluded that comprehensive interventions were more effective than single-focus interventions. (*cont.*)

Table 13.5 (*cont.*) Effect of different interventions on treatment compliance	
Overview	Conclusion
Szilagy *et al.* (2000)	Review of the effects of patient reminder systems on immunisation rates, comprising 41 studies, which showed that these were effective in 80% of the studies, irrespective of baseline immunisation rates, patient age, setting or vaccination type. Increases in immunisation rates through reminders ranged from 5 to 20 percentage points.
Van Eijken *et al.* (2003)	Review of interventions to improve medication compliance in older patients, which included 14 randomised trials of 23 interventions. Less than half of the interventions were effective. Multifaceted interventions and tailored interventions seemed to be more effective than single and generalised interventions.
Yabroff *et al.* (2003)	Review of interventions to increase cervical smear use, which included 24 studies of patient mediations. Behavioural interventions (e.g. mailed or telephone reminders) increased smear use by up to 18.8%; cognitive and sociological interventions were only marginally effective.

ment compliance (Roter *et al.* 1998) distinguished between education (oral or written information transfer), behaviour modification (skills training, reinforcement, reminders and arrangements) and affective interventions (counselling, support and home visits). These three types of interventions, and combinations of them, were all partly effective, but there was a large variation within each category. The direct effects, weighted for study size, proved to be highest for affective counselling and lowest for behaviour modification. The size of the intervention effects was small to moderate. Another review examined the effect of financial incentives and showed that these could be effective (Giuffrida and Torgerson 1997), and Balas *et al.* (1996) and Szilagy *et al.* (2000) showed that patient reminders can enhance the uptake of preventive and therapeutic activities. Thus, there is a range of interventions to enhance treatment compliance, but little insight into what works in different situations.

Self-management education

Self-management education goes further than just providing information and includes goal setting, short-term action plans and strategies to overcome barriers and to build self-confidence (Steed *et al.* 2003). Self-management education is distinguishable from other types of patient education, which usually comprise information delivery only. It is also different from psychosocial interventions, which are targeted at certain mood states, such as depression, anxiety and stress. Self-management education may be targeted at individuals who have not yet contacted a health professional (*Box 13.7*), but in most situations these interventions are used with patients who have chronic illness. Examples include:

■ Individual training, for instance skills training for patients with asthma or diabetes in the appropriate use of medication and its adjustment within specified limits;

■ Group programmes, comprising both information and mutual support, aiming at more active coping with the chronic illness;

■ Patient-held records, which are used to monitor symptoms and are shared with health professionals.

A comprehensive review of self-management approaches, summarising several reviews in specific conditions, identified 72 trials on patients with diabetes, 27 trials on

Box 13.7 Self-management leaflets (van Eijken *et al.* 2003; Little *et al.* 2001)

Self-management leaflets have been used to influence patient behaviour with regard to illness. Interestingly, some studies aimed to decrease the use of healthcare, while others aimed to increase it. In one study, about 1000 patients received a booklet on minor illnesses called *What Should I Do?* In a randomised trial and over 1 year of follow-up, this group had lower attendance rates at primary care for minor illnesses compared to a control group (OR = 0.81), while total attendance was unchanged (Little *et al.* 2001).

In another study, about 350 patients aged 70 years or over received a self-management booklet, which used validated self-screening questions and suggested attending their physician for a number of health problems, such as depressive symptoms or hearing problems. In a randomised trial over a 3 month period, attendance for these health problems did not change significantly compared to a control group, but there was a trend towards increased use (OR = 1.56).

patients with asthma, 18 trials on patients with arthritis and two studies on patients with chronic illness in general (Bodenheimer *et al.* 2002). This review showed that self-management approaches improved health outcomes more than information-only patient education, but the precise determinants of success remains to be investigated. As in other patient-mediated interventions, the effects of self-management education on professional behaviour and process of care are difficult to extract from the available research literature. However, such effects do exist. Patient-held records improved preventive care in an adult population (Dickey 1993). Self-management programmes in children or adolescents with asthma reduced the number of visits to the emergency department (Guevara *et al.* 2003). So self-management interventions can have positive effects on patient outcomes (*Table 13.6*), and the ways in which these interventions contribute to the implementation of innovations can legitimately be considered.

FEEDBACK ON PROFESSIONAL PERFORMANCE AND CARE DELIVERY

After a contact with a care provider or organisation, or after an episode of care, patients can reflect on the care they have received. Their experiences and evaluations of care can be reported to healthcare workers and organisations, which may help to achieve change. Asking patients to comment on an innovation can, for instance, support its implementation. In the evaluation of patients' complaints, professional guidelines or standards are often taken into account, so that complaint procedures can support their implementation (Garnick *et al.* 1991). Other examples of feedback on the care received are:

- Periodic surveys among samples of patients to monitor the change of patient evaluations over time;
- Reports of patients' evaluations of a specific care provider along with comparative figures relating to a larger group;
- The collection and analysis of comments and complaints that have been expressed in open questions within written questionnaires, letters and conversations with patients;
- A group of 5–10 patients who meet periodically to provide feedback on the care received and possible improvements on it (Williamson 1998).

There are no well-designed research studies on the effects of complaint procedures or patient participation groups, so it is unclear what effects they may have (Crawford *et al.* 2002). In general, feedback on patient evaluations of care may induce behaviour change or promote the implementation of innovations (Scott and Smith 1995), but it is unclear whether the implementation of a specific innovation can be enhanced. There are few studies on the impact of returning feedback from surveys of patients (*Box 13.8*). Many of these studies have methodological limitations, such as the absence of a control group.

CONCLUSIONS

A range of interesting and promising methods involve patients in healthcare delivery, and these may (also)

Table 13.6 Effects of interventions to enhance self-management in patients	
Dickey (1993)	Review of patient-held mini records to promote preventive care, comprising seven trials, which showed that their use can lead to improved preventive care for the general adult population.
Guevara *et al.* (2003)	Review of 32 trials of self-management programmes in children or adolescents with asthma. The programmes were associated with positive patient outcomes, such as improved lung function (standardised mean difference, 0.50) and self-efficacy (0.36), as well as the number of visits to an emergency department (−0.21).
Scott *et al.* (2001)	Review of eight trials of providing recordings (e.g. audiotapes) or summaries (e.g. letter with reminder of key points) of consultations to people with cancer, or to their families. In most studies most participants felt that the recording or summaries were helpful, but the outcome measures varied widely. No effects on anxiety or depression were found; effects on survival or quality of life were not examined.
Steed *et al.* (2003)	Review of 36 comparative studies of diabetes care, including seven randomised trials of self-management programmes. Quality of life improved most after self-management interventions, while feelings of depression particularly improved after psychosocial interventions.

Box 13.8 Effects of feedback on patient evaluations of care (Vingerhoets *et al.* 2001)

Each of 60 practitioners conducted a survey of 100 patients who attended their surgery (achieving a 70% response rate). The questionnaire was composed of questions on evaluations of different aspects of the care provided. 30 practitioners were allocated randomly to a group who received a report that compared the results of their patients with the results of the whole group. The other 30 practitioners were a control group and did not receive any feedback. The results showed that patients' evaluations of care did not differ between the two groups 1 year after the feedback. Nevertheless, physicians in the feedback group reported many (small) changes in the organisation of their practice or the communication with patients as a result of the feedback.

influence the uptake of innovations in practice. These methods may serve different aims, including increased responsiveness to patients' needs, improving health outcomes and better implementation of innovations and improvements (Entwistle *et al.* 1998). Our insight into the effects of most interventions on the process of care is limited, as the available knowledge focuses on effects on patient outcomes rather than on the implementation of innovations. There is, however, substantial evidence that patients can be involved to modify healthcare processes. The example of DTC advertising shows that the adverse effects of patient-mediated interventions need to be considered. Further research is needed on the effects of different patient-mediated interventions on the implementation of guidelines and innovations.

Recommended references

Wensing M and Elwyn G (2002). Research on patient views in evaluation and improvement of quality of care. *Qual Saf Health Care* **11**:153–157.

Wensing M and Grol R (2003). Patients' role in quality improvement. In: Jones R, Britten N, Culpepper L, *et al.* (eds), *Oxford Textbook on Primary Medical Care*, pp. 496–500. Oxford: Oxford University Press.

References

Ashenden R, Silagy C and Weller D (1997). A systematic review of the effectiveness of promoting life style change in general practice. *Fam Pract.* **14**:160–176.

Badger LW and Rand EH (1988). Unlearning psychiatry: A cohort effect in the training environment. *Int J Psychiatr Med.* **8**:123–135.

Balas EA, Austin SM, Mitchell JA, Ewigman BG, Bopp KD and Brown GD (1996). The clinical value of computerized information services. A review of 98 randomized clinical trials. *Arch Fam Med.* **11**:584–590.

Bessell TL, McDonald S, Silagy CA, Anderson JN, Hiller JE and Sansom LN (2002). Do internet interventions for consumers cause more harm than good? A systematic review. *Health Expect.* **5**:28–37.

Bodenheimer T, Lorig K, Holman H and Grumbach K (2002). Patient self-management of chronic disease in primary care. *JAMA* **288**:2469–2475.

Buxton J, White M and Osoba D (1998). Patients' experiences using a computerized program with a touch-sensitive video monitor for the assessment of health-related quality of life. *Qual Life Res.* **7**:513–519.

Campbell SM and Roland MO (1996). Why do people consult the doctor? *Fam Pract.* **13**:75–83.

Centre for Reviews and Dissemination (2002). *Improving the Recognition and Management of Depression in Primary Care.* Effective Health Care Bulletin, Vol. 7(5). York: University of York.

Cherkin DC, Deyo RA, Street JH, *et al.* (1996). Pitfalls of patient education. Limited success of a program for back pain in primary care. *Spine* **21**:345–355.

Coulter A, Entwistle V and Gilbert D (1999). Sharing decisions with patients: Is the information good enough? *BMJ* **318**:318–322.

Crawford MJ, Rutter D, Manley C, *et al.* (2002). Systematic review of involving patients in the planning and development of health care. *BMJ* **325**:1263–1265.

Dickey LL (1993). Promoting preventive care with patient-held minirecords: A review. *Pat Educ Couns.* **20**:37–47.

Division of Research and Education (2000). *Review of Existing Models of Reporting to Consumers on Health Service Quality. Summary Report and Guidelines.* Melbourne: Health Issues Centre and Consumers in Health Counselling.

Domenighetti G, Luraschi P, Casabianca A, *et al.* (1988). Effect of information campaign by the mass media on hysterectomy rates. *Lancet* **ii**:1470–1473.

Edwards A, Unigwe S, Elwyn G and Hood K (2002). Personalised risk communication in health screening programs. Cochrane Library, Issue 2. Oxford: Update Software.

Elwyn G, Edwards A and Kinnersley P (1999). Shared decision-making in primary care: The neglected second half of the consultation. *Br J Gen Pract.* **49**:477–482.

Elwyn G, Edwards A, Hood K, *et al.* (2004). Achieving involvement: Process outcomes from a cluster randomised controlled trial of shared decision making skill development and use of risk communication aids in general practice. *Fam Pract.* **21**:337–346.

Entwistle VA, Sowden AJ and Watt IS (1998). Evaluating interventions to promote patient involvement in decision-making: By what criteria should effectiveness by judged? *J Health Serv Res Policy* **3**:100–107.

Eijken M van, Tsang S, Wensing M, De Smet PAGM and Grol R (2003). Interventions to improve medication compliance in older patients living in the community: A systematic review of the literature. *Drugs Aging* **20**:229–240.

Foster P and Hudson S (1998). From compliance to concordance: A challenge for contraceptive prescribers. *Health Care Anal.* **6**:123–130.

Garnick DW, Hendricks AM and Brennan TA (1991). Can practice guidelines reduce the number and costs of malpractice claims? *JAMA* **266**:2856–2860.

Giuffrida A and Torgerson DJ (1997). Should we pay the patient? Review of financial incentives to enhance patient compliance. *BMJ* **315**:703–707.

Gottlieb S (2002). A fifth of Americans contact their doctor as a result of drug advertising. *BMJ* **325**:854.

Greenfield S and Kaplan S (1985). Expanding patient involvement in care. Effect on patient outcomes. *Ann Int Med.* **102**:520–528.

Greenhalgh J and Meadows K (1999). The effectiveness of the use of patient-based measures of health in routine practice in improving the process and outcomes of patient care: A literature review. *J Eval Clin Pract.* **5**:401–416.

Grilli R, Ramsay C and Minozzi S (2001). Impact of mass media on health services utilisation. The Cochrane Library, Issue 3. Oxford: Update Software.

Grol R, Wensing M, Mainz J, *et al.* (1999). Patients' priorities with respect to general practice care: An international comparison. *Fam Pract.* **16**:4–11.

Guevara JP, Wolf FM, Grum CM and Clark NM (2003). Effects of educational interventions for self management of asthma in children and adolescents: Systematic review and meta-analysis. *BMJ* **326**:1308–1314.

Gyorkos TW, Tannenbaum TN, Abrahomowicz M, *et al.* (1994). Evaluation of the effectiveness of immunization delivery methods. *Can J Public Health* **85**:S14–S30.

Harrington J, Noble LM and Newman SP (2004). Improving patients' communication with doctors: A systematic review of intervention studies. *Pat Educ Couns.* **52**:7–16.

Haynes RB, Montage P, Oliver T, McKibbon KA, Brouwers MC and Kanani R (2002). Interventions for helping patients to follow prescriptions for medications. Cochrane Library, Issue 1. Oxford: Update Software.

Herrin J (2002). Presentation of empirical evidence about health. Cochrane Library, Issue 1. Oxford: Update Software.

Hibbard JH and Jewtt JJ (1997). Will quality report cards help consumers? *J Health Affairs* **16**:218–228.

Jacobs JE, Lisdonk EH van de, Smeele I, *et al.* (2001). *Management of Patients with Asthma and COPD: The Correlation between Patients' Perceived Quality of Life and Subsequent GP Interventions.* Unpublished report. Nijmegen: WOK.

Jacobson TA, Thomas DM, Morton FJ, *et al.* (1999). Use of a low-literacy patient education tool to enhance pneumococcal vaccination rates. A randomized controlled trial. *JAMA* **282**:646–650.

Kok G, Borne B van den and Mullen PD (1997). Effectiveness of health education and health promotion: Meta-analyses of effect studies and determinants of effectiveness. *Pat Educ Couns.* **30**:19–27.

Lassen LC (1991). Connections between the quality of consultations and patient compliance in general practice. *Fam Pract.* **8**:154–160.

Little P, Somerville J, Williamson I, *et al.* (2001). Randomised controlled trial of self management leaflets and booklets for minor illness provided by post. *BMJ* **322**:1–5.

Macharia WM, Leon G, Rowe BH, Stephenson BJ and Haynes RB (1992). An overview of interventions to improve compliance with appointment keeping for medical services. *JAMA* **267**:1813–1817.

Mandelblatt J and Kantsky PA (1995). Effectiveness of interventions to enhance physician screening for breast cancer. *J Fam Pract.* **40**:162–171.

Marshall M, Shekelle P, Leatherman S, *et al.* (2000). The public release of performance data: What do we expect to gain? *JAMA* **283**:1866–1874.

McDonald HP, Garg AX and Haynes RB (2002). Interventions to enhance patient adherence to medication prescriptions. Scientific review. *JAMA* **288**:2868–2879.

Mead N and Bower P (2000). Patient-centredness: A conceptual framework and review of the empirical literature. *Soc Sci Med.* **51**:1087–1110.

Meadows KA, Rogers D and Greene T (1998). Attitudes to the use of health outcome questionnaires in the routine care of patients with diabetes: A survey of general practitioners and practice nurses. *Br J Gen Pract.* **48**:1555–1559.

Mintzes B (2002). For and against: Direct to consumer advertising is medicalising normal human experience. *BMJ* **324**:908–909.

Murray E, Davis H, Tai SS, Coulter A, Gray A and Haines A (2001). Randomised controlled trial of an interactive multimedia decision aid on hormone replacement therapy in primary care. *BMJ* **323**:1–5.

Newhouse JP (1993). *Free for all? Lessons from the RAND Health Insurance Experiment.* Cambridge MA: Harvard University Press.

O'Connor AM, Rostom A, Fiset V, *et al.* (2003). Decision aids for patients facing health treatment or screening decisions. Cochrane Library, Issue 1. Oxford: Update Software.

Osoba D (1993). Self-rating symptom checklists: A simple method for recording and evaluating symptom control in oncology. *Cancer Treat Rev.* **19**:S43–S51.

Reuben DB, Frank JC, Hirsch SH, McGuigan KA and Maly RC (1999). A randomized clinical trial of outpatient comprehensive geriatric assessment coupled with an intervention to increase adherence to recommendations. *J Am Geriatr Soc.* **47**:269–276.

Roter DL, Hall JA, Merisca R, *et al.* (1998). Effectiveness of interventions to improve patient compliance. A meta-analysis. *Med Care* **36**:1138–1161.

Scott A and Smith R (1995). Keeping the customer satisfied: Issues in the interpretation and use of patient satisfaction surveys. *Int J Qual Health Care* **6**:353–359.

Scott JT, Entwistle VA, Sowden AJ and Watt I (2001). Giving tape recordings or written summaries of consultations to people with cancer: A systematic review. *Health Expect.* **4**:162–169.

Stewart MA (1984). What is a successful doctor–patient interview? A study of interactions and outcomes. *Soc Sci Med.* **19**:167–175.

Sullivan FM and MacNaughton RJ (1996). Evidence in consultations: Interpreted and individualised. *Lancet* **348**:941–943.

Szilagy PG, Bordley C, Vann JC, *et al.* (2000). Effect of patient reminder/recall interventions on immunization rates. A review. *JAMA* **284**:1820–1827.

Steed L, Cooke D and Newman S (2003). A systematic review of psychosocial following education, self-management and psychosocial interventions in diabetes mellitus. *Pat Educ Couns*. **51**:5–15.

Vingerhoets E, Wensing M and Grol R (2001). Educational feedback on patients' evaluations of general practice: A randomised trial. *Qual Health Care* **10**:224–228.

Wensing M and Grol R (1998). What can patients do to improve health care? *Health Expect*. **1**:37–49.

Williamson C (1998). The rise of doctor–patient working groups. *BMJ* **317**:1374–1377.

Yabroff KR, Mangan P and Mandelblatt J (2003). Effectiveness of interventions to increase Papanicolauou Smear use. *J Am Board Fam Pract*. **16**:188–203.

Chapter 14

Multifaceted interventions

Michel Wensing and Richard Grol

KEY MESSAGES

- Combinations of interventions may be more effective than single interventions in changing professional behaviour. However, no specific combination provides a guarantee for success – even combinations of many different strategies may not be effective.
- The effectiveness of a combined strategy is determined by the effectiveness of separate interventions that make up the strategy and by the interaction between the different interventions, which can increase or reduce the total effect.
- Combined strategies, which include outreach visits by trained visitors who provide information, instruction, support, feedback and reminders, are often effective.
- The costs of combined strategies have to be considered, as these may be higher compared to those of single interventions.

Box 14.1 Improvement of hand hygiene in hospitals (Larson *et al.* 1997)

Care providers in the hospital should disinfect their hands frequently to reduce hospital infections. A surgery department in an Australian hospital used a combined strategy to improve handwashing:

▪ Barriers and needs of staff members were assessed in group meetings in the department, organised during both days and nights to involve as many care providers as possible;

▪ In the group meetings information was given orally and by video on the relevance of hand hygiene and on the use of supplies and the technique of disinfecting;

▪ Group meetings were used to ensure the implementation plan was shared;

▪ Four washbasins that provided water, soap and tissues automatically on the basis of infrared signals were introduced – to become used to these washbasins the level of automatic functioning was increased in three phases to fully automatic;

▪ Regular feedback on the level of hand washing was provided to healthcare workers in the department;

▪ The management of the department supported the implementation of handwashing actively and visibly.

Despite this carefully designed combined strategy, no change was achieved with respect to handwashing and no difference was detected in the comparison with a control group.

INTRODUCTION

The interventions used to implement innovations, guidelines or best practices described in previous chapters are often used in various combinations. A large systematic review found that 178 out of 235 studies (222 out of 309 comparisons) concerned multifaceted interventions (Grimshaw *et al.* 2004). It is plausible within our theoretical model that multifaceted interventions are more effective than single interventions, because more barriers to change can be addressed and there is, in most cases, a range of relevant barriers. If education can solve a lack of knowledge and feedback a lack of insight into professional performance, then a combination of these interventions should have the potential to solve both barriers to change. The effect of a combination of interventions on process and outcomes of healthcare might be larger than the effect of the interventions separately. This chapter focuses in more detail on combinations of implementation strategies described in previous chapters, their effectiveness and the potential to optimise the effectiveness.

TYPES OF MULTIFACETED INTERVENTIONS

Combinations of interventions comprise two or more single interventions, although it may be arbitrarily labelled as a single intervention. For instance, we may consider outreach visits to be a single intervention, but these often include different activities such as instruction, feedback, support, reminders and organisational change. We distinguish between specific activities, such as participation in an educational group or receiving feedback on practice patterns, following the Cochrane Effective Practice and Organisation of Care (EPOC) list of interventions where possible (see Chapter 8). In cases where an implementation strategy comprises two or more of these specific interventions, we consider it to be a combined strategy.

It is also possible to document the diversity of interventions on the basis of a classification of their content. A well-known taxonomy has been suggested by Green *et al.* (1988), which has been applied to implementation strategies by Davis *et al.* (1999). Green distinguishes between interventions targeted at:

- Predisposing factors – knowledge, attitude, opinions and values (Davis translated this into educational strategies);
- Enabling factors – skills and availability of resources (Davis also included in this category the provision of resources and organisational change);
- Reinforcing factors – opinions and behaviours of others (Davis included feedback, reminders, use of opinion leaders and other interventions in this category).

A different classification of the content of strategies, which relates more closely to the EPOC categorisation of interventions, is as follows (Wensing *et al.* 1998):

- Provision of information unrelated to behaviour – written education material, large-scale continuing education;
- Provision of information related to behaviour – feedback and reminders;
- Provision of information with the use of social influence – educational outreach visits by colleagues or experts, small-scale interactive continuing education, local consensus meetings, peer review groups and quality circles;
- Organisational change – revision of professional roles, multiprofessional collaboration, disease management, quality management, use of information and computer technology (ICT), formal regulations, provision of materials and financial incentives.

Many combined strategies include some type of information or education targeted at health professionals. In the areas of test ordering and prevention many combined strategies include feedback and reminders. However, few studies of interventions use organisational change or financial incentives to enhance the implementation of innovations. The following combinations are most prevalent in the research literature:

- Combinations of different types of education – educational material, large-scale education (courses, etc.) and/or small-scale education;
- Combinations of feedback on behaviour and education of care providers, sometimes combined with organisational change;
- Combinations of reminders and education of care providers, sometimes combined with organisational change;
- Combinations of many different interventions, such as continuing education, feedback, organisational change and financial incentives.

EFFECTS

At least 18 literature reviews summarise the effects of combined strategies (*Table 14.1*). The conclusions of the authors varied between moderately positive and very positive with respect to the effects, which provides a positive view of the effectiveness of combined strategies. However, this does not necessarily mean that multifaceted strategies are more effective than specific, single strategies. In addition, the combinations are very heterogeneous, so that it is difficult to draw conclusions as to the effectiveness of specific combinations of interventions. Furthermore, some reviews do not distinguish between different types of combinations, but only draw conclusions on the total group of multifaceted interventions. Although combined strategies are predominantly effective, it is not possible to choose which specific combinations will provide guarantees for success. Even the use of several different interventions is not always successful. One large review of 235 studies of guideline implementation did not find a relationship between the number of intervention components and effects (Grimshaw *et al.* 2004), which challenges the assumption of the effectiveness of multifaceted interventions. We describe a number of combinations in more detail below.

Table 14.1 Overview of reviews of controlled studies of combined interventions

Overview	Conclusion
Davis *et al.* (1992)	12 studies were identified on the basis of a combination of predisposing interventions (different types of education of care providers) and enabling interventions (supply of guidelines, protocols, algorithms, patient education materials, feedforwards of patient information). Nine of the ten studies with process outcomes showed positive effects. Furthermore, 31 studies focused on a combination of predisposing interventions (education) and reinforcing factors (feedback or reminders). 18 out of 26 studies with process outcomes showed positive changes and six out of nine studies with patient outcomes showed positive changes. Finally, 16 combinations of predisposing, enabling and reinforcing interventions were identified. Four of 14 studies showed positive changes on process outcomes, while five out of nine studies showed positive changes of patient outcomes.
Davis *et al.* (1995)	The review included 39 studies on a combination of two interventions, of which 25 showed positive effects, 12 no effect or negative effects, and three studies varying effects. Of the 39 other studies on three or more interventions, 31 showed positive effects, five no effect or a negative effect. Three studies showed varying effects.
Davis *et al.* (1999)	This review comprised seven studies on single types of continuing education (between 2 and 6 hours), of which two showed positive effects on physician behaviour. There were ten studies on combined or long-term types of education, for instance a series of meetings. Of these studies seven had positive effects on the performance of physicians.
Gill *et al.* (1999)	This review on change of medication prescribing included 43 studies with combinations of two or more interventions. Such combinations were effective in 21 studies.
Grimshaw *et al.* (2004)	This review comprised 235 studies (309 comparisons) on all possible interventions. Of the comparisons, 73% evaluated multifaceted interventions, but no specific combination of interventions was studied more frequently than 11 times. This makes it difficult to draw general conclusions. There was no relationship between the number of component interventions and the effects of multifaceted interventions.
Gyorkos *et al.* (1994)	This review contained three studies on a combination of reminders for care providers and reminders for patients to improve preventive care. The average effect was 17% for influenza vaccination and 13% for pneumonia vaccination.
Hulscher *et al.* (1999)	This review on prevention in primary care included 18 studies on feedback in combination with other strategies. The changes in preventive care varied between –2 and +57% compared to control groups that did not receive an intervention. In addition, the review included 15 studies on reminders combined with other strategies. Changes in preventive care varied between 4 and 35% compared to control groups without interventions. Finally, there were 11 studies on different combinations of interventions. The changes varied in this category between –5 and +26% compared to control groups without intervention.
Lancaster *et al.* (1998)	This review on stop-smoking activities of general practitioners (GPs) describes three studies on combinations of education and reminders for physicians. The probability that the smokers stopped was larger [average odds ratio (OR) = 2.37] compared to the control groups. The review also included eight studies on a combination of training, reminders and supply of nicotine chewing gum. This type of combined intervention did not result in a significant improvement in the probability that smokers stopped compared to training or reminders only.
Mandelblatt and Kanetsky (1995)	This review focused on screening for breast cancer and it contained eight studies on combinations of interventions targeted at care providers and patients. The change in the percentage of women screened varied between +0.3% and +28%.
Oxman *et al.* (1995)	This review included 15 studies on combined interventions, which led to change of professional behaviour, according to the authors, and less consistently to change of patient outcomes. (*cont.*)

Table 14.1 (cont.) Overview of reviews of controlled studies of combined interventions

Overview	Conclusion
Snell and Buck (1996)	This review focused on cancer screening in primary care. The effects of a number of interventions were (the number of studies is unclear, effect size is expressed as a standardised effect measure which varies between 0 and 1): 0.006–0.69 for a combination of reminders, education and feedback; 0.06–0.62 for reminders and education; 0.38 for reminders and feedback; 0.10 for education and feedback. The effect of combinations of strategies targeted at physicians and patients was 0.05. The effect of combinations of two strategies was on average 0.25; in three strategies this was 0.68 and in four strategies –0.01.
Solomon et al. (1998)	This review focused on change of diagnostic test ordering. Combinations of education and feedback (predisposing and reinforcing strategies) were effective in six out of seven studies. Combinations of feedback and organisational interventions (reinforcing and enabling interventions) were effective in nine of the 12 cases. Combinations of education, feedback and organisational interventions were effective in all eight included studies.
Stone et al. (2002)	Review with 81 studies on interventions to increase adult immunisation and cancer-screening services. Meta-regression analysis suggested that the most effective intervention components were organisational change (OR varied from 2.5 to 17.6), followed by patient-directed financial incentives (OR, 1.8 to 3.4) and patient reminders (OR, 1.7 to 2.8).
Thomson et al. (1997b,c)	This review contained 15 studies of combinations of feedback with educational materials or educational meetings. The relative change varied between 25 and 62%, but it was small in absolute terms. In 11 studies of feedback as part of a combined strategy the relative change varied between 13 and 56%, but it was small in absolute terms.
Thomson et al. (1997a)	Combinations of outreach visits by an external person with other interventions led to relative changes between 15 and 68% in 12 out of 13 studies.
Van der Weijden et al. (2000)	This review focused on the use of diagnostic tests. Eight studies focused on a combination of written educational material and a lecture. The absolute difference in change between intervention group and control group varied between –11 and +6% with respect to the number of requests and there was a 7–15% improvement in the quality of test ordering. Combinations of small-scale quality improvement and lectures led to a 13–15% reduction in test ordering (two studies). Combinations of small-scale quality improvement and feedback led to 0–1% improvement of test ordering (two studies). One study showed 4% absolute reduction.
Wensing et al. (1998)	This review focused on the implementation of change in general practice care. Combinations of feedback or reminders with education and/or information delivery was effective in four cases, partly effective in four cases and not effective in 12 cases (20 studies). Individual instruction or peer-review groups combined with information delivery was assessed in eight studies, of which four showed positive effects, three partly positive effects and one no positive effect. Supply of materials, incentives or regulations combined with information delivery was effective in three cases, partly effective in three cases and not effective in one case (seven studies).
Worrall et al. (1997)	This review focused on the implementation of innovations in primary medical care. Combinations of interventions were effective in one out of two studies.
Yabroff et al. (2003)	Review on interventions to increase Papanicolauou smear taking, which included 46 studies, of which 12 focused on interventions that targeted both patients and providers. It appeared that these were not more effective than interventions targeted to either patients or providers alone.

Combinations of education

A combination of formal continuing education and interactive education proved to be an effective implementation strategy in general practice care (Wensing *et al.* 1998). It is plausible that this combination is also effective in other healthcare sectors. Formal education may provide a foundation for behaviour change by improving knowledge and understanding, while interactive education directly affects behaviour because barriers and needs of participants can be targeted (*Box 14.2*). An example of an effective intervention was a combination of written information, the provision of individual instruction in short outreach visits and patient education material to influence the prescribing behaviour of physicians (Soumerai and Avorn 1986). Another successful intervention comprised a symposium, newsletter, skills training and personal tutor to improve mammography screening (Lane *et al.* 1991).

Combinations with feedback

Combinations with feedback are used mainly to change diagnostic test ordering and improve prevention. Care providers receive, for instance, figures on the number of tests or preventive procedures in combination with some type of continuing education (*Box 14.3*). This combination has often been effective, particularly to improve prevention in primary care, although the size of the effects varied (Hulscher *et al.* 1999). Effective interventions often comprise several activities, such as monthly supply of a list of patients who need preventive care, full financial reimbursement of prevention, delegation of tasks to trained nurses and use of written protocols (Morrissey *et al.* 1995). Solomon *et al.* (1998) and Van der Weijden *et al.* (2000) found that combinations of education and feedback and combinations of feedback and organisational change often had an effect on the volume of tests ordered (laboratory tests,

---

Box 14.2 Dyspepsia management in primary care (Banait *et al.* 2003)

Studies suggested that the prescribing of acid-suppressing drugs for dyspepsia and referral for gastrointestinal endoscopy could be improved. A multifaceted strategy to implement dyspepsia management in primary care comprised postgraduate education workshops with 4–8 GPs, chaired by local hospital specialists. Each seminar consisted of a 15 minute presentation that described the guidelines, followed by an hour of discussion. All the attending GPs received a copy of the text used during the discussion, as well as contact details for enquiries. A reinforcement visit was made by one member of the research team. A cluster randomised controlled trial compared this multifaceted educational intervention with postal guideline dissemination alone – a total of 111 general practices were followed up. The study showed, among other findings, that the proportion of appropriate referrals was higher in the intervention group (64% versus 50%). Also, an increase in overall expenditure of acid-suppressing drugs occurred (+8% versus +2%). The latter result was not intended.

Box 14.3 Small–scale multidisciplinary continuing education and feedback to improve prescribing for asthma and urinary tract infections (Veninga 2000)

Two meetings of existing educational groups of primary care physicians and a pharmacist focused on asthma and urinary tract infection (UTI). The clinical guidelines for asthma recommend anti-inflammatory therapy if patients use bronchodilators continuously and an increase of inhaled corticosteroids if exacerbations are not controlled. In the UTI programme the main focus was on prescribing first-choice drugs for uncomplicated cases. The researcher supplied an educational programme and background information to the group facilitator, who was one of the members of the group. In the first meeting, guidelines were briefly described and decisions on medication were discussed by means of 18 patient vignettes. In the second meeting participants received individual feedback on prescribing behaviour, which was discussed in the group meeting. Figures were supplied by the pharmacist. The effect of these interventions was assessed in a randomised trial with crossover design: 12 groups received education on asthma and 12 other groups were given the intervention (education and feedback) on UTI, but data on both asthma and UTI were collected from both groups. About 90% of the GPs attended the first meeting and 80% the second meeting. A number of changes in prescribing were found. In asthma patients, inhaled corticosteroids and oral steroids for exacerbations were prescribed more often than in the control condition. In UTI shorter prescriptions were given, but the first-choice medication did not change.

radiographs). Thomson *et al.* (1997b,c) concluded that combinations of feedback with education or other combinations in which feedback was included often led to the desired changes, but that the size of change was small and not always clinically relevant. A study on change of diagnostic tests showed that adding reminders did not provide additional effectiveness compared to feedback only (Tierney *et al.* 1986). In many cases, the effects of such combined interventions on patient outcomes were limited, although this was assessed in only some of the studies.

Combinations with reminders

Combined strategies that include reminders can help to implement preventive guidelines (Hulscher *et al.* 1999). The combinations of reminders for physicians and patients had good results (*Box 14.4*). A further example is a strategy to improve mammography, which comprised reminders for physicians, information for patients, a telephone line for making appointments, reminder postcards for patients and telephone contacts with, and financial reimbursement to, patients (Burack *et al.* 1994). Combinations of reminders or feedback and formal continuing education were only partly effective in another review, even less effective than feedback or reminders

only (Wensing *et al.* 1998). An explanation of this finding may be that combined strategies were applied in areas in which change is more difficult to achieve. As relapse into old routines is an important problem for implementation, the use of reminders after, for instance, a course or meeting is potentially a good idea.

Combinations with outreach visits

Combinations with outreach visits by trained visitors, who provide information, support, instruction, feedback and reminders, have been studied less often, but they are often remarkably successful (*Box 14.5*). A review that focused on these interventions found effects in 12 out of 13 studies (Thomson *et al.* 1997a). In nine of these studies medication prescribing was studied and eight showed positive effects. In a number of these studies outreach visits were combined with social marketing techniques, an approach similar to that of the physician visitors used by the pharmaceutical industry (Avorn *et al.* 1992). Educational outreach visits can also be combined with feedback, reminders or patient-orientated interventions. For instance, pharmacists gave advice and feedback to physicians on the decreasing use of (more expensive) analgesics and offering alternatives, which proved to be effective (Stergachis 1987 *et al.*).

Box 14.4 Computer support and paper–based risk tables to prevent cardiovascular diseases (Montgomery *et al.* 2000)

Current knowledge suggests that the risk of cardiovascular diseases cannot be assessed on the basis of blood pressure alone, but that other factors should be considered as well, such as age, gender, smoking, cholesterol and blood glucose. A physician cannot be expected to learn the risks of different patient groups, so he or she needs tools to use in patient care. Paper-based risk tables have been developed to assess individual risks on cardiovascular diseases, given a number of patient characteristics, but these are difficult to use. Therefore, computer programmes were developed that show the risk after a number of values have been entered. The ultimate aim of the risk assessment is that more adequate preventive care is provided, which results in reduced (risks of) cardiovascular diseases. An experiment compared paper-based risk tables with computer support and paper-based risk tables. The physicians in the group with computer support received training in the use of the computer for risk assessment. It was found that none of the strategies resulted in a lower risk of cardiovascular diseases compared to a control group that received usual care. It was also found that patients of physicians who had received only the paper-based risk tables had lower blood pressure and used more medication for cardiovascular diseases at 12 months compared to patients whose physicians had also received the computer support.

Box 14.5 Prevention of cancer (Dietrich *et al.* 1992)

To improve ten types of prevention of cancer in primary care (cervix screening, blood tests, etc.) two interventions were tested, both including outreach visits. The first intervention combined these with reminders – after 12 months patients had received on average 64.4% of the preventive care compared to 51.6% in the control group, who had not received an intervention (Thomson *et al.* 1997a). The second intervention combined outreach visits with lectures and reminders. The effect in this group was 61.3% on average of the desired preventive care (Thomson *et al.* 1997a).

Box 14.6 Programme to improve quality of ambulatory care for depression (Wells *et al.* 2000)

A comprehensive strategy was applied to enhance the implementation of guidelines of depression in primary care:
- The healthcare provider formally committed to promote the implementation of the guidelines and it paid half of the costs of the implementation programme;
- Local experts (GP, nurse, psychiatrist) were selected and trained in 2 day workshops;
- The experts provided lectures (attended by 80% of the physicians), distributed a handbook, gave individual instruction (used by 48% of the doctors) and feedback on individual performance (to 60% of the practitioners);
- Specialised nurses were trained to monitor and educate patients with depression;
- Potentially depressed patients were screened when they visited the practice and for the next 5–7 months.
- The specialist nurses saw patients 2 weeks after screening and assessment for treatment by the practitioner.

In one study group patients received medication, and monitoring and follow-up by the specialised nurse, while in the other study group patients were referred to a psychotherapist who was trained to provide 12–16 individual or group sessions (the costs were partly borne by the organisation instead of the patient). Compared to a control group, patients in the intervention groups, at 6 months, had engaged in more contacts with a physician related to mental problems, more often received medication against depression and more often attended a psychiatrist or psychotherapist, and had fewer depressive symptoms. On these measures the intervention groups scored 10% higher than the control group. The effects were slightly more positive for the group who received medication and who were seen by the nurse. The total number of visits to a physician was equal in both groups.

Combinations of many different interventions

Earlier reviews claimed that combinations of many different interventions are often effective (Solomon *et al.* 1998; Wensing *et al.* 1998; Davis *et al.* 1992; Ornstein *et al.* 1991). Such comprehensive implementation strategies are also expensive, so the higher effectiveness should be related to the higher costs (*Box 14.6*). A more recent review has challenged the effectiveness of multifaceted interventions, as it found that a higher number of intervention components was not related to greater effectiveness (Grimshaw *et al.* 2004; *Table 14.2*).

It seems plausible that combined interventions are only more effective than single interventions if these address factors that are actually related to professional performance. For instance, if there is no lack of knowledge, then educational interventions are unlikely to contribute to the effectiveness of a multifaceted implementation strategy. Furthermore, specific single interventions (such as reminders or outreach visits) were highly effective in certain conditions. A limitation of this review is that the number of organisational interventions was relatively small – most interventions were targeted at professionals.

DETERMINANTS OF THE EFFECTIVENESS

The remarks in previous chapters on the determinants of the success of single interventions are also relevant if these are part of a multifaceted intervention. Combinations of interventions may be more effective if they address a larger variety of barriers for change. In other words, a combination of different types of education is probably less effective than a combination of education and organisational change. The first combination only addresses a lack of knowledge, while the second combination also addresses organisational problems. Of course, the intensity and duration of different interventions are relevant as well.

There is little insight in the added value of combining interventions. Thomson *et al.* (1997b,c) identified four studies that assessed the added value of feedback compared to other interventions. These studies focused on

Table 14.2 Effect sizes of multifaceted interventions versus no intervention (Grimshaw *et al.* 2004)

Number of intervention components	Median (%)absolute effect size across studies (*n* = number of studies)
1	10.2 (*n* = 52)
2	7.4 (*n* = 36)
3	11.0 (*n* = 25)
4	4.0 (*n* = 11)
5	21.8 (*n* = 4)
6	15.0 (*n* = 1)

local consensus development for the medical treatment of haemoglobin values, reminders for preventive care, reminders for medical treatment for hyperlipidaemia and invitations sent to patients for breast-cancer screening. In three of these studies feedback did not lead to an additional effect; the fourth study showed a non-significant improvement. Stone *et al.* (2002) used meta-regression to explore which intervention components were most influential in improving prevention. They found that organisational interventions were most relevant – the use of separate clinics devoted to prevention (*Box 14.7*), designation of non-physician staff to carry out specific prevention activities, teamwork and collaboration. The next most effective intervention components were patient-directed financial incentives and patient reminders.

A determinant that is particularly relevant to multifaceted interventions is the interaction between different strategies. The effect of a combined intervention does not necessarily equal the sum of the effects of the single interventions that comprise it. On the one hand, different interventions can result in the same direction of effect as when used alone, but of a smaller magnitude, so the overall effect is less than the sum of the individual parts. For instance, in one study both reminders and feedback influenced preventive care, but the combination did not result in a larger effect than the interventions separately (Tierney *et al.* 1986). On the other hand, different interventions can support each other, so the total effect may be larger than the effects of the interventions separately. For instance, new insights gained from a course may only be applicable if the organisation has been changed. This emphasises again the importance of a careful documentation of the most important barriers to improvement and the systematic development of an implementation plan.

DISCUSSION AND CONCLUSIONS

Multifaceted interventions may be more effective than single interventions, but it is not possible to specify which combinations of strategies are most effective in which situations. Even combinations of interventions are not effective in some situations. Furthermore, the higher likelihood of successful implementation should be balanced with the higher costs of multifaceted interventions. A multifaceted intervention with many activities that are not carefully related to the relevant factors is an unfocused intervention – it is likely to be partly unnecessary or not effective.

An alternative is a tailored strategy for a specific group of care providers, patients, practices or organisations. This tailored intervention should relate to the relevant barriers and the needs of the target group, so it may be cheaper and simpler. Educational outreach visits have more or less the character of a tailored intervention, which may explain their effectiveness. However, it requires time and money to document barriers and needs and it may be unclear which intervention can be applied to overcome a specific barrier. Research evidence to support the effectiveness and efficiency of tailored implementation interventions is scarce and not consistently positive.

Recommended literature

Grol R and Grimshaw J (2003). From best evidence to best practice: Effective implementation of change in patients' care. *Lancet* **362**:1225–1230.

Grimshaw JM, Shirran L, Thomas R, *et al.* (2001). Changing provider behavior. An overview of systematic reviews of interventions. *Med Care* **39**:S2–S45.

Box 14.7 Improvement of the management of alcohol problems in primary care (Anderson *et al.* 2004)

Evidence suggests that the detection and management of alcohol problems in primary care is effective, but primary care physicians find managing alcohol problems difficult. A systematic review focused on interventions to implement the improved management of alcohol problems in primary care. 12 trials on 15 implementation programmes were found, which examined various interventions such as outreach visits, educational workshops, patient-directed interventions and office support. The weighted mean-effect size (0.73) was associated with significant heterogeneity. Regression analysis using a weighted random-effects model (because of heterogeneity) found a significant effect for alcohol-specific programmes as opposed to general prevention programmes in which alcohol was included, and for multifaceted programmes as opposed to single-faceted programmes. No difference in the improvement of management of alcohol problems was found between professionally based interventions and organisationally based interventions.

References

Avorn J, Soumerai SB, Everitt DE, *et al.* (1992). A randomized trial of a program to reduce the use of psychoactive drugs in nursing homes. *N Engl J Med.* **327**:168–173.

Anderson P, Laurant M, Kaner E, Grol R and Wensing M (2004). Engaging general practitioners in the management of hazardous and harmful alcohol consumption: Results of a meta-analysis. *J Stud Alcohol* **65**:191–199.

Banait G, Sibbald B, Thompson D, Summerton C, Hann M and Talbot S (2003). Modifying dyspepsia management in primary care: A cluster randomised controlled trial of educational outreach compared with passive guideline dissemination. *Br J Gen Pract.* **53**:94–100.

Burack RC, Gimotty PA, George J, *et al.* (1994). Promoting screening mammography in inner-city settings: A randomized controlled trial of computerized reminder as a component of a programme to facilitate mammography. *Med Care* **32**:609–624.

Davis DA, Thomson MA, Oxman AD, *et al.* (1992). Evidence for the effectiveness of CME. A review of 50 randomized controlled trials. *JAMA* **268**(9):1111–1117.

Davis DA, Thomson MA, Oxman AD, *et al.* (1995). Changing physician performance. A systematic review of the effect of continuing medical education strategies. *JAMA* **274**:700–705.

Davis D, O'Brien MA, Freemantle N, *et al.* (1999). Impact of formal continuing medical education: Do conferences, workshops, rounds, and other traditional continuing education activities change physician behavior or health care outcomes? *JAMA* **282**:867–874.

Dietrich AJ, O'Connor CT, Keller A, *et al.* (1992). Cancer: Improving early detection and prevention. A community practice randomised trial. *BMJ* **304**:687–691.

Gill PS, Mäkelä M, Vermeulen KM, *et al.* (1999). Changing doctor prescribing behaviour: A review. *Pharm World Sci.* **21**(4):158–167.

Green LW, Eriksen MP and Schor EL (1988). Preventive activities by physicians: Behavioral determinants and potential interventions. *Am J Prev Med.* **4**:S101–S107.

Grimshaw JM, Thomas RE, MacLennan G, *et al.* (2004). Effectiveness and efficiency of guideline dissemination and implementation strategies. *Health Technol Assess.* **8**(6):1–84.

Gyorkos TW, Tannenbaum TN, Abrahamowicz M, *et al.* (1994). Evaluation of the effectiveness of immunization delivery methods. *Can J Public Health* **85**(Suppl. 1):S14–S30.

Hulscher MEJL, Wensing M, Grol RPTM, *et al.* (1999). Interventions to improve the delivery of preventive services in primary care. *Am J Public Health* **89**(5):737–746.

Lancaster T, Silagy C, Fowler G, *et al.* (1998). Training health professionals in smoking cessation. The Cochrane Library, Issue 4. Oxford: Update Software.

Lane DS, Polednak AP and Bung MA (1991). Effect of continuing medical education and cost reduction on physician compliance with mammography screening guidelines. *J Fam Pract.* **33**:359–368.

Larson EL, Bryan JL, Adler LM, *et al.* (1997). A multifaceted approach to changing handwashing behavior. *Am J Infect Control* **25**:3–10.

Mandelblatt J and Kanetsky PA (1995). Effectiveness of interventions to enhance physician screening for breast cancer. *J Fam Pract.* **40**(2):162–171.

Montgomery AA, Fahey T, Peters TJ, *et al.* (2000). Evaluation of computer based clinical decision support system and risk chart for management of hypertension in primary care: Randomised controlled trial. *BMJ* **320**:686–690.

Morrissey JP, Harris RP, Kincade-Norburn J, *et al.* (1995). Medicare reimbursement for preventive care. Changes in performance of services, quality of life, and health care costs. *Med Care* **33**:315–331.

Ornstein SM, Garr DR, Jenkings RG, *et al.* (1991). Computer-generated physician and patient reminders. Tools to improve population adherence to select preventive services. *J Fam Pract.* **32**:82–90.

Oxman AD, Thomson MA, Davis DA, *et al.* (1995). No magic bullets. A systematic review of 102 trials of interventions to help health care professionals deliver services more effectively or efficiently. *Can Med Assoc J.* **153**(10):1423–1431.

Snell J and Buck EL (1996). Increasing cancer screening: A meta-analysis. *Prev Med.* **25**:702–707.

Solomon DH, Hashimoto H, Daltroy L, *et al.* (1998). Techniques to improve physicians' use of diagnostic tests. *JAMA* **280**(23):2020–2027.

Soumerai SB and Avorn J (1986). Economic and policy analysis of university-based drug detailing. *Med Care* **24**:313–331.

Stergachis A, Fors M, Wagner EH, *et al.* (1987). Effect of clinical pharmacists on drug prescribing in a primary-care clinic. *Am J Hosp Pharm.* **44**:525–529.

Stone EG, Morton SC, Hulscher ME, *et al.* (2002). Interventions that increase use of adult immunization and cancer screening services: A meta-analysis. *Ann Intern Med.* **136**:641–651.

Thomson MA, Oxman AD, Davis DA, *et al.* (1997a). Outreach visits to improve health professional practice and health care outcomes. The Cochrane Library, Issue 3. Oxford: Update Software.

Thomson MA, Oxman AD, Davis DA, *et al.* (1997b). Audit and feedback to improve health professional practice and health care outcomes (Part I). The Cochrane Library, Issue 3. Oxford: Update Software.

Thomson MA, Oxman AD, Davis DA, *et al.* (1997c). Audit and feedback to improve health professional practice and health care outcomes (Part II). The Cochrane Library, Issue 3. Oxford: Update Software.

Tierney WM, Hui SL and McDonald CJ. (1986). Delayed feedback of physician performance versus immediate reminders to perform preventive care. Effects on physician compliance. *Med Care* **24**:659–666.

Veninga CC, Denig P, Zwaagstra R, *et al.* (2000). Improving drug treatment in general practice. *J Clin Epidemiol.* **53**(7):762–772.

Wells KB, Sherbourne C, Schoenbaum M, *et al.* (2000). Impact of disseminating quality improvement programs for depression in managed primary care. A randomized controlled trial. *JAMA* **283**:212–220.

Weijden T van der, Wensing M, Giffel M, *et al.* (2000). *Interventions Aimed at Influencing the Use of Diagnostic Tests.* Report. Maastricht: WOK.

Wensing M, Weijden T van der and Grol R (1998). Implementing guidelines and innovations in general practice: Which interventions are effective? *Br J Gen Pract.* **48**:991–997.

Worrall G, Chaulk P and Freake D (1997). The effects of clinical practice guidelines on patient outcomes in primary care: A systematic review. *Can Med Assoc J.* **156**(12):1705–1712.

Yabroff KR, Mangan P and Mandelblatt J (2003). Effectiveness of interventions to increase Papanicolauou smear use. *J Am Board Fam Pract.* **16**:188–203.

Part V

Organisation

Chapter 15

Effective organisation of the implementation

Richard Grol

KEY MESSAGES

- Good planning of the implementation activities (when, where, how and by whom?) is of great importance to the successful introduction of innovations, guidelines, new procedures and changes in care processes in practice.
- Begin small, test the plan on a small scale using motivated groups and gradually expand.
- In making the plan, consider:
  - A cost-effective mixture of interventions of proven value;
  - Implementation activities in all phases of the process of change, so the plan is for both dissemination and implementation;
  - Implementation activities at the correct or multiple levels (central, local group, team/department, practice and individual);
  - Good planning time management;
  - Involvement of the target group in designing and executing the plan;
  - Incorporation of the plan into existing activities for communication and teaching of the target group;
  - Adequate budgetary and other support;
  - Incorporate periodic evaluation in the plan;
  - Consider organisational aspects that promote or retard implementation, such as leadership, the role of physicians, collaboration, teaching of quality methods and organisation culture.

Box 15.1 Implementation projects in England (Evans and Haines 2000)

An analysis was conducted of 17 projects set up within the framework of a national research programme in the area of 'implementation of evidence'. Success factors and lessons from the experiences in these projects were listed. In summary, 10 central lessons were found:

- Seek individuals and organisations willing and able to begin the implementation;
- Seek subjects for which the change can be established;
- Seek a suitable project co-ordinator;
- Form an effective team from individuals with the necessary expertise;
- Localise the implementation project to the setting in which the changes must take place;
- Integrate continuous evaluation of the activities and progress made from the start of the project;
- Build ahead and make use of existing channels and structures for training, making improvements in quality and contacts within the target group;
- Ensure the genuine commitment of key figures;
- Return to the plan repeatedly and determine whether everything is on the right track;
- Remain flexible and focus efforts on problems in the implementation that may arise during the project.

INTRODUCTION

As we have outlined in previous chapters (*Figure 15.1*) on the process of introducing innovations and changes in patient care, the first requirement is a good basis for change. This may be new scientific knowledge, or problems in the provision of care noted by the group itself, or good experience gained with a particular procedure in practice ('best practices').

Figure 15.1 Implementation of guidelines and changes

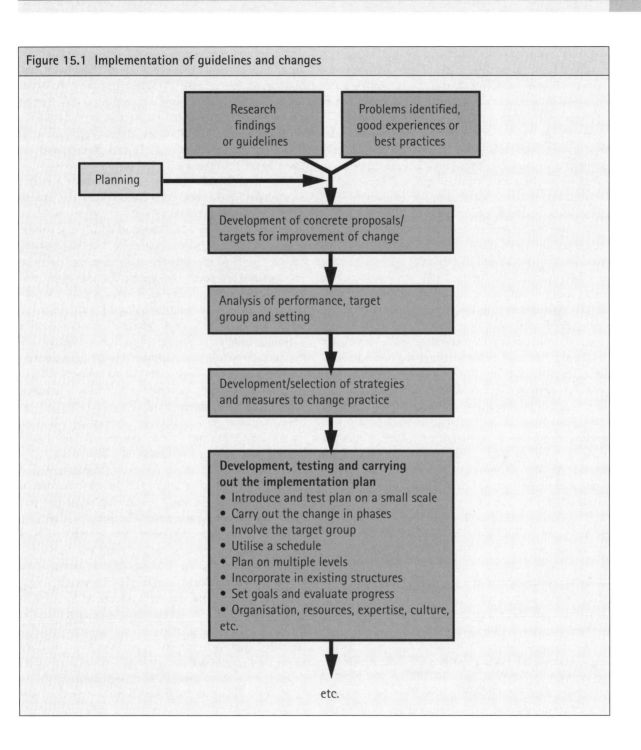

A diagnostic analysis of the target group and setting must then reveal who is to be involved in the introduction or who will be affected by it, which aspects of the care are most in need of improvement, and which promoting and hindering factors will play a role in effective implementation. Such an analysis usually yields a variety of bottlenecks. The next step is to develop or select methods, strategies and measures able to remove these bottlenecks. Ideally, these will be interventions that have proved to be cost effective. Which interventions work best in particular situations is not yet clear. What is clear is that a combination of interventions and measures is often indicated. However, exactly what must be done in a concrete situation is not always obvious beforehand. This often requires careful preparation and necessitates the development of an *implementation plan* specifically compatible with the target group and the setting in which the implementation or change will take place. Finally, successful implementation of improvements in patient care appears to also be a question of good management. These issues of planning and management of the implementation activities are considered further in this chapter.

Planning to implement innovations is obviously different for the implementation of a national clinical guideline on stroke than for optimising antibiotic policy in a hospital or introducing a new care pathway or process for an outpatient clinic for mammary or vascular diseases. It also differs between the situation of a group of physicians or a neighbourhood nursing care team who want to bring treatment more into agreement with a local protocol, or the situation of a practice wanting to implement an appointment system that has been tested elsewhere. All of these cases concern the implementation of potentially valuable changes in patient care. However, the scale on which one or another occurs, the ambitions involved and the investment of time, staff and materials differ greatly. The principles involved in the planning are, however, generally the same and are illustrated below. They address:

- Development and testing of the plan;
- Planning according to phases in the change process;
- Adapting to and involving the target group;
- Scheduling;
- Planning on different levels;
- Incorporating the plan into existing activities;
- Setting goals for evaluation;
- Organising the implementation – structures, materials, personnel and organisation culture.

DEVELOPMENT AND TESTING OF THE PLAN

The first question is what will form the final combination of strategies and measures to enable putting the changes into practice. In the choice of interventions to be incorporated into the plan, different considerations may play a role. For example, the question of which interventions have a *proved value* within the setting, for both the target groups of the implementation and for the changes desired. In previous chapters we show that feedback and reminders are often used with success in improving preventive care, influencing medication

decisions and requesting diagnostic tests. In contrast, for multidisciplinary care processes in a hospital, a total quality management (TQM) approach (process redesign and quality improvement projects) may be preferable. It is advisable to make use of the available, continually growing literature in this area, such as in the Cochrane Effective Practice and Organisation of Care (EPOC) database.

The choice is also influenced by the *available budget* and the required effort by staff and volunteers, as well as by considerations concerning *cost effectiveness*. There is an optimum (*Figure 15.2*) beyond which many more resources are required to achieve a small additional effect (A) or beyond which the effect may even decrease (B). The latter can occur, for example, because the plan evokes a negative reaction in the target group, which does not want to be continually faced with initiatives for change. In a study of the effectiveness of the effort of trained outreach visitors to improve preventive care in general practice, there appeared to be a great difference between practices in terms of numbers of visits to the practices, but a greater number of visits was not associated with more changes (Hulscher *et al.* 1997). Data on the cost effectiveness of diverse intervention activities are still largely lacking – the first studies in this are now beginning to appear (see further in Chapter 20).

The scientific literature concerning implementation usually offers little assistance to the introduction of changes, so it is necessary to develop strategies and measures for doing so oneself. In this situation, it is important to *begin small*: choose a few concrete changes and an implementation strategy, and test these in a small, motivated group. The small-scale *testing of the plan* and its components can thereby be seen as a crucial element in preparing the implementation (Cretin 1998; Green *et al.* 1989). What has been developed at the desk, or in a group, of experts usually turns out differently when it is put into practice. We know, for example, that the use of outreach visitors is an effective way to make changes in some aspects of care delivery, but who can best fill this role, how often the visits must be made, what materials the visitor must utilise and what position he or she should have in the team that the innovation must adopt cannot be determined in advance. This must be tried out on a small scale and then gradually built up on the basis of the first experiences (as an example, see the PDSA cycle in *Box 15.2*). The 'triability' of an innovation is, according to Rogers (1995), one of the characteristics of successful implementation.

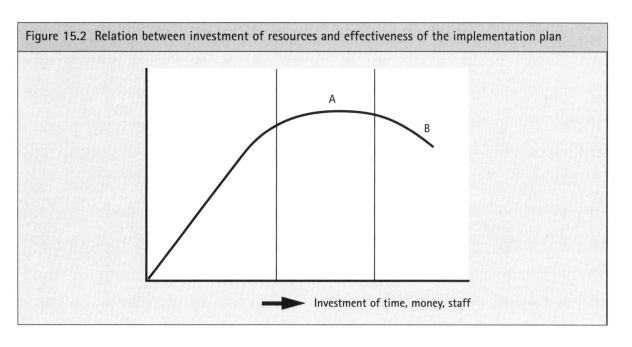

Figure 15.2 Relation between investment of resources and effectiveness of the implementation plan

A

B

Investment of time, money, staff

However, one must realise that not everything can be planned in advance. The plan must often be *flexible* and amenable to repeated readjustment and adaptation, tailoring it to the requirements or qualities of the target group. This means that the plan must be able to offer help with concrete introduction problems in specific care settings and in seeking alternatives when a given approach does not appear to work well.

PLANNING BY PHASES IN THE CHANGE PROCESS

In Chapter 3 we show there is consensus that implementation often requires a process in which change for care providers and teams occurs in different steps. We summarise that process in five steps in Chapters 3 and 8:

- Orientation:
  - Promote awareness of the innovation;
  - Stimulate interest and involvement;
- Insight:
  - Create understanding;
  - Develop insight into own routines;
- Acceptance:
  - Develop a positive attitude, a motivation to change;
  - Create positive intentions or decisions to change;
- Change:
  - Promote actual adoption in practice;
  - Confirm benefit value of change;
- Maintenance:
  - Integrate new practice into routines;
  - Embed new practice within the organisation.

Box 15.2 Testing and introduction of a plan for change (Plsek 1999)

Changing is a cyclic process in which a number of steps are taken time and again. The PDSA cycle is a practical model, having as steps:
- Plan – set goals and generate ideas about how the goals can best be achieved;
- Do – carry out the plan and record what has been done;
- Study – analyse data, reflect on the lessons that can be learned;
- Act – continue, adapt or change the activities, formulate new ideas for the plan, etc.

The starting point is always *to test the changes on a small scale* and repeatedly go through the cycle, adding or sharpening ideas (*Figure 15.3*). Multiple cycles are planned to test the changes before the real implementation begins. Begin on a small scale and gradually expand. In each cycle data are collected on the principle that ideas can be added. Ideally, the test is carried out in different surroundings, under different conditions.

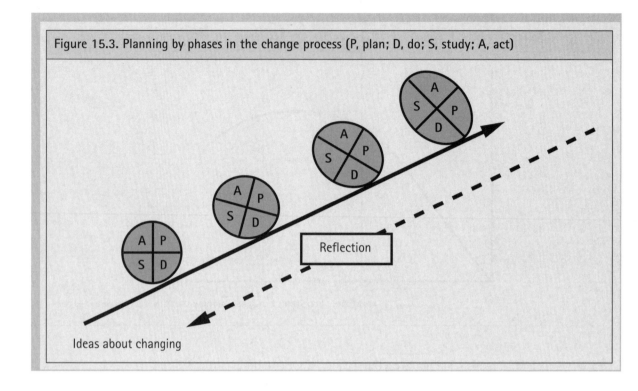

Figure 15.3. Planning by phases in the change process (P, plan; D, do; S, study; A, act)

A plan to disseminate and implement a new procedure or improvement in care must, in principle, give adequate attention to each of these steps, of course depending on the scale and dimension of the implementation activity, the nature of the innovation and any implementation problems encountered. For instance, in the implementation of a new multidisciplinary guideline for stroke with recommendations for treatment from a large number of disciplines, initial attention must be given to developing a good *dissemination plan*. This must ensure that all of those involved are well-informed about the guideline and its key recommendations, and be used to carry out local discussions and make agreements about the guidelines. If there is an institutional consensus that the percentage of postoperative wound infections is unacceptably high and it is intended to bring this in line with the performance of the best hospitals in the area, much more emphasis must be placed on the actual *plan to change routines* with, for example, a change in the existing care processes and the setting up of a continuous monitoring and feedback system. It is therefore important that both a good *dissemination plan* and a good *implementation and change plan* are made.

The steps in the process of changing do not all require the same attention, and the planned sequence will not always be followed. However, different steps do, to some degree, necessitate other actions. It is prudent, in setting up a plan to introduce changes in practice, to consider these steps and to anticipate possible problems (see further in Chapter 8).

INVOLVING THE TARGET GROUP IN THE PLAN

As it is difficult to understand fully a given setting in advance, it is impossible to involve representatives from the target group in the selection of strategies and measures to accomplish the change and in developing a plan for its introduction. This can be done by previously described methods, such as interviews or group meetings. People from the target group are asked what kind of activities and measures are attainable, will be accepted and are likely to work best. The involvement of certain representatives or key individuals from the target group in the actual introduction of the implementation can also be discussed.

Usually, the group of those concerned (for whom the implementation has consequences) is much greater than initially imagined (Lomas 1997). Often the implementation is found to affect not only clinicians, but also patients, the management or directors of the institution, colleague care providers, insurers, politicians and policy makers, and sometimes people from the business world who must provide materials for the implementation. A list of all those people and organisations whose co-operation, in one form or another, is desirable, for whom specific information or supporting materials must eventually be prepared and for whom a separate strategy must be developed and introduced, can be useful at such a moment. Consider the example of a *sounding board group* composed of different kinds of concerned individuals, who discuss together the development of an effective plan (NHMRC 2000).

Experience in many projects has shown that it is best to start with a *small group* of enthusiastic care providers, practices or institutions (Evans and Haines 2000). This means seeking individuals or organisations prepared to start an implementation or change and who meet certain conditions. For example, for a project to implement guidelines for the prevention of cardiac and vascular diseases in primary care, a search was first made for motivated practices with a satisfactory computer system and enough assistants, because these points were considered preconditions for the implementation (Lobo *et al.* 2002a, 2002b). These motivated individuals or organisations next functioned as examples for others. In the introduction of small local quality circles of general practitioners (GPs) in the 1980s, a start was made with teachers involved in training for general practice. Then teachers from peripheral training practices were approached, after which the programme was offered to 'normal' physicians and was implemented widely with the help of participants of the early groups (Grol 1987).

SCHEDULING THE ACTIVITIES

The different interventions and measures that concern the implementation must also be planned according to a schedule. Among the important considerations are:

- The activities cannot all be offered at the same time, as this could overwhelm the target group and overtax the organisation. A *logical order* must be introduced – what is the most important to do first, and what later? Sometimes specific measures help to start a spontaneous process of change, which does not require much extra intervention.
- The plan should be *divided* into a number of well-organised and manageable components that can be introduced and evaluated separately.
- The sequence of these can be determined by the different *steps in the change process* that the care providers and teams undergo (see Chapter 8 and Planning by phases in the change process, above).

For new guidelines, processes and procedures it is advisable to make both a 'dissemination plan' and an 'implementation plan' and schedule these.

- The major problem or the most important opportunities for change, as revealed by the analysis of the target group and setting, obviously receive the greatest attention.
- *Evaluation and feedback* at regular intervals are also incorporated into the plan. This is necessary to respond to problems in the introduction, to new priorities, to the needs of the target group and to stagnation of progress. Therefore, a plan for evaluation is made at the outset. The methods for this are described in the following chapters.
- It should be realised that the full course of most implementations requires *sufficient time* (sometimes years). Experience in many projects has shown that the time required was a disappointment. 'Progress is not linear, but three steps forward and two steps back' (Wye and McClenahan 2000). However, it has to be realised that changes proceed slowly, but at the same time a certain speed and boldness are necessary to prevent the loss of momentum. Those in the target group generally want quick success, once they have committed themselves to a new way of working. Otherwise it is back again to the old way.

PLANNING ON DIFFERENT LEVELS

Assuming that a combination of interventions, adapted to the target group, is most effective, the question is which interventions and measures should be targeted and carried out at what level. National implementation programmes require different activities than does the introduction of changes in a nursing department, in a care team or in a primary care practice of GPs, midwives or physiotherapists. Mittman *et al.* (1992) distinguished three types of situations, each of which requires a different strategy:

- *Small groups* (2–3 people) – strategies include, particularly, face-to-face instruction by trained personnel, individual consultation by 'experts', training in master–assistant relations and personal contact between colleagues;
- *Middle-size groups* (e.g. members of a department, care team, health centre or local groups of physicians or paramedics) – strategies here are the efforts of opinion leaders and key figures, interactive study groups, preparing consensus agreements, clinical audit and quality circles;

■ *Large groups* (e.g. all leaders of professional groups, all care providers in a region or all hospitals in a country) – an important strategy is the use of mass media. For the effective introduction of an innovation, it is sometimes necessary to work on multiple levels at the same time, especially when it concerns programmes on a national or regional scale or all employees in an institution or home-care organisation. The activities on different levels (central, local, department/practice or individual) then have different goals and contents (*Table 15.1*):

■ *Central* – on a central level, professional organisations, policy makers and financiers can provide support by creating good preconditions for the implementation of the innovation and by providing the necessary infrastructure, provisions and regulations. By contributing a definite, positive point of view about the change, they can make their influence felt peripherally.

■ *Local or institution* – local organisations of care providers or an institution can help with the realisation of a successful change by making local agreements among all of those involved to support a new procedure and include it in their policy, to clearly communicate this to the target group and to assist in the achievement of the necessary organisational and structural conditions.

■ *Department, team or practice* – at the level of a department of an institution, a team or a practice, there is usually a multidisciplinary group of care providers who must accept and apply the change or innovation. Various methods discussed in previous chapters can facilitate the change.

■ *Individual professional* – finally, the individual care provider must become informed and motivated, and for this he or she must participate in education, audit, feedback programmes and similar activities.

INTEGRATING THE PLAN INTO EXISTING ACTIVITIES

Experience in numerous implementation projects has shown the great importance of *integrating the implementation plan into existing structures and channels* for contact with, training of and improving the quality of the target group. The advice is to make use of what is already available (Wye and McClenahan 2000) – regular team meetings, educational meetings, audit and visiting procedures, and existing communication channels. In other words, use the media with which the target group is already familiar, which they trust and can use without extra effort. For the various levels, this can be slightly different:

■ Central – scientific and professional journals for professionals, as well as newsletters from professional organisations;

■ Local groups – for example, for dentists their local study groups, for community nurses the meetings of their care teams, for GPs their continuing medical education (CME) courses and local group meetings;

■ Institute – existing quality programmes, quality committee meetings, accreditation programmes and monitoring systems;

■ Team – visiting programmes, clinical audit, department-related quality improvement projects and team meetings;

■ Practice – practice meetings and clinical audit projects;

■ Individual – re-registration programmes and educational initiatives.

SETTING GOALS FOR EVALUATION

A component of the planning and performance of the procedure of implementation, continuing on into the next step in the implementation cycle (Evaluation, see Part VI), is the formulation of *concrete measurable goals* with which the progress and success of the activities

Table 15.1 Introducing changes on multiple levels	
Level	Methods
Central	Publications in journals Mailing and/or internet Development of instructional materials and introductory programmes Financial incentives Issuing regulations
Local or institution	Local courses Local consensus and protocol development Use of key people and opinion leaders Quality projects in institutions
Department, team, practice	Setting goals for department or practice Setting up protocol, making work agreements Setting up quality projects with data collection Involving consultants and/or experts Outreach visits
Individual professional	Self-study, courses Audit, feedback Reminders Skill training

can be measured. Evaluation activities are ideally integrated into the change process from the very beginning. For this purpose it is necessary to formulate specific goals. These must be ambitious and very concrete, as well as attainable within the setting of implementation (Schellekens 2000). A goal such as 'lowering the number of Caesarean sections' is insufficiently concrete. 'Reducing the number of Caesarean sections by 15% within 1 year' contains points against which success can be evaluated. The goals must be sufficiently ambitious to get real changes started, such as 25% fewer postoperative wound infections, 80% shorter time to perform certain procedures, 40% fewer amputations in diabetics or 70% fewer medication errors (Schellekens 2000). There must also be clear deadlines for achievement of these goals.

It is clear that when ambitious goals are set, evaluation of progress towards them cannot be delayed to the end of the project. A finger must be kept on the pulse and the implementation plan must be reconsidered repeatedly – is it still suitable for stimulating changes or does it need adaptation? Begin small, check to be sure everything is on the right track, improve the plan, expand to other segments of the target group – a cyclic process that closely fits the model for making changes presented in TQM (see the example of the PDSA cycle in *Box 15.2*).

ORGANISATION OF THE IMPLEMENTATION: STRUCTURES, MEANS AND PERSONNEL

To carry out the implementation activities well, it is usually necessary that a *team or small group* steer, co-ordinate and communicate the activities and, where necessary, provide support. How such a team is made up depends largely on the scale of the implementation (national, local, team or practice?) and the budgetary possibilities. It is generally preferable to include different kinds of expertise in such a group:

- *Leadership expertise* – someone who is seen by the target group as an authority in the field of the change and who fills a central role in communicating the message and involving the target group in the implementation;
- *Co-ordination expertise* – someone who keeps close watch on the normal organisation of all activities and directs others;
- *Technical expertise* – one or more individuals who have specific knowledge or skills that are advantageous to the process of implementing change, such as familiarity with data collection, computers or data analysis;

- *Administrative expertise* – one or more individuals who prepare materials, send invitations, prepare meetings and plan social activities.

The team makes a plan in which the different tasks and responsibilities are worked out carefully and written down.

Few implementation or change plans succeed if they are completely dependent on the voluntary, unpaid efforts of many different kinds of people. An adequate *budget* (obviously different for a national, local, department-related or practice-related plan) with sufficient financial resources and available personnel is usually a precondition for success. Such a budget must be negotiated with the government, insurer, directors of the institute or leaders of a team or practice. Depending on the objectives and scale of the project, the budget contains provision for such items as:

- Co-ordination;
- Supporting personnel;
- Computers, equipment and supplies;
- Reimbursement for extra work in the target group.

ORGANISATION CULTURE

In achieving change in patient care, a certain *organisational culture* in an institute or within a professional group can be highly beneficial (see also Chapters 2 and 12). Although this does not offer a direct opportunity for making changes, elements of such a culture can be so advantageous to effective implementation that specific attention to it may be a part of the plan. Concepts, experience and research from organisation and management theory support the importance of attention to the culture in a practice or institute in the implementation of changes (*Box 15.3*). For example, a study by Shortell *et al.* (1995) in 61 hospitals revealed that a flexible, risk-taking organisational culture strongly related to a successful implementation of quality care activities. This appeared to have more influence than the available number of formal quality-of-care structures.

In the literature about a good organisational context for the implementation of guidelines, protocols and new procedures, some of the items that come to the fore are:

- Leadership;
- Central role of physicians;
- Collaboration;
- Quality culture and training.

Leadership

Involvement of directors and top management in the implementation of improvements is seen as being very important (Berwick *et al.* 1990; Berwick 1989). Leaders of an institute or professional group are often seen to radiate enthusiasm at the beginning and to take the initiative to make changes start, but then delegate the actual implementation and show no further interest. This does not seem to work. A consistent viewpoint about the change proposal, the proposal of concrete and ambitious goals, managing strict deadlines and setting an example are important in such leadership (Schellekens 2000). A study was carried out in 2193 hospitals on the effect of the style of leadership on participation by physicians in quality improvement and the formation of improvement teams and projects on the work floor. Top management taking a clear leadership role appeared to be a significant factor and, especially if physicians assume the leadership, more projects are undertaken to improve quality (Weiner *et al.* 1997).

Central role of physicians

The central role of physicians is being emphasised to an increasing degree in achieving change in patient care (*Box 15.4*; Berwick and Nolan 1998; Weiner *et al.* 1997; Boerstler *et al.* 1996; Lammers *et al.* 1996; Ovretveit 1996). When physicians are brought in later, progress is usually much slower. Many physicians are still unfamiliar with or sceptical about quality improvement, for several reasons (Berwick 1998; Blumenthal and Kilo 1998; Shortell *et al.* 1998):

- The evidence of its effectiveness is limited;
- Little is published about it in the clinical journals that physicians read;
- It is managers who have introduced quality care into the institution, with the accompanying jargon.

According to Ovretveit (1996) it is untrue that physicians are disinterested in quality improvement. Most continually strive to introduce useful improvements in their management of health problems and to attend courses, but they see the new approaches of quality

---

Box 15.3 Lessons from 'organisational development' theory (Garside 1998, 1999)

'Learning organisations' have a clear vision of where they want to go and all employees are continually busy to detect faults, attend courses, introduce improvements, integrate new ideas and adapt new work processes. To achieve real changes, the following aspects are important:
- A clear, consistent perception of optimal quality of care, expressed by the directors of an organisation;
- An open, change-oriented culture, to be achieved by involving everyone, constantly training employees and ensuring mutual communication;
- Management of change processes proceeds most effectively by:
  - Engaging persons who work devotedly on the change;
  - Establishing a project team in which all of those concerned take part;
  - Quickly demonstrating success;
  - Taking time to achieve the proposed changes;
  - Providing an adequate budget.

Box 15.4 How can continuous quality improvement be undertaken in an institution? (Blumenthal and Kilo 1998)

A 'report card' on continuous quality improvement (CQI) at present reveals the following recommendations for its broad application and to create conditions to implement changes in care:
- Involve physicians in the programme right from the start;
- Place emphasis on clinical, patient-oriented improvements;
- Invest in quality development – it costs money and the invested time and extra work must be reimbursed;
- Avoid jargon;
- Train people only when improvement projects begin;
- Invest in information systems – accurate data about the care provided are essential;
- Involve the managers and directors in the activities.

improvement and evidence-based medicine as 'management fashions' and 'disguised strategies for cutting costs'. Some quality concepts and methods do not immediately appeal to them because they are derived from industry. Many physicians are also ambivalent about giving guidance to others and about quality improvement – this is discussed as the personal responsibility of care providers. According to Ovretveit (1996), to be more successful the quality programme must provide an answer to the problems of physicians and the physicians must see that the programme really produces something of value for the patients as well as for the care providers themselves. In addition, support is needed in the form of good measurement and data systems. Training in quality improvement can best be related to actual improvement activities and be fitted into the limited time available. Jargon and an overzealous approach to management should be avoided (Box 15.5).

Collaboration

Achieving good results in health care is partly dependent on individual expertise and performance. However, most care providers work in groups and teams, and depend on others for the effectiveness of their own performance. This also applies to the implementation of innovations in practice. To improve processes in care, it is often necessary to first improve interaction and communication between those involved in these processes (Clemmer et al. 1998; Firth-Cozins 1998). Leaders in an institution or organisation, who are often physicians, must stimulate this co-operation. In other disciplines (such as economics and psychology) a good deal of study is carried out on the elements of effective co-operation. Especially in the sphere of safety and effectiveness, co-operation appears to be crucial. A large proportion of aeroplane accidents appear to be partly

the result of communication errors in the cockpit. Clemmer et al. (1998) set out in a review article how leaders in health care can stimulate co-operation:

- Develop a joint objective (e.g. to improve a certain important part of the care);
- Provide an open, safe atmosphere in which everyone can participate;
- Involve everyone who has something to do with achieving the goal;
- Encourage the expression of diverse opinions;
- Learn how to manage and yet achieve a consensus;
- Urge honesty and equality between participants.

Quality culture and training

Mention has already been made of the resistance and scepticism of many care providers with regard to quality improvement and implementation plans. According to Blumenthal and Kilo (1998), this is related to the great autonomy that care providers and teams themselves have in shaping core processes in patient care. Hence they are not so easily guided into taking part in time-intensive courses on implementation of change. Even if they are in favour, they often lack the necessary knowledge and skill to deal well with a project (Solberg et al. 1998). In many hospitals an attempt has been made to train the entire staff, but many participants later found it difficult to translate what they had learned into concrete improvement activities. In other words, an institution or professional group has to foster a positive culture about quality improvement and also provide sufficient skill to be able to implement the changes. For this it is important to avoid jargon and to use language that is in keeping with the language with which clinicians are familiar (Batalden and Mohr 1998). Training in methods of improvement should be delayed until a concrete change is underway, and then the train-

Box 15.5 Continuous quality improvement in a primary care clinic in the USA (Solberg et al. 1998)

A survey was conducted into the attitudes and experiences with CQI of 647 of 988 involved care providers in 44 primary care clinics. Most were positive about this approach, but knowledge about and experience with it appeared to be limited. Of the 44 clinics, 20 had carried out at least one quality improvement project. A total of 89 teams were working on a quality improvement subject, and 60% of the team members found the experience very worthwhile. There was concrete information for about 12 projects. The teams appeared to have the greatest difficulty with:

- Arranging to meet together every other week;
- Making and carrying out a plan to measure success in the project;
- Collecting data about the achievement of goals.

Only five projects completed the entire improvement cycle.

Box 15.6 Quality development in hospitals (Ovretveit 1996)

Experience in six Norwegian hospitals with continuous quality development led to the following conclusions:
- It costs time to introduce a quality programme and to disseminate quality-improvement approaches;
- Involvement of management and physicians is crucial;
- Models for CQI and/or TQM that are not adapted to the clinical care are refused;
- Working in small teams on a project according to fixed steps can result in measurable changes, provided that sufficient training and support are provided;
- Training in quality methods is only useful when people are actually involved in a concrete project;
- Data collection and monitoring of quality usually appear to be the greatest weakness in the quality programme, and thus much support must be given to these.

ing must be pinned to the kinds of problems that are relevant to the target group (Ovretveit 1996). An example is 'cascade training', in which leaders from a higher hierarchical level always train those in the next level down in the organisation. This also means that top management must receive the same training; in any case, the measurement and analysis of data must be a part of quality training. This is, as shown by many projects (Geboers *et al.* 1999a, 1999b; Solberg *et al.* 1998; Ovretveit 1996), the most difficult part of many quality improvement projects (*Box 15.6*).

CONCLUSIONS

The successful implementation of innovations in the practice of patient care requires good preparation and planning. This is especially true when implementation activities are being selected and when they are being carried out. Although the scientific literature in the field of planning of implementation is limited, there is now extensive experience in setting up implementation and change programmes in many different sectors of health care. The analysis of multiple projects to identify the determinants of effective implementation is being carried out more often (e.g. Evans and Haines 2000; Gustafson *et al.* 1997; Ovretveit 1996). Such analyses continually indicate the importance of good planning. Ideally, a start is made on a small scale and the activities are expanded gradually. The target group is involved intensively in the activities in all phases of the implementation. A realistic schedule is made (usually more time is required than anticipated). Arrangements are made for an adequate budget and use of staff, and the plan is incorporated into the normal activities of the target group. Continuing evaluation is carried out to add to the plan where necessary. The implementation of innovations will approach expectations far better in a setting in which the management stands behind the changes, good co-operation exists among disciplines, practices and departments, and a 'quality culture' predominates.

Recommended literature

Evans D and Haines A (2000). *Implementing Evidence-Based Changes in Health Care*. Abingdon: Radcliffe Press.

References

Batalden P and Mohr J (1998). Building knowledge of health care as a system. *Qual Manage Health Care* **6**:57–62.

Berwick DM (1989). Continuous improvement as an ideal in health care. *N Engl J Med.* **320**(1):53–56.

Berwick DM (1998). Developing and testing changes in delivery of care. *Ann Intern Med.* **128**:651–656.

Berwick DM and Nolan TW (1998). Physicians as leaders in improving health care. *Ann Intern Med.* **128**:289–292.

Berwick D, Godfrey B and Roessner J (1990). *Curing Health Care*. San Francisco: Jossey-Bass Publications.

Blumenthal D and Kilo CM (1998). A report card on continuous quality improvement. *Milbank Q.* **76**:625–648.

Boerstler H, Forster R, O'Connor E, *et al.* (1996). Implementation of total quality management: Conventional wisdom versus reality. *Hosp Health Serv Adm.* **41**:143–159.

Clemmer T, Spuhler V, Berwick D, *et al.* (1998). Cooperation: The foundation of improvement. *Ann Intern Med.* **128**:1004–1009.

Cretin S (1998). *Implementing Guidelines: An Overview*. Report. Santa Monica: RAND.

Evans D and Haines A (2000). *Implementing Evidence-Based Changes in Health Care*. Abingdon: Radcliffe Press.

Firth-Cozins J (1998). Celebrating teamwork. *Qual Health Care* **7**(Suppl.):S3–S7.

Garside P (1998). Organisational context for quality: Lessons from the field of organisational development and change management. *Qual Health Care* **7**(Suppl.):S8–S15.

Garside P (1999). The learning organisation: A necessary setting for improving care? *Qual Health Care* **8**:211.

Geboers H, Grol R, Bosch W van den, *et al.* (1999a). A model for continuous quality improvement in small scale practices. *Qual Health Care* **8**:43–48.

Geboers H, Horst M van der, Mokkink H, *et al.* (1999b). Setting up improvement projects in small scale primary care practices: Feasibility of a model for continuous quality improvement. *Qual Health Care* 8:36–42.

Green L, Gottlieb N and Parcell G (1989). Diffusion theory extended and applied. In: *Advances in Health Education and Promotion*, Volume 3. Greenwich: JAI Press.

Grol R (1987). *Kwaliteitsbewaking in de Huisartsgeneeskunde. Effecten van Onderlinge Toetsing [Quality Improvement in General Practice. Effect of Peer Review]*. Thesis. Nijmegen: KUN.

Gustafson D, Risberg L, Gering D, *et al.* (1997). *Case Studies from the Quality Improvement Support System*. AHRQ-Publications 97-0022. Rockville: Agency for Healthcare Research and Quality.

Hulscher MEJL, Drenth BB van, Wouden JC van der, *et al.* (1997). Changing preventive practice: A controlled trial on the effects of outreach visits to organize prevention of cardiovascular disease. *Qual Health Care* 6:19–24.

Lammers J, Cretin S, Gilman S, *et al.* (1996). Total quality management in hospitals. *Med Care* 34:463–478.

Lobo CM, Frijling BD, Hulscher MEJL, *et al.* (2002a). Improving quality of organizing cardiovascular preventive care in general practice by outreach visitors: A randomized controlled trial. *Prev Med.* 35:422–429.

Lobo CM, Frijling BD, Hulscher MEJL, *et al.* (2002b). Organizing cardiovascular preventive care in general practice: Determinants of a successful intervention. *Prev Med.* 35:430–436.

Lomas J (1997). *Beyond the Sound of Hand Clapping: A Discussion Document on Improving Health Research Dissemination and Update*. Sydney: University of Sydney.

Mittman BS, Tonesk X and Jacobson PD (1992). Implementing clinical practice guidelines: Social influence strategies and practitioner behaviour change. *QRB* 18:413–422.

NHMRC (2000). *How to Put the Evidence into Practice: Implementation and Dissemination Strategies*. Canberra: National Health Medical Research Council.

Ovretveit J (1996). Medical participation in and leadership of quality programmes. *J Manage Med.* 10:21–28.

Plsek PE (1999). Section 1: Evidence-based quality improvement, principles, and perspectives. Quality Improvement methods in clinical practice. *Pediatrics* 103:203–214.

Rogers E (1995). *Diffusion of Innovations*. New York: Free Press.

Schellekens W (2000). Een passie voor patiënten [A passion for patients]. *Med Contact* 55:412–414.

Shortell S, O'Brien J, Carman J, *et al.* (1995). Assessing the impact of continuous quality improvement/total quality management: Concept versus implementation. *Health Serv Res.* 30:377–401.

Shortell SM, Bennett CL and Byck GR (1998). Assessing the impact of continuous quality improvement on clinical practice: What it will take to accelerate progress. *Milbank Q.* 76(4):593–624.

Solberg L, Brekke M, Kottke T, *et al.* (1998). Continuous quality improvement in primary care: What's happening? *Med Care* 36:625–635.

Weiner B, Shortell S and Alexander J (1997). Promoting clinical involvement in hospital quality improvement efforts: The effects of top management, board and physician leadership. *Health Serv Res.* 32(4):491–510.

Wye L and McClenahan J (2000). *Getting Better with Evidence*. London: King's Fund.

Part VI

Evaluation

Chapter 16

Measuring changes in patient care: development and use of indicators

Jozé Braspenning, Stephen Campbell and Richard Grol

KEY MESSAGES

- How to measure change depends on the purpose of the evaluation. There are three distinct purposes – internal quality measurement, external quality measurement and research.
- A rigorous systematic procedure is needed to develop valid and reliable quality indicators – different methods are available.
- Indicators should be integrated within implementation programmes.

Box 16.1 Improving diabetes care by introducing a 'diabetes passport' (Dijkstra and Braspenning 2001)

Patient-centred care based on evidence-based guidelines was expected to improve the quality of diabetes care delivered in hospitals. The tool developed to achieve this goal was a patient-held record, a 'diabetes passport', in which was recorded not only glucose levels, but also blood pressure, serum lipids, results of feet and eye examinations and the Quetelet index. This passport, owned by the patient, gives information on his or her actual health status and can be used for appropriate management. It also provides an overview of the necessary performance based on national evidence-based clinical guidelines. The diabetes passport was introduced in four hospitals with five hospitals as controls. The implementation programme started off with local meetings led by key individuals in diabetes care to introduce the national guidelines and the use of the diabetes passport. Different meetings were arranged for the professionals and the patients. Professionals were given feedback on their actual performance to identify aspects of care in need of improvement. After 6 months the intervention group again received feedback on actual performance based on 15–20 patients. The intervention period was 12 months, after which a second measurement was performed. The data collection was based on two sources, a search in the medical records and a patient questionnaire about the care delivered. To measure (changes in) care provision a set of indicators was derived from the national guidelines. Some examples are presented here.

Performance in diabetes care by 59 internists in 13 hospitals (Dijkstra *et al.* 2004)		
	Adherence (%)	Range
Blood pressure measured once a year	98	94–100
Eye examination once a year	84	70–95
Urine examination once a year	74	41–97
Feet examination once a year, or sooner	40	18–72
Target value HbA1c attained	23	15–34

INTRODUCTION

An important step in the implementation of innovations in patient care involves the evaluation of the results or effects of the implementation process. For example, we need to know if the targets have been achieved or to what extent the implementation of a guideline, a new procedure or change in a care process was successful. Evaluation of the care provided to patients and the changes made in that care is a crucial step in the implementation process that often receives insufficient attention. Data on actual care provision in relation to the innovation are required throughout the implementation process to determine where changes are most needed and whether the investments led to success.

Evaluation is important to determine current care provision and to identify important gaps in performance. Ongoing evaluation of the progress made during, or as a consequence of, the implementation of a new activity is vital (*Figure 16.1*) and can help to:

▨ Improve the proposal for change – when targets are not achieved easily (unrealistically high) or are achieved too easily (unrealistically low), they can be adapted;

▨ Further analyse problems in changing care – when targets are not met a further analysis of the barriers and facilitating factors may be needed to better focus the implementation strategies;

▨ Alter strategies and measures for change – when targets are not achieved other, potentially more effective, strategies may be selected;

▨ Alter the implementation plan – not achieving the aims of an implementation may be caused by failures in the implementation process.

Such an evaluation is not and should not be just the final step in an implementation programme. Continuous monitoring is required and the project or programme needs to be adapted continuously on the basis of such monitoring. The exact nature of an evaluation depends largely on the type of project or programme: whether it is concerned with a small-scale, local, single-site (one hospital, one team or one practice) project, with a large-scale national or regional programme or with a carefully designed implementation study. However, to know the extent to which changes occur we need measurements – quality indicators or review criteria. Methods

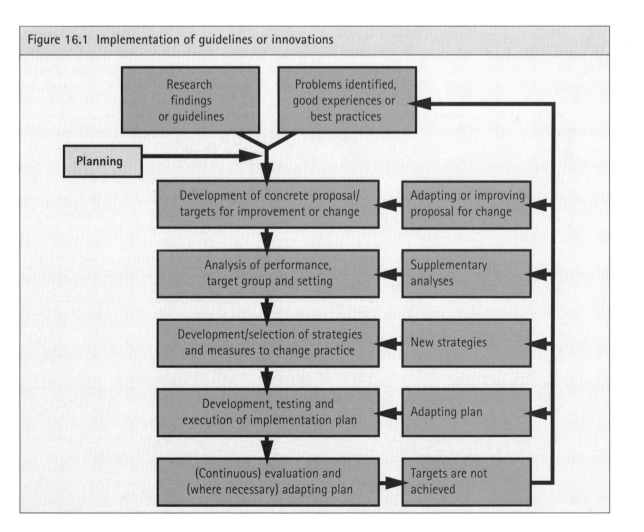

Figure 16.1 Implementation of guidelines or innovations

of developing indicators are addressed in this chapter. Their use in the evaluation of implementation projects and programmes is presented in subsequent chapters.

AIMS OF EVALUATION

The aims of an evaluation need to be clear and specific. Three types of aims can be distinguished:

■ Short-term aims – have the conditions for a successful change been achieved, is the target group aware of the innovation and does it accept the changes?

■ Intermediate aims – is the innovation applied in practice and have the necessary changes been integrated in normal routines?

■ Long-term aims – have the targets of the innovation been achieved, and has it resulted in better health outcomes or more satisfaction in patients or reduced costs of health care?

The aims of the evaluation and how the measurement will be conducted will depend, to a large extent, on the purpose of the evaluation itself (*Table 16.1*); for example, whether it is for internal quality improvement, for external quality assessment and accountability, or for research purposes (Solberg *et al.* 1997).

The use of data, the type of data collected, the time frame, measuring possible confounders (such as the age of patients or type of diabetes) and the confidentiality of the data differ between these three types of evaluation and subsequent measurement of (changes in) the quality of patient care (*Table 16.1*). The project described in *Box 16.1* was both a form of internal quality improvement for the participating hospitals and research into the best strategy to implement the nation-

al guidelines. Therefore, a broad measurement strategy was developed utilising both retrospective and prospective data.

The topic of the quality measurement – what is to be measured – relies very much on the perspective of the stakeholder (Ovretveit 1992; Donabedian 1980). Health professionals usually focus on professional guidelines, health outcomes and efficiency. Patients usually relate quality to a pleasant demeanour and good communication skills, but also to good clinical performance by professionals. Managers are often more interested in data on efficiency, patients' satisfaction and their accessibility to care. Quality indicators can be developed to measure all these aspects of care.

INDICATORS: DEFINITION, TYPOLOGY AND NORMS

Definition

A quality indicator is "a measurable element of practice performance for which there is evidence or consensus that it can be used to assess the quality, and hence change in the quality of care provided" (Lawrence and Olesen 1997). A quality indicator measures the quality of the performance of professional practice. The different aspects of practice performance can be expressed most simply as a numerator and a denominator. The denominator usually describes the target group in absolute numbers and the numerator represents the actual performance within the target group. For example, an indicator for (appropriate) use of radiographs in patients with low back pain might be:

Table 16.1 Characteristics of measurement according to three different aims of data collection – internal, external or scientific quality transparency (Solberg *et al.* 1997)

	Internal quality measurement	External quality measurement	Research
Aim	Quality improvement	Accountability	Knowledge
Data collection	Few items and simple	Very few items and complex	Many items and very complex
Description	Approximately	Exact and valid	Very exact and valid
Type	Mostly process descriptions	Mostly patient outcomes	Description of structure, care processes and patient outcomes
Time frame	Short term, prospective	Long term, retrospective	Long term, retro- and prospective
Confounders	Hardly measured	Describe and try to measure	Measure and control
Confidentiality needs	Very high	None, comparison is the objective	High, especially for individual participants

Number of radiographs of patients with low back pain in general practice (numerator)

Number of patients with low back pain in general practice (denominator)

By defining an indicator and expressing it in a numerator and a denominator the quality of care can be described explicitly as a percentage between 0 and 100. Moreover, transforming indicators into a percentage allows different indicators to be compared, although it can be argued that weighting (e.g. based on prevalence) should precede such comparison.

Typology

Quality indicators can refer to structures, processes (interpersonal or clinical) or outcomes of care (*Table 16.2*; Campbell *et al.* 2000a). Structural indicators focus on organisational aspects of service provision, such as the availability of diabetes or asthma clinics, appointment or recall systems, equipment or the skills of staff. Process indicators focus on the actual care delivered to and negotiated with patients, as well as communication with patients. Outcome indicators specify the ultimate goal of the care given and can relate either to health status or patient evaluations of care.

There has been much debate about whether processes or outcomes should be measured in quality assessment. There are advantages and disadvantages to measuring both processes and outcomes and the decision rests with the aims of the research or assessment. It is neither necessary nor helpful to 'take sides' in any generalised sense. Internal quality improvement often focuses on process indicators and external quality measurement usually relies more on outcome indicators. Eddy (1998) described several problems with outcome

indicators. Firstly, patient outcomes cannot always be attributed on a one-to-one basis to the management of individual patients. For example, some people get better after the appropriate treatment, but others do not; it is also true that some people get better (and some people remain ill) after inappropriate treatment. Even if there is enough scientific evidence to expect a given outcome, this does not mean that it will occur for all patients, because known or unknown confounders, such as the patient's age or sex, lifestyle choices, risk factors, compliance and health status may prevent an expected outcome. A second problem with outcome indicators is that their occurrence is sometimes so rare that reliable statements are difficult to make or can only be made after very long periods of time. Thirdly, some outcomes refer to the prevention of illness in the future, but proxies may be needed now. For instance, HbA1c is a valuable proxy for many complications of diabetes mellitus (coronary heart diseases, lower limb amputation, blindness and renal insufficiency). Finally, caution is required when using outcome indicators because (unknown) confounders may play a role, which makes reliable and valid measurement difficult.

Process indicators are easier to formulate and are less affected by confounders, but their relationship with specific patient outcomes may be less certain. However, the results from process indicators offer concrete information to guide improvement programmes and change interventions. Many have argued that process data should be the primary object of assessment for the vast majority of medical conditions (Brook *et al.* 2000; Palmer 1997; Donabedian 1980).

Brook *et al.* (1996) distinguishes between explicit and implicit assessment methods of measuring care. Implicit assessments involve no pre-determined prior standards about what constitutes good or bad care. Data are reviewed and assessed according to the subjective judgement of individuals based on their expertise and experience. Implicit assessment is unreliable because such judgements vary greatly among reviewers and therefore are used rarely. Explicit approaches involve process data or outcome data being reviewed and assessed against pre-determined, objective criteria and are most frequently used in quality assessments (Brook *et al.* 1996; Irvine 1990). An example of such an explicit norm is "the percentage of patients with high blood pressure in a practice should be reduced from 20% to 5% within 6 months".

In consequence, process measures implemented against pre-determined explicit standards or targets have been the primary focus of quality assessment.

Table 16.2 General examples of indicators	
Indicators	Measures
Structure indicators	Number of professionals (full time equivalents) per 1000 patients Special clinics rates
Process indicators	Referral rates Prescription rates Vaccination rates
Outcome indicators	Hospital re-admission rates Post-operative wound infections rates

METHODS OF DEVELOPING QUALITY INDICATORS

Quality indicators can be developed in systematic or unsystematic ways (Campbell *et al.* 2002a). Non-systematic approaches can often occur just because data are available; they can be very valuable in terms of assessing or improving quality of care, but little is known about the reliability and validity of the indicators used and non-systematic approaches do not tap into the evidence base of health care (*Box 16.2*).

Systematic approaches are preferable as they help maximise the accuracy of quality measurement. Whenever possible indicators should be based directly upon published scientific evidence, such as rigorously conducted (trial-based) empirical studies (Hearnshaw *et al.* 2001). The stronger the evidence that specific care processes are linked to patient outcomes, the greater the potential for the indicators to reflect true reductions in morbidity and mortality or improvements in the health status of patients. For example, in the UK sets of evidence-based indicators have been developed for use in primary care organisations (McColl *et al.* 1998).

However, many areas of health care have a weak, or non-existent, published evidence base. To cope with this, systematic methods have been developed that combine evidence and expert opinion using consensus techniques (Campbell *et al.* 2002a; Black *et al.* 1999; Murphy *et al.* 1998; Jones and Hunter 1995). As experts often disagree on the interpretation of evidence, rigorous methods are needed to assess the level of agreement. Consensus methods are group facilitation techniques designed to quantify the level of consensus among a group of experts by synthesising and clarifying individual expert opinion so that individual opinions are aggregated into refined aggregated opinion.

The experts can be health professionals, patients or policy makers. Since their views on important quality aspects differ it is necessary to decide beforehand which perspectives should be included in any given evaluation. Where views are diverse, separate groups are recommended (Krueger 1988).

Consensus techniques are characterised by three aspects – the ratings or judgements of experts are anonymous, they are iterative processes with feedback and individual responses are synthesised and aggregated into a group judgement (Normand *et al.* 1998). Group judgements are preferred to individual judgements because they are more consistent and less prone to personal bias or lack of reproducibility. Below we describe in more detail three of the most commonly used consensus techniques that combine evidence and expert opinion.

Delphi technique

The Delphi technique is a structured, interactive method that involves the repeated administration of confidential postal questionnaires, usually over two or three rounds (Linstone and Turoff 1975); panels rarely meet face-to-face. The main stages include:

- Identifying a (research) problem;
- Developing questionnaire statements to rate;
- Selecting appropriate panellists;
- Conducting anonymous iterative postal questionnaire rounds;
- Feeding back results (analysed statistically, qualitatively or both) between rounds;
- Summarising and feeding back the findings.

The absence of any face-to-face meeting prevents panel discussion of potentially different viewpoints, but this postal method is less costly than face-to-face

---

Box 16.2 Non-systematic approach: contraceptives and adolescents (Pringle 2000)

A 13-year old girl having a termination of pregnancy led to a team meeting in an English general practice. Her medical record showed two occasions when contraceptives could have been discussed. Practice members formed a group that reviewed the literature and conducted a survey in two local schools. The results culminated in three changes in practice management:

- Adolescents (13 years and older) were included in the administrative systems recording processes on smoking behaviour, alcohol consumption and usage of contraceptives;
- Posters on contraception were displayed in the practice, the schools and youth centres.
- A special 1 hour clinic, early in the evening, was introduced for adolescents to talk about lifestyle, safe sex, contraceptives, vaccinations and cervical smears.

To measure the effects of the changes the practice staff developed a quality indicator on the coverage of advice about lifestyle and risk factors. The practice was satisfied with the extra service as judged by an increase in the number of visits by adolescents.

meetings and enables a larger panel of experts from a more geographically diverse population to be involved.

The Delphi technique has been used to generate indicators for more than just clinical care. It has been used to develop:

- Prescribing indicators (*Box 16.3*; see also Campbell *et al.* 2000b);
- Managerial indicators (Hasson *et al.* 2000);
- Indicators of practitioners' and health managers' perspectives of quality in primary care (Campbell *et al.* 1998);
- Indicators for cardiovascular disease (Normand *et al.* 1998);
- Key attributes of a general practice trainer (Munro *et al.* 1998).

RAND appropriateness method

In the USA. the Agency for Healthcare Research and Quality (AHRQ, formerly AHCPR) used the RAND appropriateness method (Dalkey 1969) to develop guidelines and quality indicators. The method has been developed on an ongoing basis and has been used extensively (Shekelle *et al.* 1998; Brook 1986). This approach combines systematic literature reviews and expert panels. Preliminary indicators are extracted from the literature. In the first round, panellists are sent the literature review and indicator rating sheets by post. They are asked to read the review and then rate the indicators according to how necessary they are for high-quality care. The second round involves a face-to-face meeting, at which the ratings from the first round are fed back and the panel members discuss all the indicators and then re-rate them. Only second round ratings are used to derive indicators.

The RAND method has been used to develop quality indicators in primary and secondary care for many conditions, for example coronary artery bypass (Leape *et al.* 1996), care of the vulnerable elderly (Shekelle *et al.* 2001), coronary revascularisation (Hemingway *et al.* 2001), angina, asthma and type 2 diabetes (Campbell *et al.* 1999, 2002b). In contrast to the Delphi technique, the RAND method focuses strongly on the idea that panellists make use of the scientific information in the systematic review. This increases the opportunities for panel members to ground their opinions in the scientific evidence.

There has been criticism of this method, especially on the definition of appropriate care and the lack of user and/or patient involvement (Ayanian *et al.* 1998;

Box 16.3 Prescribing indicators in primary care (Cantrill *et al.* 1998)

Nine opinion leaders and prominent scientists took part in a nominal group technique to discuss the meaning of appropriate prescribing in primary care. This group came up with 103 items that could be used in answering the question "How to screen medical files for (in)appropriate prescribing?". These items were discussed and individuals ranked their top ten that, after aggregation, resulted in 34 items. Physicians (66) and pharmacists (75) next judged the 34 items in a Delphi survey by answering the question "Are these items suitable for determining appropriate prescribing?". A postal questionnaire was sent twice; in the second round the group received the feedback (separately for physicians and pharmacists) from the first round. This resulted in the selection of 18 indicators. Half of these were not used subsequently in an audit study, because the feasibility or the reliability of the data collection was felt to be questionable.

Indicators for appropriate prescribing

1. The indication for the drug is recorded and supported in the *British National Formulary* (BNF).
2. The reason for prescribing a drug of limited value is recorded and valid.
3. Compared with alternative treatments in the same therapeutic class, which are just as safe and effective, the drug prescribed is either one of the cheapest or a valid reason is given for using an alternative.
4. A generic product is prescribed if one is available.
5. If a potentially hazardous drug–drug combination is prescribed, the prescriber shows knowledge of the hazard.
6. If the total daily dose is outside the range stated in the BNF, the prescriber gives a valid reason.
7. If the dosing frequency is outside the range stated in the BNF, the prescriber gives a valid reason.
8. If the duration of treatment is outside the range stated in the BNF, the prescriber gives a valid reason.
9. Prescribing for hypertension adheres to the evidence-based guidelines in the BNF.

The indicators described are not very detailed, meaning that there was some room for interpretation for the researcher who subsequently collected the data in the practices. Extracting the medical files proved to be very time-consuming, but the process was valued by the primary care physicians.

Hicks 1994). While the reliability of the rating procedure (see Chapter 5 for more detail) is weak in terms of Kappa values, it has better reliability than many widely accepted clinical procedures (e.g. reading of mammograms). The reliability of the method increases when using a higher cut-off point to determine consensus within a panel (an overall panel median rating of 8 out of 9; see Shekelle *et al.* 1996, 1998). The RAND procedure involves a group discussion. While there are practical reasons for restricting the number of panellists to about 12, a review of studies using consensus methods suggested that including more participants seldom changed the overall ratings (Murphy *et al.* 1998).

Guideline-driven indicators

The availability of evidence-based clinical guidelines also makes it possible to derive quality indicators. Review criteria on heart failure, for example (*Box 16.4*) have been derived from clinical guidelines (Hadorn *et al.* 1996).

The National Institute for Clinical Excellence (NICE) in the UK has started to publish summaries of clinical guidelines, including a set of review criteria, for instance on the management of type 2 diabetes (NICE 2002). In the Netherlands, where guidelines for primary care are developed by the Dutch College of General Practitioners, several research projects have generated indicators and review criteria from guidelines following an 'iterated consensus rating procedure' (Braspenning *et al.* 2001). Indicators are developed based on the impact of guideline recommendations on the outcomes of care, using professional experts who

study the guideline and suggest key recommendations to be discussed in a broader panel (*Table 16.3*).

For example, in a study on low back pain (Schers *et al.* 2000), an expert group first discussed the key recommendations of the national guidelines. The main question was, "What are the most important guideline recommendations that will really make a difference to the quality of care in general practice?". The expert group decided, on the basis of scientific evidence in the guideline, that patients benefited most from advice to stay active and that costs can be saved by not referring to the physiotherapist when the patient has had symptoms for less than 6 weeks. This was the basis for a further selection of recommendations and development of indicators. In another study, this same procedure was used to select quality indicators for all 70 guidelines developed by the Dutch College of General Practitioners (Braspenning *et al.* 2001). The first round generated a pre-selection of suitable recommendations based on all the available Dutch guidelines for general practice. Two general practitioners read the 70 guidelines and discussed suitable items. Selection was based on the two criteria of relevance to patients' health and reduction of unnecessary performance (reduction of possible harm and cost). If the two experts agreed, the item was added to the pre-selection. The pre-selection contained 182 recommendations from 63 guidelines (no recommendations were produced for seven of the guidelines).

In the second round, a panel of eight physicians assessed these 182 recommendations. They rated the items for relevancy and reduction of unnecessary performance using five point rating scales from zero (not

---

Box 16.4 Review criteria for heart failure (Hadorn *et al.* 1996)

In 1992 the AHCPR (now AHRQ) developed a clinical practice guideline on the management of heart failure. The 16-member multidisciplinary expert panel was subsequently re-convened to translate the 34 guideline recommendations into review criteria and to determine standards of performance.

Two members of the expert panel rated the 34 recommendations on the basis of their importance to quality of care and feasibility of monitoring using a four point rating scale (1 being 'not important' or 'not feasible' and 4 being 'very important' or 'very feasible'); 20 recommendations were submitted to a six-member sub-committee of the full heart failure guideline panel, who reduced the number of recommendations to 16. In discussion concerns were raised in three areas – documentation difficulties (e.g. diet education), feasibility of monitoring (the whole medical file would have

to be searched to find the correct answer) and disagreement with the recommendation (level of evidence was too low). On the basis of the panellists' comments, six criteria were retained for further consideration and were resubmitted to the full panel (16 members), which increased the final number to eight.

When developing the standards of care the discussion focused on acceptable alternative scenarios to each criterion. However, the panel concluded that recommendations should not be a laundry list of possibilities that might occur in clinical practice and therefore no alternative scenarios were incorporated into the standards, but instead the standard of performance was fixed at something less than 100% adherence. For six criteria the standard of performance was set at 90–95% and for the other two criteria it was set at 75–80%.

Table 16.3 Iterated consensus rating procedure for deriving indicators from guidelines

Round	Aim	People, measurements involved	Selection criteria
1	Deriving key recommendations from guidelines	Small expert group	Strength of linkage to patients' outcomes and cost
2	Rating and adding key recommendations	Expert panel (8–10 people) using rating scales	Cut-off score (e.g. above midpoint of rating scale)
3	Determining inter- and intra-rater reliability	Ratings and re-ratings	Kappa, rho
4	Developing set of potential indicators	Small expert group Research team	Combination of the three above
5	Testing set of indicators in practice: data collection, analysis	Professional opinion Routine performance data	Feasibility, acceptability, clinimetric characteristics

relevant) to four (extremely relevant). *Table 16.4* shows 15 recommendations from five of the guidelines and their relevancy scores on both criteria. The panel was encouraged to add recommendations to be used to develop clinical indicators, resulting in 203 recommendations from all (*n* = 70) guidelines. In the third round, one-third of the recommendations (randomly selected) were judged again, and this set was extended with all the added items. The reliability of assessment was determined by calculating the inter- and intra-rater correlations. Since test–retest reliability showed considerable variation, a relatively low cut-off point was chosen (a score above the mean on one of the two criteria), which enabled all the relevant items to be part of the selection. In the fourth round the set of potential indicators was chosen. A total of 154 recommendations from 66 guidelines were selected in this way.

Table 16.4 The mean relevancy scores (0–4) from eight panel members on both criteria for the recommendations from five different guidelines

Condition	Recommendation	Health outcome		Possible harm, cost	
		Mean	Standard deviation	Mean	Standard deviation
Diabetes, type 2	Prevalence rate	3.63	0.74	2.63	1.19
	Number of hospital admissions	2.13	1.64	2.86	1.07
	Testing HbA1c	3.50	0.53	2.13	1.13
	Testing creatinine	2.63	1.06	–	–
	Referral for eye examination	3.38	0.74	2.50	1.20
	% high blood pressure	3.25	1.06	2.88	0.64
	% high cholesterol	2.75	0.74	2.50	0.76
Alcohol abuse	Prevalence rate	2.63	1.06	3.00	0.93
Acute sore throat	Prevalence rate	–	–	2.38	0.74
	Prescribing antibiotics	2.25	0.89	–	–
	First choice antibiotics	2.25	0.71	–	–
Urinary tract infection	First choice antibiotics	2.50	0.53	2.13	0.99
	Duration of treatment	–	–	2.13	1.13
Low back pain	Radiograph	–	–	2.88	1.25
	Referral to physiotherapist	–	–	3.25	0.71

– Means that the mean rating on this criterion for this recommendation was not above the midpoint of the rating scale.

The panel judgements were discussed within the research team, which resulted in five items being added to the selection. Consequently, a total of 159 items from 67 guidelines were available for transforming into a numerator and denominator, a task performed by the research team. The set of indicators was next tested in practice, both by asking the opinion of professionals on their value and by testing them against the availability of routine performance data. This resulted in a final set of 104 indicators that met criteria of reliability, availability of data, etc.

This third method of developing sets of indicators shares some similar characteristics with the RAND procedure. However, the literature from the systematic reviews that underlies the guidelines is not a direct part of the procedure. The assumption is that the guideline developers have interpreted the literature appropriately and transferred the necessary information to the guidelines. Another difference is that group discussion is replaced by written ratings, as in the Delphi method. The final set of indicators is based on these ratings, but a heavily weighted final interpretation is required from a small group of experts.

Which method is best for developing indicators?

Although no research that systematically compared these different methods of developing indicators, some issues relate equally to all three systematic approaches (*Table 16.5*). For example, irrespective of the method used, the result depends on the panel composition.

Using indicators from existing sources

While it is possible, and sometimes necessary, to develop indicators *de novo*, it is also possible to make use of indicators that are already available. There are many published sets of indicators for a wide variety of clinical problems or aspects of health care delivery. For example, an important set of indicators has been created in the USA HEDIS programme (Health Plan Employer Data and Information Set). Marshall *et al.* (2002) developed indicators for 19 common conditions presented in primary care. Kotsanos (1997) described indicators for seven chronic diseases, developed using an expert panel (*Table 16.6*).

An added advantage of using existing indicators is that reference data may be available. The disadvantage is that the original purpose of these indicators may not match the current need. For example, some indicators have been described at a population level, but not at a patient level (see Campbell *et al.* 1998). It is also not necessarily appropriate to use indicators developed in one country in other countries without testing their validity and relevance first (Marshall *et al.* 2003).

INDICATOR REQUIREMENTS

Quality measures need to be valid and reliable, as well as sensitive to change, acceptable, feasible and communicable (AQUA 2002; Campbell *et al.* 2002a; Marshall *et al.* 2002; Eddy 1998; McGlyn and Asch 1998; Streiner and Norman 1995). These attributes can be tested by evaluating the clinimetric properties of indicators (statistical analysis) and assessing their value in daily practice (process evaluation).

Validity and reliability

Measuring quality of care accurately, using quality indicators, requires that the indicators be valid and reliable. The validity of the quality indicators is usually described in terms of content and construct validity. The content validity of an indicator is strongly related to the method chosen to develop quality indicators. The more the indicator is grounded within evidence-based data on best practice, the stronger the content validity.

Table 16.5 Possible factors influencing the quality of the indicators	
Subjects	**Factors that influence quality**
Panel members	Knowledge, coherence of panel view, dominant individuals, focussing on different aspects of quality, number of panellists
Rating procedure	Rating scale, selection criteria, possibility of adding free-text information
Consensus procedure	Method of feedback, cut-off point, face-to-face meeting or postal survey

Construct validity can be established by relating the measurement to actual quality of health care. The measurement must be able to discriminate between different aspects of quality and different target groups with different levels of quality. So far, little attention has been given to the construct validity of quality indicators, but it is necessary to link the quality indicators as strongly as possible to the aspects of quality that are addressed.

Criterion validity is hard to determine for many measurement tools. The critical question to be answered is, can quality indicators predict good patient outcomes (health, quality of life, etc.)? Since good outcomes are determined not only by providing good care, but also by many other factors, criterion validity is hard to establish.

The reliability can be expressed by a test–retest procedure. An example of this type of testing is the inter- and intra-rater reliability (see *Table 16.3*).

Sensitivity to change

Alongside validity and reliability, sensitivity to change is an important clinimetric property. A quality indicator should be sensitive to changes in the quality of care (Mant and Hicks 1995), because the purpose of measurement is quality improvement and therefore it should capture changes in behaviour or setting. Time series and longitudinal analyses can be used to learn more about the sensitivity to change of indicators (see Chapter 18 for more details).

Acceptability and feasibility

Acceptability can be part of the development of an indicator during a consensus procedure, and it also can be established later when the indicator is being applied. It may take time for some stakeholders to accept indicators as being relevant and valid measurements for quality of care. Time allocated to go through this process should be protected, because acceptance in an early stage enhances usage over a longer period. The feasibility of the indicators, or more precisely of the data collection, depends on the data source.

Simple and communicable

Using indicators that can be communicated easily and understood by the target group enhances their acceptance and application. Eddy (1998) claims that process indicators are easier to communicate than outcome

Table 16.6 Performance indicators for seven chronic diseases (Kotsanos 1997)

Condition	Measurement
Chronic obstructive pulmonary disease (COPD)	Smoking cessation rate Influenza vaccination rate Adequacy of oxygen supplementation in COPD patients Hospitalisation rates
Chronic stable angina	Stress test and risk-factor profile recording rates Hospital admission rate Appropriate use of pharmacotherapy Stability or improvement in quality of life
Depression	Depression screening rate Rate of suicides and suicide attempts Rate of continuation of treatment of depression
Diabetes mellitus	Rate and average value of glycosylated haemoglobin tests Annual rate of diabetes education Self-monitoring of blood glucose Dilated ophthalmoscopic examination rates Foot examination rate Hospitalisation rate of diabetes patients
Hypercholesterolaemia	Identification of adults with hypercholesterolaemia Identification of adults with recent hospitalisation for atherosclerotic cardiovascular disease and hypercholesterolaemia Adequacy of management of hypercholesterolaemia Identification of children with hypercholesterolaemia
Hypertension	Essential hypertension incidence Essential hypertension prevalence Latency period to control of blood pressure Proportion of patients who comply with treatment Percentage of utilisation by hypertensive patients Hypertensive patients satisfaction
Rheumatoid arthritis	Rate of monitoring of acute-phase reactions

indicators. A discussion on the number of eye examinations for diabetics has relatively more to offer in terms of quality improvement than a discussion on morbidity rates.

USING INDICATORS

Using measurements to implement innovation and improve patient care is not new. Florence Nightingale managed to make notes about hospital deaths during the Crimean war and Ernest Codman tried at the beginning of the 1900s to collect data systematically on surgical hospital outcomes and to make them available to the public. Ideally, indicators should be introduced within a quality programme that has an implementation strategy from the onset to cover issues such as the feasibility and availability of data collection, feedback and a process to evaluate success or failure.

When applying quality indicators, data can be gathered by using routinely available sources or, if necessary, by developing new information systems. Routine data to assess the quality of care is becoming more available, sometimes even electronically, and information systems are increasingly based on patient data. These case-based information systems centred on clinical encounters (with diagnosis codes, prescription codes, referral codes, laboratory codes, etc.) make data searches easier. While such information systems offer much promise for accurate data collection, several caveats require consideration (Powell *et al.* 2003).

Firstly, when interpreting comparative data it is necessary to be aware of the measurement properties of the routinely collected data. For instance, a blood pressure measurement is reliable if it has been measured three times in a row, but routinely collected data shows only one measurement and we do not know if this one is based on three or fewer measurements. As another example, it is more common to make notes about the smoking habits for smokers than for non-smokers, which means that no information on smoking habits in the records can have different meanings – never asked,

asked and does not smoke or asked but not recorded. Some electronic medical record systems have a default on 'non-smoking'.

Quality measurement needs accurate and consistent information systems. Administrative data at macro- (health insurance company) or microlevel (individual medical files) are often constrained by inconsistent and unreliable data (Craddock *et al.* 2001; Baker 2000; Enthoven 2000; McColl *et al.* 1998).

Secondly, confounders based on case mix or other relevant factors have to be made clear and be taken into account. Thirdly, some variation in quality might be natural and not attributable to change. Lastly, the data should be of high quality (complete and accurate). All these issues can alter the interpretation of the comparative data (*Box 16.5*).

CONCLUSION

Measuring (change or improvement in) patient care requires an evaluation. A key question in each evaluation concerns the purpose of the evaluation: is it quality improvement, accountability or a scientific interest in effective innovations or implementation strategies? The exact measurement approach undertaken should correspond to the aim. Indicators of quality of care are used increasingly as part of such measurements, focusing upon structure, process or outcome indicators. Outcome indicators are usually used for external accountability; process indicators are more often applied in quality improvement and implementation of change projects. Indicators can be found in the published literature or on the internet, but often they have to be developed *de novo* or modified in the light of the purposes of the evaluation. Different systematic types of development methods can be used, such as the RAND procedure, the Delphi technique or the iterated consensus rating procedure. Indicators should be tested for their validity, reliability, acceptability, feasibility, sensitivity to change and how communicable or understandable they are.

Box 16.5 Using quality indicators in daily practice (McColl *et al.* 2000)

Quality indicators were developed for primary care using an evidence-based approach that resulted in 26 indicators. Data collection took place across 18 primary care groups. However, data across all the primary care groups was only available for seven of the 26 indicators. Information on patient education was particularly hard to find in medical records; for example, weight and smoking behaviour are only found in medical records if the caregiver plans to act on it.

Websites

www.rand.org
www.ahcpr.gov (Conquest)
www.newcastle.ac.uk/qip (Maryland)
www.npcrdc.man.ac.uk

Recommended literature

AHCPR (1995). *Using Clinical Practice Guidelines to Evaluate Quality of Care.* AHCPR Publication No. 95-0045. Rockville: US Department of Health and Human Services.

Brook RH, McGlynn EA and Shekelle PG (2000). Defining and measuring quality of care: A perspective from US researchers. *Int J Qual Health Care* 12:281–295.

Campbell SM, Braspenning J, Hutchinson A and Marshall M (2002). Research methods used in developing and applying quality indicators in primary care. *Qual Saf Health Care* 11(4):358–364.

Grol R, Baker R and Moss F (2003). *Quality Improvement Research. Understanding the Science of Change in Health Care.* London: BMJ Books.

References

AQUA (2002). *Qualitätsindikatoren der AOK für Arztnetze [Quality Indicators of AOK for GP Networks].* Göttingen: Aqua Institut für angewandte Qualitätsförderung und Forschung im Gesundheitswesen.

Ayanian JZ, Landrum MB, Normand SLT, Guadagnoli E and McNeil BJ (1998). Rating the appropriateness of coronary angiography – do practising physicians agree with an expert panel and with each other? *New Engl J Med.* 338:1896–1904.

Baker R (2000). Managing quality in primary health care: The need for valid information about performance. *Qual Health Care* 9:83.

Black N, Murphy M, Lamping D, *et al.* (1999). Consensus development methods: A review of best practice in creating clinical guidelines. *J Health Serv Res Policy* 4:236–248.

Braspenning J, Drijver R and Schiere AM (2001). *Quality Indicators for General Practice [Kwaliteits – en Doelmatigheidsindicatoren voor het Handelen in de Huisartspraktijk.]* Nijmegen/Utrecht: Centre for Quality of Care Research/Dutch College of General Practitioners,.

Brook RH (1986). The RAND/UCLA appropriateness method. In: McCormick KA, Moore SR and Siegel RA (eds). *Methodology Perspectives*, pp. 59–70. AHCPR Pub No 95-009. Rockville: Public Health Service, US Department of Health and Human Services.

Brook RH, McGlynn EA and Cleary PD (1996). Measuring quality of care. *N Engl J Med.* 335:966–970.

Brook RH, McGlynn EA and Shekelle PG (2000). Defining and measuring quality of care: A perspective from US researchers. *Int J Qual Health Care* 12:281–295.

Campbell SM, Roland MO, Quayle JA, Buetow SA and Shekelle PG (1998). Quality indicators for general practice. Which ones can general practitioners and health authority managers agree are important and how useful are they? *J Public Health Med.* 20:414–421.

Campbell SM, Roland MO, Shekelle PG, Cantrill JA, Buetow SA and Cragg DK (1999). Development of review criteria for assessing the quality of management of stable angina, adult asthma, and non-insulin dependent diabetes mellitus in general practice. *Qual Health Care* 8(1):6–15.

Campbell SM, Roland MO and Buetow S (2000a). Defining quality of care. *Soc Sci Med.* 51:1611–1625.

Campbell SM, Cantrill JA and Richards D (2000b). Prescribing indicators for UK general practice: Delphi consultation study. *BMJ* 321:1–5.

Campbell SM, Braspenning J, Hutchinson A and Marshall M (2002a). Research methods used in developing and applying quality indicators in primary care. *Qual Saf Health Care* 11(4):358–364.

Campbell SM, Hann M, Hacker J and Roland MO (2002b). Quality assessment for three common conditions in primary care: Validity and reliability of review criteria developed by expert panels for angina, asthma and type 2 diabetes. *Qual Saf Health Care* 11(2):125–130.

Cantrill JA, Sibbald B and Buetow S (1998). Indicators of the appropriateness of long term prescribing in general practice in the United Kingdom: Consensus development, face and content validity, feasibility and reliability. *Qual Health Care* 7:130–135.

Craddock J, Young A and Sullivan G (2001). The accuracy of medical record documentation in schizophrenia. *J Behav Health Ser Res.* 28:456–466.

Dalkey NC (1969). *The Delphi Method: An Experimental Study of Group Opinion.* Santa Monica: The Rand Corporation.

Dijkstra R and Braspenning J (2001). Implementation of effective guidelines. [Implementatie van doelmatige richtlijnen. In: *Effecten en Kosten van de Herziene Richtlijnen voor Diabetes. Diabetische Retinopathie. Diabetische Nefropathie, Diabetische Voet, Diabetische Controle*, Niessen LW, Casparie AT (eds), pp. 75–82.] Utrecht: IMTA, NDF, CBO.

Dijkstra RF, Braspenning JCC, Huijsmans Z, *et al.* (2004). Patients and nurses determine variation in adherence to guidelines at Dutch hospitals more than internists or settings. *Diabetes Med.* 21:586–591.

Donabedian A (1980). *Explorations in Quality Assessment and Monitoring. Volume 1: The Definition of Quality and Approaches to its Assessment.* Ann Arbor: Health Administration Press.

Eddy DM (1998). Performance measurement: Problems and solutions. *Health Affairs* 17:7–26.

Enthoven AC (2000). Modernising the NHS: A promising start, but fundamental reform is needed. *BMJ* 320:1329–1331.

Hadorn DC, Baker DW, Kamberg CJ and Brook RH (1996). Phase II of the AHCPR-sponsored heart failure guideline: Translating practice recommendations into review criteria. *Jt Comm J Qual Improv.* 22:266–275.

Hasson F, Keeney S and McKenna H (2000). Research guidelines for the Delphi survey technique. *J Adv Nurs.* 32:1008–1015.

Hearnshaw HM, Harker RM, Cheater FM, Baker RH and Grimshaw GM (2001). Expert consensus on the desirable characteristics of review criteria for improvement of health quality. *Qual Health Care* 10:173–178.

Hemingway H, Crook AM, Feder G, *et al.* (2001). Underuse of coronary revascularization procedures in patients considered appropriate candidates for revascularization *N Engl J Med*. **344**:645–654.

Hicks NR (1994). Some observations on attempts to measure appropriateness of care. *BMJ* **309**:730–733.

Irvine D (1990). Managing for quality in general practice. London: Kings Fund Centre.

Jones JJ and Hunter D (1995). Consensus methods for medical and health services research. *BMJ* **311**:376–380.

Kotsanos JG (1997). Development of performance measures for seven chronic diseases. Health Outcomes Workgroup of the Pharmaceutical Research and Manufacturers of America. *Jt Comm J Qual Improv*. **23**(3):150–161.

Krueger RA (1988). *Focus Groups: A Practical Guide for Applied Research*. Thousand Oaks: Sage Publications.

Lawrence M and Olesen F (1997). Indicators of quality in health care. *Eur J Gen Pract*. **3**:103–108.

Leape LL, Hilborne LH, Schwartz JS, *et al*. (1996). The appropriateness of coronary artery bypass graft surgery in academic medical centres. *Ann Intern Med*. **125**:8–18.

Linstone HA and Turoff M (1975). *The Delphi Survey. Method, Techniques and Applications*. Reading: Addison-Wesley.

Mant J and Hicks N (1995). Detecting differences in quality of care: The sensitivity of measures of process and outcome in treating acute myocardial infarction *BMJ* **311**:793–796.

Marshall M, Campbell SM, Hacker J and Roland MO (2002). *Quality Indicators for General Practice: A Practical Guide for Health Professionals and Managers*. London: Royal Society of Medicine.

Marshall MN, Shekelle PG, McGlynn EA, Campbell SM, Brook RH and Roland MO (2003). Can health care quality indicators be transferred between countries? *Qual Saf Health Care* **12**:8–12.

McColl A, Roderick P, Gabbay J, Smith H and Moore M (1998). Performance indicators for primary care groups: An evidence-based approach. *BMJ* **317**:1354–1360.

McColl A, Roderick P, Smith H, *et al*. (2000) Clinical governance in primary care groups: The feasibility of deriving evidence-based performance indicators. *Qual Health Care* **9**:90–97.

McGlynn EA and Asch SM (1998). Developing a clinical performance measure. *Am J Prev Med*. **14**:14–21.

Munro N. Hornung RI and McAteer S (1998). What are the key attributes of a good general practice trainer? A Delphi Study. *Educ Gen Prac*. **9**:263–70.

Murphy MK, Black NA, Lamping DL, *et al*. (1998). Consensus development methods and their use in clinical guideline development. *Health Technol Assess*. **2**(3):1–88.

NICE (2002). *Management of Type 2 Diabetes: Renal Disease – Prevention and Early Management*. London: National Institute for Clinical Excellence.

Normand S-LT, McNeil BJ, Peterson LE, *et al*. (1998). Eliciting expert opinion using Delphi technique: Identifying performance indicators for cardiovascular disease. *Int J Qual Health Care* **10**(3):247–260.

Ovretveit J (1992). *Health Service Quality: An Introduction to Quality Methods for Health Services*. Oxford: Blackwell Scientific Publications.

Palmer RH (1997). Process-based measures of quality: The need for detailed clinical data in large health care databases. *Ann Intern Med*. **127**:733–738.

Powell AE, Davies HTO and Thomson RG (2003). Using routine comparative data to assess the quality of health care: Understanding and avoiding common pitfalls. *Qual Saf Health Care* **12**:122–128.

Pringle M (2000). Clinical governance in primary care. Participating in clinical governance. *BMJ* **321**:737–740.

Schers H, Braspenning J, Drijver R, Wensing M and Grol R (2000). Low back pain in general practice: Reported management and reasons for not adhering to the guidelines in the Netherlands. *Br J Gen Pract*. **50**:640–644.

Shekelle PG, Kahan JP, Park RE, *et al*. (1996). Assessing appropriateness by expert panels: How reliable? *J Gen Intern Med*. **10**(Suppl.):81.

Shekelle PG, Kahan JP, Bernstein SJ, Leape LL, Kamberg CJ and Park RE (1998). The reproducibility of a method to identify the overuse and underuse of procedures. *N Engl J Med*. **338**:1888–1895.

Shekelle PG, MacLean CH, Morton SC and Wenger NS (2001). Assessing care of vulnerable elders: Methods for developing quality indicators. *Ann Intern Med*. **135**:647–652.

Solberg LI, Moser G and McDonald S (1997). The three faces of performance measurement: Improvement, accountability and research. *Jt Comm J Qual Improv*. **23**:135–147.

Streiner DL and Norman GR (1995). *Health Measurement Scales: A Practical Guide to Their Development and Use*. Oxford: Oxford Medical Publications.

Chapter 17

Experimental evaluations of change and improvement strategies

Martin Eccles, Jeremy Grimshaw, Marion Campbell and Craig Ramsay

---

KEY MESSAGES

- Quantitative designs should be used within a sequence of evaluation, building as appropriate on preceding theoretical, qualitative and modelling work.
- There are a range of more or less complex randomised designs.
- Whatever design is chosen, it is important to minimise bias and maximise generalisability.
- When using randomised designs it is important to consider the appropriate use of cluster, rather than individual, randomisation. This has implications for both study design and analysis.
- Where randomised designs are not feasible, non-randomised designs can be used, although these are more susceptible to bias.

Box 17.1 A randomised controlled trial (Eccles *et al.* 2002a)

This study was a before-and-after pragmatic cluster randomised controlled trial (RCT) that utilised a two-by-two incomplete block design and was designed to evaluate the use of a computerised decision support system (CDSS) in implementing evidence-based clinical guidelines for the primary care management of asthma and angina in adults. It was based in 60 general practices in the north east of England and the participants were general practitioners (GPs) and practice nurses in the study practices and their patients aged 18 years or over with angina or asthma. The practices were randomly allocated to two groups. The first group received computerised guidelines for the management of angina and provided intervention patients for the management of angina and control patients for the management of asthma. The second received computerised guidelines for the management of asthma and provided intervention patients for the management of asthma and control patients for the management of angina. The outcome measures were adherence to the guidelines, determined by recording of care in routine clinical records and any subsequent impact measured by patient-reported generic and condition-specific measures of outcome. There were no significant effects of CDSS on consultation rates, process of care measures (including prescribing) or any quality-of-life domain for either condition. Levels of use of the CDSS were low.

INTRODUCTION

Evaluation of the effects of implementation activities is very important, but may use different methods and designs depending on the goals. Different evaluation designs are used depending on whether one wants to test progress and changes in care processes in a hospital or practice or one wants to provide generalisable information on the value of a new strategy or improvement programme (*Table 17.1*). In the latter case it is very important that the effects can be attributed confidently to the intervention, while in the former case the main

aim is to establish if the desired changes have been achieved. Such 'practical' projects can be either single site (one hospital or department, one team or one practice working on the implementation of a new routine or process) or large scale (all hospitals or practices in a district or region).

These different settings and their designs are addressed in two different chapters. This chapter focuses primarily on the setting of research to evaluate the effectiveness of specific quality improvement and implementation interventions in which the main aim is to make internally valid statements on their value

Table 17.1 Characteristics of different types of implementation projects and studies

	Small-scale improvement project	Large-scale implementation project	Implementation research
Aim of evaluation	Test of change in performance	Determining if goals are achieved	Determining value of intervention
Population	All care providers	Sample of providers, teams, hospitals and patients	Sample of providers, teams, hospitals and patients
Design	Monitoring, audit, statistical process control	Monitoring, time-series analysis, community, intervention trial	RCT, non-experimental study (controlled before and/or after, time-series analysis)
Data collection	Simple, few key indicators	Complex, some key indicators	Complex, detailed
Generalisability	Not important	Often possible	Key issue

and generalisability to a wider population or to other settings – a range of research designs and methodological considerations are presented. In Chapter 18 (Observational evaluations of implementation strategies) the focus is on small-scale improvement projects and large-scale implementation projects.

There is a substantial literature about the design, conduct and analysis of evaluations of relatively simple healthcare interventions such as drugs. However, the methods of evaluating complex interventions, such as quality improvement interventions, are described less well. Evaluation informs the choice between alternative interventions or policies by identifying, estimating and, if possible, valuing the advantages and disadvantages of each (Russell 1983).

A number of quantitative designs could be used to evaluate quality improvement interventions (*Box 17.2*).

All of these designs attempt to establish general causal relationships across a population of interest. The choice of design is dependent upon the purpose of the evaluation and the degree of control the researchers have over delivery of the intervention(s). In general, researchers should choose a design that minimises

potential bias (any process at any stage of inference that tends to produce results or conclusions that differ systematically from the truth – also referred to as internal validity) and maximises generalisability [the degree to which the results of a study hold true for situations other than those pertaining to the study, in particular for routine clinical practice – also referred to as external validity (Shadish *et al.* 2002; Campbell and Stanley 1966)].

A FRAMEWORK FOR EVALUATING IMPLEMENTATION INTERVENTIONS

Campbell *et al.* (2000a) have suggested that the evaluation of complex interventions should follow a sequential approach, which involves:

- Development of the theoretical basis for an intervention;
- Definition of components of the intervention (using modelling, simulation techniques or qualitative methods);
- Exploratory studies to develop the intervention further and plan a definitive evaluative study (using a variety of methods);
- Definitive evaluative study (using quantitative evaluative methods, predominantly randomised designs).

This framework demonstrates the inter-relation between quantitative evaluative methods and other methods; it also makes explicit that the design and conduct of quantitative evaluative studies should build upon the findings of other quality improvement research. However, it represents an idealised framework and, in some circumstances, it is necessary to undertake evaluations without sequentially working through the earlier stages (e.g. when evaluating policy interventions that are being introduced without prior supporting evidence).

> ## Box 17.2 Quantitative evaluative designs for implementation research
>
> Randomised designs:
> - Individual patient RCTs;
> - Cluster RCTs.
>
> Non-randomised designs:
> - Uncontrolled before-and-after studies;
> - Controlled before-and-after studies;
> - Time-series designs.

In this chapter we describe quantitative approaches for the evaluation of implementation interventions that focus on methods to estimate the magnitude of the benefits. We also focus on the evaluation of interventions within systems rather than evaluations of whole systems. We discuss several study designs, including a range of randomised designs and three non-randomised or quasi-experimental evaluative designs.

RANDOMISED DESIGNS

RCTs are the gold standard method for evaluating healthcare interventions (Cochrane 1979). They estimate the impact of an intervention through direct comparison with a randomly allocated control group that receives either no intervention or an alternative intervention (Pocock 1983). The randomisation process is the best way to ensure that both known and (particularly importantly) unknown factors (confounders) that may independently affect the outcome of an intervention are likely to be distributed evenly between the trial groups. As a result, differences observed between groups can be ascribed more confidently to the effects of the intervention rather than to other factors. The same arguments that are used to justify RCTs of clinical interventions, such as drugs, are at least as salient to the evaluations of quality improvement and implementation interventions. In particular, given our incomplete understanding of potential confounders relating to organisational or professional performance, it is even more difficult to adjust for these in non-randomised designs.

Cluster randomisation

While it is possible to conduct randomised trials of quality improvement interventions that randomise individual patients, this may not always be ideal. If there is a possibility that the treatment given to control individuals is affected by an organisation's or professional's experience of applying the intervention to other patients in the experimental or control group, there is a risk of contamination. For example, Morgan *et al.* (1978) investigated the effects of computerised reminders for antenatal care. Patients were randomised and physicians received reminders for intervention patients, but not control patients. Compliance in intervention patients rose from 83% to 98% over 6 months, while compliance in control patients rose from 83% to 94% over 12 months. This is a probable contamination effect.

If such contamination is likely, the researcher should consider randomising organisations or healthcare professionals rather than individual patients, although data may still be collected about the process and outcome of care at the individual patient level. Such trials, which randomise at one level (organisation or professional) and collect data at a different level (patient), are known as cluster randomised trials (Donner and Klar 2000; Murray 1998). Cluster randomisation has considerable implications for the design, power and analysis of studies, but has frequently been ignored.

Design considerations

The main design considerations concern the level of randomisation and whether to include baseline measurement. Frequently, researchers need to trade off the likelihood of contamination at lower levels of randomisation against decreasing numbers of clusters and increasing logistical problems at higher levels of randomisation. For example, in a study of an educational intervention in secondary care settings, potential levels of randomisation should include the individual clinician, the ward, the clinical service or directorate, and the hospital. Randomisation at the level of the hospital minimises the risk of contamination, but dramatically increase the size and complexity of the study because of the greater number of hospitals required. Randomisation at the level of the individual clinician, however, decreases the number of hospitals required, but there may then be a risk of contamination across clinicians who work in the same wards or specialty areas.

In situations where relatively few clusters (e.g. hospitals) are available for randomisation there is an increased danger of imbalance in performance between the study and control groups because of the play of chance. Baseline measurements can then be used to assess the adequacy of the allocation process, and are also useful because they provide an estimate of the magnitude of a problem. Low performance scores prior to the intervention may indicate that performance is poor and there is much room for improvement, whereas high performance scores may indicate that there is little room for improvement (ceiling effect). In addition, baseline measures could be used as a stratifying or matching variable or could be incorporated into the analysis to increase statistical power (see below). These potential benefits have to be weighed against the increased costs and duration of studies that incorporate baseline measurements and concerns about testing effects [introduction of a potential bias through sensitisation of the study subjects during the baseline measurement (Campbell and Stanley 1966)].

Sample-size calculation

A fundamental assumption of the standard statistics used to analyse patient-randomised trials is that the outcome for any individual patient is completely unrelated to that for any other patient – they are said to be 'independent'. This assumption is violated, however, when cluster randomisation is adopted, because two patients within any one cluster are more likely to respond in a similar manner than are two patients from different clusters. For example, the management of patients in a single hospital or primary care practice is more likely to be consistent than the management of patients across a number of hospitals. The primary consequence of adopting a cluster randomised design is that it is not as statistically efficient as and has lower statistical power than a patient-randomised trial of equivalent size.

Sample sizes for cluster randomised trials therefore need to be inflated to adjust for clustering. A statistical measure of the extent of clustering is known as the 'intra-cluster correlation coefficient' (ICC), which is based on the relationship of the between-cluster to within-cluster variance (Donner and Koval 1980).

Experience has taught us that, as a rule of thumb, ICCs for measures of the process of care tend to be higher than those for measures of patient-based outcomes, and ICCs for measures of the process of care in secondary care settings tend to be higher than those for similar measures in primary care settings. A database of ICCs across a range of activities and settings is available from http://www.abdn.ac.uk/hsru/epp/cluster.shtml. *Table 17.2* shows, as an example, a number of ICCs from a primary care study of computerised guidelines for patients with either asthma or stable angina. In general, the ICCs for prescribing are low. However, the ICCs for the recording of risk factors and management are higher, as high as 0.15 for checking compliance with treatment in patients with asthma.

Both the ICC and the cluster size influence the inflation required – the sample size inflation can be considerable, especially if the average cluster size is large. The extra numbers of patients required can be achieved by increasing either the number of clusters in the study [the more efficient method (Diwan *et al.* 1992)] or the number of patients per cluster (*Box 17.3*). In general, little additional power is gained by increasing the number of patients per cluster above 50. Researchers often have to trade off the logistic difficulties and costs

---

Box 17.3 An example of a sample size calculation (Eccles *et al.* 2000)

In the context of a RCT of computerised guidelines for the primary care management of two chronic conditions (see *Box 17.1*), the following sample size calculation was performed. The trial used a before-and-after incomplete block design. There are no published tables to calculate the sample size needed for a 'before-and-after incomplete block'. The simplest approach is to regard the design as two embedded randomised trials (one of guidelines for angina, the other of guidelines for asthma in adults) and determine the sample size for each trial separately.

It is felt that, for both conditions, doctors in the practices who receive the computerised prompt will adhere more closely to the guidelines than those in practices who receive the paper versions. It is required that each trial should have 80% power to detect a 10% difference in adherence (e.g. between 45 and 55%) using a significance level of 5%. Adherence to the guidelines is determined by measures of process recorded in the patients' medical records. As the unit of randomisation is the practice rather than the patient, it is necessary to take into account the lack of independence between observations on different patients within a single practice. It is estimated that the ICCs for measures of process will be 0.06. Using methods proposed by Donner and Klar (2000), it can be

demonstrated that it is necessary to sample records from 57 patients with each condition in each of 60 practices. Different measures of process may have different ICCs. If the average ICC were 0.1, we would need to sample an average of 86 patients with each condition in each of 60 practices to give 80% power to detect a difference of 12% (44 to 56%). Were the ICC 0.15, we would need to sample 40 patients in each of 60 practices to give 80% power to detect a difference of 15% (42.5 to 57.5%).

Patient-based outcomes were also assessed in this trial using a range of generic and condition-specific measures. Typically, these measures take the form of a summated Likert scale and can be considered as continuous variables with a normal distribution. Again, it is necessary to take into account the clustering of patients within practices. An ICC of 0.06 is assumed here as well. Application of standard methods indicate that if we sample 35 patients from each of 60 practices we would have 90% power to detect an effect size of 0.25 with a significance of 5% (or 80% power to detect an effect size of 0.22); 61 patients from each of 60 practices would give 90% power to detect an effect size of 0.23 with a significance of 5%.

Table 17.2 ICCs for medical record and prescribing data for angina and asthma (Eccles *et al.* 2002b, 2003)

Angina	ICC	Asthma	ICC
Patient consultation rates			
Number of consultations	0.04	Number of consultations	0.03
Number of consultations for angina	0.16	Number of consultations for asthma	0.05
Recording of risk factors and management			
Was blood pressure recorded?	0.04	Compliance checked?	0.15
Was exercise level or advice about exercise recorded?	0.08	Inhaler technique checked?	0.10
Any advice about Mediterranean diet or oily fish?	0.01	Lung function recorded?	0.08
Weight or advice about weight recorded?	0.10	Asthma education recorded?	0.12
Smoking status recorded?	0.10	Smoking status recorded?	0.09
		Smoking advice and/or education recorded?	0.03
Investigations			
Electrocardiogram (ECG) recorded?	0.01		
Thyroid function recorded?	0.01		
Blood glucose or HbA1c recorded?	0.03		
Cholesterol or other lipids recorded?	0.04		
Haemoglobin recorded?	0.05		
Exercise ECG recorded?	0.02		
Prescription of drugs			
Was verapamil prescribed?	0.01	Was short acting beta-2 agonist prescribed?	0.02
Was beta-blocker prescribed?	0.01	Inhaled corticosteroids	0.02
Short-acting glyceryl trinitrate (GTN)	0.01	Long-acting beta-2 agonists	0.01
Modified-release GTN	0.01	Oral corticosteroids	0.02
Transdermal GTN	0.02	Oral bronchodilators	0.02
Isosorbide dinitrate [short-acting (SA) and modified	0.07	Prescribing of inhaled corticosteroids	0.04
release (MR)]		for subjects who were prescribed a	
Isosorbide mononitrate (SA and MR)	0.02	mean daily dose of more than 6 puffs	
Diltiazem	0.02		
Ca channel blocker	0.01		
Statins	0.02		
Beta-blocker plus dinitrate	0.04		
Calcium blocker plus dinitrate	0.04		
Nitrate, calcium blocker plus beta-blocker	0.02		

associated with recruitment of extra clusters against those associated with increasing the number of patients per cluster (Flynn *et al.* 2002).

Assume a situation in which a trial is being designed to promote adherence to a national guideline for the use of statins in the management of patients with ischaemic heart disease. The current rate of prescription is 60%. A programme to implement the guidelines aims to increase adherence by at least 15% to 75%. With a 5% level of significance (alpha of 0.05) and 80% power (beta of 0.80), the number of practices (clusters) needed for the study and the number of patients per

practice (and thus the number of patients in the trial) varies with different assumptions about the ICC. *Table 17.3* shows the number of practices (clusters) needed in the trial.

If this was a patient RCT rather than a cluster RCT, it would require 304 patients. Assuming an ICC for the primary effect measure (prescription of a statin) of 0.05 the trial needs 46 practices to provide 10 patients each (460 patients); if the trialists have only 30 practices available, they can still run the study, but each cluster has to recruit 20 patients (600 patients in total). If the trial had to be powered on an outcome that required an ICC of

Table 17.3 The number of practices (clusters) needed in the trial for different ICCs and cluster sizes

ICC	Number of practices (clusters) needed in the trial			
	5 patients per practice	10 patients per practice	15 patients per practice	20 patients per practice
0.05	74	46	36	30
0.10	86	58	50	46
0.15	98	72	64	60

0.1 then, for the same assumptions, 46 practices would need to recruit 20 patients each (920 patients).

Analysis of cluster randomised trials

There are three general approaches to the analysis of cluster randomised trials – analysis at cluster level, the adjustment of standard tests and advanced statistical techniques using data recorded at both the individual and cluster level (Donner 1998; Murray 1998; Turner *et al.* 1991). Cluster level analyses use the cluster as the unit of randomisation and analysis. A summary statistic (e.g. mean, proportion) is computed for each cluster and, as each cluster provides only one data point, the data can be considered to be independent, which allows standard statistical tests to be used. Patient level analyses can be undertaken using adjustments to simple statistical tests to account for the clustering effect. However, this approach does not allow adjustment for patient or practice characteristics. Recent advances in the development and use of new modelling techniques to incorporate patient-level data allow the inherent correlation within clusters to be modelled explicitly, and thus a 'correct' model can be obtained. These methods can incorporate the hierarchical nature of the data into the analysis. For example, in a primary care setting, we may have patients (level 1) treated by GPs (level 2) nested within practices (level 3), and may have covariates measured at the patient level (e.g. patient age or gender), the GP level (e.g. gender, time in practice) and at the practice level (e.g. practice size). Which of the methods is better to use is still a topic of debate. The main advantage of such sophisticated statistical methods is their flexibility. However ,they require extensive computing time and statistical expertise, both for the execution of the procedures and in the interpretation of the results.

No consensus exists as to which approach should be used. The most appropriate analysis option depends on a number of factors, including:
- The research question;
- The unit of inference;
- The study design;
- Whether the researchers wish to adjust for other relevant variables at the individual or cluster level (covariates);
- The type and distribution of outcome measure;
- The number of clusters randomised;
- The size of cluster and variability of cluster size;
- Statistical resources available in the research team.

Campbell *et al.* (2000b) and Mollison *et al.* (2000) present worked examples that compare these different analytical strategies (*Box 17.4*).

Possible types of cluster randomised trials

Two-arm trials

The simplest randomised design is the two-arm trial in which each subject is randomised to study or control groups (*Box 17.5*). Observed differences in performance between the groups are assumed to result from the intervention. Such trials are relatively straightforward to design and conduct and they maximise statistical power (half the sample is allocated to the intervention and half to the control). However, they only provide information about the effectiveness of a single intervention compared to control (or the relative effectiveness of two interventions without reference to a control).

Multiple arm trials

The simplest extension to the two-arm trial is to randomise groups of professionals to more than two groups (e.g. two or more study groups and a control group). Such studies are relatively simple to design and allow head-to-head comparisons of interventions or levels of intervention under similar circumstances. These benefits are, however, compromised by a loss of statistical power – for example, to achieve the same power as a two-arm trial, the sample size for a three-arm trial needs to be increased by up to 50%. *Box 17.6* shows an example of a three-arm trial.

Box 17.4 The impact of different analytical approaches to the same data (Campbell *et al.* 2000b)

The URGE study evaluated the effectiveness of a guideline-based open-access 'fast-track' investigation service for two common urological problems, benign prostatic hyperplasia (BPH) and microscopic haematuria. Practices were allocated randomly to two groups – one group received guidelines for the appropriate referral of BPH patients for the open-access 'fast-track' system while the other group acted as a control for BPH patients (but did receive guidelines for microscopic haematuria). Using data from this study, Campbell *et al.* (2000b) illustrated the impact of difference analytical approaches to the comparison of waiting times between intervention and control groups. The significance of the results varies considerably between analyses:

Comparison of waiting times[a] between intervention and control groups				
Statistical test	Test statistic	P-value	Effect size	95% CI
Aggregated analysis				
t-test	3.99	0.0003	0.65	0.53–0.81
Weighted t-test	4.72	0.00003	0.65	0.54–0.78
Individual patient				
Unadjusted t-test	5.11	0.000001	0.65	0.55–0.77
Adjusted t-test	4.09	0.00006	0.65	0.52–0.80
Multilevel modelling	4.08	0.0001	0.66	0.54–0.81
Multilevel modelling[b]	2.71	0.01	0.70	0.55–0.91

[a]Waiting times were log transformed.
[b]The analysis was conducted on all patients (pre- and post-intervention cohorts) and the model contained a correction for baseline, intervention and intervention phase interaction.

Factorial designs

Factorial designs allow the evaluation of the relative effectiveness of more than one intervention compared with a control. For example, in a 2×2 factorial design that evaluates two interventions against a control, participants are randomised to each intervention (A and B) independently. In the first randomisation, the study participants are randomised to intervention A or control. In the second randomisation, the same participants are randomised to intervention B or control. This results

Box 17.5 An example of a two-arm trial (Lobo *et al.* 2002)

The trial aimed to assess whether the quality of cardiovascular preventive care in primary care could be improved through a comprehensive intervention implemented by an educated outreach visitor. After baseline measurements, 124 general practices (in the southern half of the Netherlands) were randomly allocated to either intervention or control. The intervention, based on the educational outreach model, comprised 15 practice visits over a period of 21 months and addressed a large number of issues around task delegation, availability of instruments and patient leaflets, record keeping and follow-up routines. Post-intervention measurements were performed 21 months after the start of the intervention. The difference between ideal and actual practice in each aspect of organising preventive care was defined as a deficiency score. The primary outcome measure was the difference in deficiency scores before and after the intervention. All practices completed both baseline and post-intervention measurements. The difference in change between intervention and control groups, adjusted for baseline, was statistically significant ($p < 0.001$) for each aspect of organising preventive care. The largest absolute improvement was found for the number of preventive tasks performed by the practice assistant.

Box 17.6 An example of a three-arm trial (Scheel *et al.* 2002)

Active sick leave (ASL) is an option provided by the Norwegian National Insurance Administration that enables employees to return to modified duties at the workplace with 100% of normal wages. In a cluster RCT design, Scheel *et al.* (2002) evaluated the effects of two strategies to increase the use of ASL among patients with low back pain (LBP) on improved return to work and quality of life.

Sixty-five municipalities in Norway were randomly assigned to a passive intervention, a proactive intervention or a control group. The interventions, which were designed to improve the use of ASL, were targeted at patients on sick leave for LBP for more than 16 days ($n = 6179$), their GPs, employers and local insurance officers. The main outcome measures were the average number of days off work, the proportion of patients returning to work within 1 year and self-reported quality of life while on sick leave.

The median number of days on sick leave was similar in the proactive intervention group (70 days), the passive intervention group (68 days) and the control group (71 days; $p = 0.8$). The proportion of patients returning to work before 50 weeks was also similar in the proactive (89%), passive (89.5%) and control groups (89.1%). Response rates for the questionnaires sent to patients were low (38%), and no significant differences were observed across the three groups for quality of life or patient satisfaction.

The authors concluded that it is unlikely that efforts to increase the use of ASL will result in measurable economic benefits or improved health outcomes at the population level. The benefits of ASL for individual patients with LBP are not known.

in four groups – no intervention, intervention A alone, intervention B alone and both intervention A and B.

During the analysis of factorial designs, it is possible to undertake independent analyses to estimate the effect of the interventions separately (Cochran and Cox 1957); essentially, this design allows the conduct of two randomised trials for the same sample size as a two-arm trial. However, these trials are more difficult to operationalise and analyse, they provide only limited power for a direct head-to-head comparison of the two interventions and the power is diminished if there is interaction between the two interventions. *Box 17.7* shows an example of a factorial design trial that was powered to be able to detect any interaction effects.

Balanced incomplete block designs

In guideline-implementation research, a number of non-specific effects may influence the estimate of the effect of an intervention. These could be positive atten-

tion effects from participants who know that they are the subject of a study, or negative demotivation effects from being allocated to a control rather than an intervention group. Currently, these non-specific effects are grouped together and termed the 'Hawthorne effect'. If these are unequal across study groups in a quality improvement trial, the resulting estimates of effects may be biased. As these effects can potentially be of the same order of magnitude as the effects that the studies are seeking to demonstrate, there is an advantage to dealing with them systematically. While these effects may be difficult to eliminate, balanced incomplete block designs can be used to equalise such non-specific effects and thereby minimise their impact (Cochran and Cox 1957). An example is shown in *Box 17.1*. As doctors in both groups in the example in *Box 17.1* were subject to the same level of intervention, any non-specific effects are equalised across the two groups, which leaves any resulting difference as caused by the intervention.

Box 17.7 Example of a factorial design trial (Eccles *et al.* 2001)

The trial evaluated the effectiveness of audit and feedback and educational reminder messages to change radiology-ordering behaviour for lumber spine and knee radiographs. The design was a before-and-after pragmatic cluster RCT using a 2×2 factorial design that involved 244 practices and six radiology departments in two geographical regions. Each practice was randomised twice, to receive or not each of the two interventions. Educational reminder messages were based on national guidelines and were provided on the report of every relevant radiograph ordered during the 12 month intervention period. For example, the lumbar spine message read "In either acute (less than 6 weeks) or chronic back pain, without adverse features, X-ray is not routinely indicated". The audit and feedback covered the preceding 6 month period and was delivered to individual practitioners at the start of the intervention period and again 6 months later. It provided practice-level information that related the number of requests made by the whole practice relative to the number of requests made by all the practices in the study. Audit and feedback led to a non-significant reduction of around 1% radiograph requests, while educational reminder messages led to a relative reduction of about 20% radiograph requests.

NON-RANDOMISED DESIGNS

Quasi-experimental designs

Quasi-experimental designs to study the effectiveness of implementation strategies are useful where there are political, practical or ethical barriers to conducting a genuine (randomised) experiment. Under such circumstances, researchers may have less or little control over the delivery of an intervention and may have to plan an evaluation for a proposed intervention. A large number of potential designs are summarised by Campbell and Stanley (1966) and Shadish *et al.* (2002). Here we discuss the three most commonly used designs in quality improvement studies – uncontrolled before-and-after studies, controlled before-and-after studies and time-series designs.

Controlled before-and-after studies

In controlled before-and-after studies, the researcher attempts to identify a control population of similar characteristics and performance to those of the study population and collects data in both populations before and after the intervention is applied to the study population. Analysis compares post-intervention performance or change scores in the study and control groups and observed differences are assumed to result from the intervention.

While well-designed before-and-after studies should protect against secular trends and sudden changes, it is often difficult to identify a comparable control group. Even in apparently well-matched control and study groups, performance at baseline often differs. Under these circumstances, 'within group' analyses are often undertaken (where change from baseline is compared within both groups separately and where the assump-tion is made that if the change in the intervention group is significant and the change in the control group is not, the intervention has had an effect). Such analyses are inappropriate for a number of reasons. Firstly, the base-line imbalance suggests that the control group is not truly comparable and may not experience the same secular trends or sudden changes as the intervention group; thus any apparent effect of the intervention may be spurious. Secondly, there is no direct comparison between study and control groups (Campbell and Stanley 1966). Another common analytical problem in practice is that researchers fail to recognise clustering of data when interventions are delivered at an organisational level and data are collected at the individual patient level (*Box 17.8*).

Time-series designs

Time-series designs attempt to detect whether an intervention has had an effect significantly greater than that of the underlying secular trend (Shadish *et al.* 2002). They are useful in quality improvement research to evaluate the effects of interventions when it is difficult to randomise or identify an appropriate control group, for example after the dissemination of national guidelines or mass media campaigns (*Box 17.9*). Data are collected at multiple time points before and after the intervention. The multiple time points before the intervention allow the underlying trend and any cyclical (seasonal) effects to be estimated. The multiple time points after the intervention allow the intervention effect to be estimated while taking account of the underlying secular trends.

The most important influence on the analysis technique is the number of data points collected prior to the intervention. It is necessary to collect enough data points to be convinced that a stable estimate of the underlying secular trend has been obtained. A number

---

Box 17.8 A controlled before–and–after study (Larson and Hargiss 1984)

The authors conducted an evaluation of the effectiveness of a core of specially trained staff nurses in the maintenance of intravenous (IV) therapy. Five staff nurses for each of two experimental units were trained for 1 month by an IV nurse educator and were expected to perform venepuncture and monitor peripheral IV care on their units. On three control units, IV therapy continued to be a shared function of all the medical house staff and nurses.

During this study, 876 IV infusions on 707 patients were studied. A decrease was found in the phlebitis rate on experimental units from baseline to study periods from 33.5 to 20.9% (relative risk, controlled for duration of the use of an IV device, 0.53, $p = 0.05$), whereas the rate on control units increased slightly (23.8 to 26.7%, $p > 0.5$). Bacterial colonisation of IV devices occurred more often on experimental units than on control units, both at baseline (12.7% versus 7.1%; $p = 0.25$) and during the study phase (19.4% versus 5.9%; $p < 0.01$). This increased colonisation occurred with IV infusions started by both physicians and nurses. Patient comfort, measured by number of sticks for each venepuncture and patient interview, was significantly improved ($p < 0.001$) on experimental units during the study phase.

Box 17.9 Time–series analysis (Matowe *et al.* 2002)

An interrupted time series using monthly data for 34 months before and 14 months after dissemination of the guidelines was used to evaluate the effect of a postal dissemination of the third edition of the Royal College of Radiologists' guidelines on GP referrals for radiography. Data were abstracted for the period April 1994 to March 1998 from the computerised administrative systems of open-access radiological services provided by two teaching hospitals in one region of Scotland. 117,747 imaging requests from general practice were made during the study period. There were no significant effects of disseminating the guidelines on the total number of requests or on requests for 18 individual tests. If a simple before-and-after study had been used, we would have erroneously concluded that 11 of the 18 procedures had significant differences.

of statistical techniques can be used, depending on the characteristics of the data, the number of data points available and whether autocorrelation is present (Shadish *et al.* 2002). Autocorrelation refers to the situation whereby data points collected close in time are likely to be more similar to each other than to data points collected far apart. For example, for any given month, the waiting times in hospitals are likely to be more similar to waiting times in adjacent months than to waiting times 12 months previously. Autocorrelation has to be allowed for in an analysis, and time-series regression models (Ostrom 1990; *Box 17.10*) and autoregressive integrated moving averages (ARIMA) modelling (Shadish *et al.* 2002) are all methods used to deal with this problem.

Well-designed time-series evaluations increase the confidence with which the estimate of effect can be attributed to the intervention, although the design does not provide protection against the effects of other events occurring at the same time as the study intervention that might also improve performance. Furthermore, it is often difficult to collect sufficient data points unless routine data sources are available. It was found that many published time-series studies were inappropriately analysed, which frequently resulted in overestimates the effect of the intervention (Grilli *et al.* 1998, 2002).

Uncontrolled before–and–after studies

Uncontrolled before-and-after studies measure performance before and after the introduction of an intervention in the same study site(s) and observed differences in performance are assumed to result from the intervention. They are relatively simple to conduct and are superior to observational studies, but they are intrinsically weak evaluative designs because secular trends or sudden changes make it difficult to attribute observed changes to the intervention. Some evidence suggests that the results of uncontrolled before-and-after studies may overestimate the effects of quality improvement-like interventions. Lipsey and Wilson (1993) undertook an overview of meta-analyses of psychological, educational and behavioural interventions. They identified 45 reviews that reported separately the pooled estimates from controlled and uncontrolled studies, and noted that the observed effects from uncontrolled studies were greater than those from controlled studies. In general, the results of uncontrolled before-and-after studies to evaluate

Box 17.10 An example of a time–series regression model (Ramsay *et al.* 2003)

In a previous RCT (see *Box 17.7*), educational reminder messages attached to radiograph reports were shown to be effective in reducing the number of radiograph requests for knee and lumbar spine radiographs. In this study, all radiology departments from the previous trial were asked for monthly referral records for the 12 month intervention period for knee and lumbar spine radiographs for each general practice. Poisson regression was used to test for a change over time in the number of referrals between control and intervention practices.

Data were obtained for 66% of the practices in the main trial. The number of referrals for both knee and lumbar spine radiographs remained consistently and statistically significantly lower in the educational reminder messages group compared to the control group (relative risk = 0.64 and 0.64 for knee and lumbar spine radiographs, respectively). There was no evidence that this difference increased or decreased throughout the 12 month period.

The effect of educational reminder messages was produced as soon as the intervention was delivered, and it was maintained throughout the intervention period. There was no evidence of the effect of the intervention wearing off.

the effectiveness of implementation strategies should be interpreted with great caution.

REFLECTION

Randomised trials of implementation strategies and interventions should only be considered when there is genuine uncertainty about the effectiveness of an intervention, when information on the effectiveness can really add to the improvement of patient care, when wide dissemination of the strategy is possible and when there is a budget for such a trial. While RCTs are the optimal design for evaluating implementation interventions, they are not without their problems. They can be logistically difficult, especially if the researchers are using complex designs to evaluate more than one intervention or if cluster randomisation, which requires the recruitment of large numbers of clusters, is planned. They are undoubtedly methodologically challenging and require a multidisciplinary approach to plan and conduct adequately. However, they can also be time consuming and expensive. In our experience, a cluster randomised trial of a quality improvement or implementation intervention can rarely be completed in less than 2 years.

Critics of randomised trials frequently express concerns that the tight inclusion criteria of the trials or the artificial constraints placed upon the participants limit the generalisability of the findings. While this is a particular concern in efficacy (explanatory) studies of drugs, it is likely to be less of a problem in quality improvement evaluations that are likely to be inherently pragmatic (Schwartz and Lellouch 1967). Pragmatic studies aim to test whether an intervention is likely to be effective in routine practice by comparing the new procedure against the current regimen; as such, they are the most useful trial design for developing policy recommendations. Such studies attempt to approximate normal conditions and do not attempt to equalise contextual factors and other effect modifiers in the intervention and study groups. In pragmatic studies, the contextual and effect-modifying factors therefore become part of the interventions. Such studies are usually conducted on a pre-defined study population and withdrawals are included within an 'intention to treat' analysis; all subjects initially allocated to the intervention group would be analysed as intervention subjects, irrespective of whether they received the intervention or not. For example, in an evaluation of CDSS as a method of delivering clinical

guidelines (see *Box 17.1*), some physicians may not have had the computing skills to apply the intervention. In an intention-to-treat analysis, data from all participants would be included in the analysis, irrespective of whether they could and did use the system or not. As a result, the estimates of effect are more likely to reflect the effectiveness of the intervention in real-world settings.

The main limitation of quasi-experimental designs is that the lack of randomised controls threatens internal validity and increases the likelihood of plausible rival hypotheses. Cook and Campbell (1979) provide a framework for considering the internal validity of the results of experiments and quasi-experiments when trying to establish causality. They suggest that:

> Estimating the internal validity of a relationship is a deductive process in which the investigator has to systematically think through how each of the internal validity threats may have influenced the data. Then the investigator has to examine the data to test which relevant threats can be ruled out. … When all of the threats can plausibly be eliminated it is possible to make confident conclusions about whether a relationship is probably causal.

Despite the potentially greater threats to internal validity and less ability to account for these within quasi-experiments, we believe that the design and conduct of quasi-experimental studies is at least as methodologically challenging as the design and conduct of randomised trials. The generalisability of quasi-experimental designs is also uncertain. Many quasi-experimental studies are conducted in a small number of study sites that may not be representative of the population to which the researcher wishes to generalise. Nevertheless, they may be the only solution for a particular set of circumstances and offer important lessons about effective implementation of change in healthcare.

CONCLUSIONS

We have considered a range of research designs for studies to evaluate the effectiveness of change and improvement strategies. Quantitative designs should be used within a sequence of evaluation, building as appropriate on preceding theoretical, qualitative and modelling work. There are a range of more or less complex randomised designs. The design chosen will reflect the needs (and resources) in any particular circumstances and also the purpose of the evaluation. The general principle that underlies the choice of evaluative design is, however, simple – those conducting such evaluations should use the most robust design possible to minimise bias and maximise generalisability. When using randomised designs it is important to consider the appropriate use of cluster, rather than individual, randomisation. This has implications for both study design and analysis. Where randomised designs are not feasible, non-randomised designs can be used, although they are more susceptible to bias and should therefore be interpreted with caution.

Recommended literature

Campbell DT and Stanley J (1966). *Experimental and Quasi-Experimental Designs for Research*. Chicago: Rand McNally.

Campbell M, Fitzpatrick R, Haines A, *et al.* (2000). Framework for design and evaluation of complex interventions to improve health. *BMJ* 321:694–696.

Donner A and Klar N (2000). *Design and Analysis of Cluster Randomization Trials in Health Research*. London: Arnold.

Turner MJ, Flannelly GM, Wingfield M, *et al.* (1991). The miscarriage clinic: An audit of the first year. *Br J Obstet Gynaecol*. 98:306–308.

References

Campbell DT and Stanley J (1966). *Experimental and Quasi-Experimental Designs for Research*. Chicago: Rand McNally.

Campbell M, Fitzpatrick R, Haines A, *et al.* (2000a). Framework for design and evaluation of complex interventions to improve health. *BMJ* 321:694–696.

Campbell MK, Mollison J, Steen N, Grimshaw J and Eccles M. (2000b). Analysis of cluster randomized trails in primary care: A practical approach. *Fam Pract*. 17(2):192–196.

Cochran WG and Cox GM (1957). *Experimental Design*, Second Edition. New York: Wiley.

Cochrane AL (1979). *Effectiveness and Efficiency: Random Reflections on Health Services*. London: Nuffield Provincial Hospitals Trust.

Cook TD and Campbell DT (1979). *Quasi-Experimentation: Design and Analysis Issues for Field Settings*. Chicago: Rand McNally.

Diwan VK, Eriksson B, Sterky G and Tomson G (1992). Randomization by group in studying the effect of drug information in primary care. *Int J Epidemiol*. 21:124–130.

Donner A (1998). Some aspects of the design and analysis of cluster randomization trials. *Appl Stat*. 47:95–113.

Donner A and Klar N (2000). *Design and Analysis of Cluster Randomization Trials in Health Research*. London: Arnold.

Donner A and Koval JJ (1980). The estimation of intraclass correlation in the analysis of family data. *Biometrics* 36:19–25.

Eccles M, Grimshaw J, Steen N, *et al.* (2000). The design and analysis of a randomised controlled trial to evaluate computerised decision support in primary care: The COGENT Study. *Fam Pract*. 17:180–186.

Eccles M, Steen N, Grimshaw J, *et al.* (2001). Effect of audit and feedback, and reminder messages on primary-care radiology referrals: A randomised trial. *Lancet* 357:1406–1409.

Eccles M, McColl E, Steen N, *et al.* (2002a). Effect of computerised evidence based guidelines on management of asthma and angina in adults in primary care: Cluster randomised controlled trial. *BMJ* 325(7370):941–944.

Eccles M, McColl E, Steen N, Rousseau N, Grimshaw J and Parkin D (2002a). *An Evaluation of Computerised Guidelines for the Management of Two Chronic Conditions*. Newcastle: Centre for Health Services Research.

Eccles M, Grimshaw J, Campbell M and Ramsay C (2003). Research designs for studies evaluating the effectiveness of change and improvement strategies. *Qual Saf Health Care* 12:47–52.

Flynn TN, Whitley E and Peters TJ (2002). Recruitment strategies in a cluster randomised trial – cost implications. *Stat Med*. 21:397–405.

Grilli R, Freemantle N, Minozzi S, Domenighetti G and Finer D (1998). *Impact of Mass Media on Health Services Utilisation*. The Cochrane Library, Issue 3. Oxford: Update Software.

Grilli R, Ramsay CR and Minozi S (2002). *Mass Media Interventions: Effects on Health Services Utilisation*. The Cochrane Library. Oxford: Update Software.

Larson E and Hargiss C (1984). A decentralized approach to maintenance of intravenous therapy. *Am J Infect Control* 12(3):177–186.

Lipsey MW and Wilson DB (1993). The efficacy of psychological, educational, and behavioral treatment: Confirmation from meta-analysis. *Am Psychol*. 48(12):1181–1209.

Lobo CM, Frijling BD, Hulscher MEJL, *et al.* (2002). Improving quality of organising cardiovascular preventive care in general practice by outreach visitors: A randomised controlled trial. *Prev Med*. 35:430–436.

Matowe L, Ramsay C, Grimshaw JM, Gilbert F, Needham G and Macleod MJ (2002). Influence of the Royal College of Radiologists' guidelines on referrals from general practice: A time series analysis. *Clin Radiol*. 57:575–578.

Mollison JA, Simpson JA, Campbell MK and Grimshaw JM (2000). Comparison of analytical methods for cluster randomised trials: An example from a primary care setting. *J Epidemiol Biostat*. 5(6):339–348.

Morgan M, Studney DR, Barnett GO and Winickoff RN (1978). Computerized concurrent review of prenatal care. *Q Rev Bull*. 4:33–36.

Murray DM (1998). *The Design and Analysis of Group Randomised Trials*. Oxford: Oxford University Press.

Ostrom CW (1990). *Time Series Analysis: Regression Techniques*. London: Sage.

Pocock SJ (1983). *Clinical Trials: A Practical Approach*. New York: Wiley.

Ramsay CR, Eccles M, Grimshaw JM and Steen N (2003). Assessing the long term effect of educational reminder messages on primary care radiology referrals. *Clin Radiol*. 58:319–321.

Russell IT (1983). The evaluation of a computerised tomography: A review of research methods. In: Culyer AJ and Horisberger B (eds). *Economic and Medical Evaluation of*

Health Care Technologies, pp. 298–316. Berlin: Springer-Verlag.

Scheel IB, Hagen KB, Herrin J, Carling C and Oxman AD (2002). Blind faith? The effects of promoting active sick leave for back pain patients: A cluster-randomized controlled trial. *Spine* **27**(23):2734–2740.

Schwartz D and Lellouch J (1967). Explanatory and pragmatic attitudes in clinical trials. *J Chron Dis*. **20**:637–648.

Shadish WR, Cook TD and Campbell DT (2002). *Experimental and Quasi-Experimental Designs for Generalized Causal Inference*. New York: Houghton Mifflin.

Turner MJ, Flannelly GM, Wingfield M, *et al*. (1991). The miscarriage clinic: An audit of the first year. *Br J Obstet Gynaecol*. **98**:306–308.

Chapter 18

Observational evaluations of implementation strategies

Michel Wensing, Martin Eccles and Richard Grol

KEY MESSAGES

- Observational evaluations include audit studies, developmental studies, descriptive case studies, comparative case studies, impact evaluations and community intervention studies.
- These studies can be used to assess the process and impact of interventions, but not to provide unbiased estimates of intervention effects.
- Their value is in supporting incremental decisions on implementation activities and helping to phrase hypotheses for potentially effective interventions.

Box 18.1 Case study of personal medical services (Campbell *et al.* 2003)

Government initiatives in the UK have sought to improve quality of care, and include fundholding, national service frameworks, clinical governance and personal medical services (PMS). PMS contracts allow practitioners to develop their services without the restrictions of standard contract regulations. A multiple case study was performed to evaluate the impact of PMS on the quality of primary mental healthcare between 1998 and 2001. The study comprised two sets of in-depth semi-structured interviews with a purposeful sample of key staff (family practitioners, nurses, managers and health authority managers) in six family practices, which had specifically planned to improve their mental healthcare. Each site was visited in April 1998 and in April 2001. The study showed that one site had met its mental health objectives successfully, one had a mixed but mostly positive experience, two had mixed but mostly negative experiences and two had essentially failed to meet their objectives. The pilots that had met all or many of their aims successfully were characterised by clear aims, a shared vision between practice staff, community trust partners and the health authority, good teamwork and effective collaboration with the health authority and secondary care providers. These factors were associated with a successful improvement in mental healthcare, which may be generalisable to initiatives that seek to improve quality of care in practices for other clinical areas and/or services.

INTRODUCTION

Chapter 17 shows that a well-performed trial provides the most robust research evidence for the effectiveness of a specific implementation strategy. Rigorous evaluations of implementation interventions are needed to obtain unbiased estimates of their effects. These estimates are particularly needed to inform major, long-term policy decisions. For instance, the decision to use outreach visits combined with education and feedback to improve prevention of cardiovascular diseases on a national scale was based partly on the results of a large cluster randomised trial (Hulscher *et al.* 1997). However, the resources to perform rigorous evaluations are lim-ited and in some circumstances it may be not possible to perform a randomised trial (Black 1996). Also, many decisions regarding implementation activities or quality improvement refer to decisions related to smaller programmes or projects, such as a quality improvement programme in one specific practice or hospital department, or smaller components of larger programmes. In many cases, evaluations that are not trials can both support such decisions and help to pose relevant hypotheses for further research. This chapter describes a range of observational methods for the evaluation of implementation interventions.

Observational evaluations have a number of specific characteristics. By definition, observational evaluations examine the natural variation among study participants to explore the effect of interventions on outcomes, and associated factors. The researcher or change agent has little or no control over the study conditions, particularly not over the allocation of study participants (patients and physicians) to intervention groups, while such control is a key feature of experimental designs (Deeks *et al.* 2003). Some non-randomised designs (see Chapter 17) may be labelled either as observational or as experimental, as the difference can be difficult to establish. This is particularly the case for controlled before-and-after studies (including prospective cohort studies), which are discussed in Chapter 17. There is a range of methods for allocating study participants to study groups, which vary from random allocation (= strictly experimental) and a purposeful selection of existing groups, to allocation to groups as preferred by participants (= strictly observational). There is more potential for confounding in observational studies compared to experimental studies, so that estimates of intervention effects should not be made or should be interpreted carefully (Deeks *et al.* 2003). However, in their favour, the non-intrusive character of observational studies may enhance their validity, because study participants behave more naturally compared to those in experimental evaluations.

In this chapter we distinguish broadly between descriptive and comparative evaluations (*Table 18.1*). While there may be overlaps between these two groups it is possible to characterise them as follows.

In *descriptive evaluations*, the main aim is to monitor and document change on relevant indicators for performance in a specific clinical setting. Documentation of and the analysis of factors perceived to be associated with change are components of many of these studies. Descriptive evaluations usually include all healthcare providers in the project and the measurements are relatively simple. These studies cannot determine 'cause and effect' relationships and their generalisability is often limited; the value of these studies lies in checking progress on the defined targets for improvement and in informing local decisions on smaller programmes.

Comparative evaluations, however, monitor and document the impact of implementation strategies and use comparisons between different subjects or settings to identify potential determinants of change. In many cases, a sample of healthcare providers is sufficient for generalisable results. The measurements tend to be more complex, because a wider range of determinants is included.

AUDIT AND MONITORING STUDIES

Audit and monitoring studies are relatively quick and low-cost evaluations that can help healthcare professionals and managers to develop strategies for improvement (Ovretveit and Gustafson 2002). They are typified as observational studies to document performance before, during and after an implementation intervention

Table 18.1 Observational evaluations of implementation strategies

	Descriptive evaluations	Comparative evaluations
Objectives	Document changes, identify which factors are perceived to be associated with changes	Document impact, suggest factors associated with change
Study population	All healthcare providers	Sample of healthcare providers
Designs	Audit and monitoring studies Developmental studies Descriptive case studies	Comparative case studies Impact evaluations Community intervention studies
Implementation strategies	Observed in practice	Observed in practice
Measurements	Relatively simple	More complex
Analysis	Mainly descriptive statistics	Comparative statistics
Causal effects	Cannot be determined because confounders are not controlled	Cannot be determined, but comparisons may suggest possible causal mechanisms
Generalisability	Limited, may not be sought	May provide generalisable descriptive information

(*Box 18.2*). If the measurements are made before and after the intervention, the evaluation may be similar to an (uncontrolled) before-and-after study (see Chapter 17), but the researcher has little or no control over the study conditions. Performance on specified aspects of the structure, process or outcomes of healthcare is measured and feedback of the findings may be provided to professionals, managers or policy makers. In quality improvement projects, such evaluation is an integral part of the process, linked as it is to an explicit assessment of the progress and effect of implementing planned changes in practice (*Box 18.3*). Audit studies have an inherent cyclical element to them, which helps to close the loop of the quality improvement cycle, an area in which many projects have been shown to fail in the past (Johnston *et al.* 2000; Eccles *et al.* 1996). They identify areas in which improvements have been achieved and those for which further interventions are needed.

The sample taken in these evaluations usually comprises all healthcare providers in a project, but in some cases it comprises a sample of all cases, in which case the sample is best selected randomly out of the total population. Indicators for measurement and assessment should be valid, reliable, feasible and enhance improvement. Where possible, validated indicators should be used (see Chapter 16). The analysis is mainly descriptive, although statistics can be used to compare subgroups and differences between measurement points (Russell and Russell 1990). Statistical procedures, such as confidence intervals or reliability analysis, can help to assess the accuracy of the measures, providing the required assumptions of these procedures are met. Time-series analysis may be used if data have been collected at sufficient points in time and have appropriate statistical properties (see Chapter 17).

If an audit study includes a range of measurements over time, 'statistical process control' may be used to monitor change (Benneyan *et al.* 2003). This statistical technique quantifies whether variation between measurement moments is caused by chance ('random variation') or potentially caused by interventions or specific events. The technique is particularly useful if relevant

---

Box 18.2   Audit on aspirin use for secondary prophylaxis of myocardial infarction (Parr *et al.* 1999)

In one district in north-east England, 52% of all patients admitted with suspected myocardial infarction during a 6 month period received 300 mg of aspirin, either from their general practitioner (GP) prior to admission or in the hospital on admission.

A high-profile publicity campaign was aimed at professionals and patients, 12 months after which physicians' performance had changed from 25% to 53% of patients admitted to hospitals being prescribed aspirin prior to admission.

After a definite myocardial infarction, 78% of patients were discharged taking 75 mg of aspirin, with no valid reason for omission in 7% of patients; 6 months after discharge 72% of patients were still taking aspirin, and 12 months later 90% of discharged patients were taking aspirin. Data for general practice prescribing showed a marked increase in prescribing 75 mg aspirin during the period.

Box 18.3   Evaluation of breakthrough collaboratives in hospitals

'Breakthrough' is a multifaceted strategy to achieve substantial improvements in the organisation and delivery of healthcare. It was originally developed by Berwick and colleagues in the USA and then spread throughout the world. The method brings together teams from a number of healthcare organisations to work on quality problems for which specific targets are set. A structured procedure is used, which includes repeated cycles of conferences, local improvement activities and performance feedback. The method aims to promote the implementation of research evidence and best practice.

The Breakthrough method was used to improve intensive care and emergency care in ten hospitals (18 teams) in the Netherlands. Support, materials and web-based communication was provided by the Quality Institute for Healthcare (CBO).

Specific targets were formulated by the teams, such as '40% reduction of artificial respiration time', 'reduction of inappropriate antibiotics use' and '90% reduction of pressure ulcer incidence rate'. Registration systems were selected or specially designed to assess hospital performance related to these targets and differences over time were tested statistically where possible (by 'statistical process control'). So, evaluation of change was integrated in the method, but comparison across hospitals would have been possible only if similar indicators had been used, which was not the case. A wide range of improvements was found regarding the targets, for example, a reduction of inappropriate hospital days from 16.5 to 5.0% in one project and a reduction of inappropriate use of antibiotics from 30 to 8%.

data are collected routinely, such as laboratory test turn-around time, surgical site infections or appointment times (Benneyan *et al*. 2003). Non-random variation, such as increased number of infections, may be associated with specific events, such as the arrival of a new surgical team (*Box 18.4*). However, such associations cannot be interpreted causally ('the new surgical team causes more infections') because the natural history is unknown (the number of infections may have increased because patients are not as healthy as before)

DEVELOPMENTAL STUDIES

An evaluation may also aim to guide and support ongoing implementation projects through feedback and advice to the project team. One such type of evaluation is 'action research', which is broadly defined as an approach to research that involves the participants actively and that has an explicit focus on promoting and facilitating change (Waterman *et al*. 2001). Within an

implementation project, developmental research may form part of a flexible intervention programme, such as a tailored educational approach to implement clinical guidelines, enabling actions to be planned on the basis of increasing insight into barriers for change (Harvey and Wensing 2003; *Box 18.5*). Community development to achieve public health objectives can also be included within this category (El Ansari *et al*. 2001). Developmental approaches to evaluation may be particularly useful within the context of organisational learning (Argyris 1992) and learning by professionals (Schon 1988). The study population comprises one project or a defined set of projects, and generalisation is not sought. Measurements should be feasible and enhance improvement, while also being as valid and reliable as possible. Similar to case studies, data can be collected in many different ways, including interviews, brainstorming, field visits, case studies and surveys. The type of knowledge generated by developmental approaches is seen to be practical and propositional, and the focus

Box 18.4 Statistical monitoring of adverse events (Spiegelhalter *et al*. 2003)

Cumulative monitoring of adverse events can be used to examine trends in quality and outcomes of healthcare services, but the challenge is to distinguish 'real' trends from random variation. For this purpose several statistical methods can be used.

A retrospective study tested one method, the classic sequential probability ratio test, which was developed in World War II. Different data sets were analysed, including the annual mortality rates for open-heart surgery on children under 1 year of age of the Bristol Royal Infirmary Inquiry (1985–1995) and the mortality rates for male and female patients aged 65 years or over in the practice list (1977–1998) of Dr Harold Shipman.

Comparative data that referred to similar sites were sought for statistical testing. The analysis of the Bristol case suggested that mortality had been higher than comparative data since 1991 ($p < 0.001$) or 1994 ($p < 0.001$), depending on the comparative data used. The analysis of the Shipman case suggested that mortality in women had been higher than national data since 1997 ($p < 0.000001$); the low p-value is chosen because the national data are based on 27,000 doctors. In both cases, statistical analysis of cumulative data on mortality could have detected the divergent performance earlier than actually happened.

Box 18.5 Wound management in community nursing (Selim *et al*. 2001)

The project was set up to establish and encourage an improved approach to wound management in a community nursing organisation in South Australia. Within this organisation about 50% of client visits were related to wound care, and hence the importance of promoting best practice in this area of care. Following an initial survey of wound-management practices, participatory action-research groups were established to address some of the issues identified.

Each group followed an action–research approach, with its three phases of planning, action and evaluation being undertaken as part of a cyclical process. One group chose to focus specifically on evidence-based practice related to the care of leg ulcers. This involved comparing the use of tap-water cleansing to an aseptic technique with sterile saline solution.

As part of the planning phase, a review of the literature was undertaken, which suggested that there was not enough evidence to conclude that tap-water cleansing was ineffective. Moving on to the action phase of the research cycle, the group examined the current cleansing practices used by their colleagues and reasons underpinning their chosen approach. This highlighted concerns around infection that influenced the choice of aseptic technique, so the group ran educational sessions to disseminate the research evidence on cleansing wounds. A repeat survey subsequently carried out showed an increase in the use of the clean tap-water technique. As a spin-off from the action–research, a randomised controlled trial was subsequently set up to compare the use of warmed sterile saline with warm tap water for cleansing chronic leg ulcers.

is on generating and refining theory through inductive processes within repeated cycles of research (Harvey and Wensing 2003). The generalisability of the knowledge generated may be limited to associations between different variables within the project under study.

DESCRIPTIVE CASE STUDIES

Case studies (case series) aim to provide detailed insight into specific projects in terms of the interventions and activities, the views of professionals, patients and other stakeholders, changes in process of healthcare delivery and the contextual factors that may have influenced the change. In methodology books, case studies are qualified as the lowest level of evidence in terms of generating generalisable results (Deeks *et al.* 2003). However, they can be particularly helpful for understanding the internal dynamics of a change process (or absence of change) and the influence of organisational, cultural and financial factors on this process. The focus is often on 'why' questions, such as why and under what conditions healthcare professionals decide to adopt an innovation or change in their clinical practice (*Box 18.6*). Descriptive case studies simply describe the programme as implemented, so that others can understand what was done and can draw lessons from the experiences.

Case studies are characterised by a large number of relevant variables compared to the number of cases. Ideally, cases are selected so that sufficient variation is achieved on relevant factors, but in reality a representative selection of cases is not always possible. Cases can be defined at different levels, such as a quality improvement project in a specific practice, a regional collaboration in the field of occupational health or a national programme to enhance mental healthcare. It

is unclear how the level of aggregation might affect the case study.

The case study approach is not characterised by any one specific method of data collection. Instead, a key feature is the use of data from a range of sources, data that are often collected using both quantitative (e.g. interviews with key informants, written surveys among stakeholders, analysis of documents) and qualitative (e.g. direct observation and audit studies that are a component of the programme) methods. Combining data from multiple sources regarding specific variables, called 'triangulation', is recommended as it increases the validity of the conclusions. It may, however, be expensive or impossible to achieve triangulation for all the variables studied. Descriptive case studies usually result in narrative reports, which should provide a balanced view on the case. Qualitative methods can be used to strengthen the validity, such as asking different researchers to write reports and having reports checked by key individuals involved in the cases.

COMPARATIVE CASE STUDIES

Comparative (or multiple) case studies aim to identify potential determinants of change through systematic comparisons between a number of similar cases (Yin 1989). Comparative case studies provide information that is more generalisable than descriptive case studies. Comparative case studies should be based on *a priori* defined hypotheses, but these should allow for the identification of potential barriers to change that were not identified beforehand (*Box 18.7*). The analysis is a systematic comparison of cases with respect to their scores on indicators for success and scores on potential determinants. Although the number of cases

---

Box 18.6 Implementation of a hospital information system (Littlejohns *et al.* 2003)

In Limpopo Province, South Africa, a large programme was set up to implement an information system in the 42 hospitals in this region. The overall goal was to improve the efficiency and effectiveness of health and welfare services through a computer system for clinical, administrative and monitoring purposes. A study was set up to evaluate the implementation as well as the benefits and costs. This study was designed as a randomised trial, but implementation of the information system failed, so a case study was performed, using qualitative and quantitative methods.

A large number of reasons for the failure were identified, including:

- Staff education focused too much on 'how' the system worked rather than on 'why' it should be used;
- Use of the system interfered with healthcare interactions and with patients' complex pathways through the healthcare system;
- Teams that oversaw the process were rarely in post for the whole period;
- There was reluctance to stop throwing good money after bad.

The authors suggest that these reasons were similar to those in other computer projects in other countries and that these lessons should be learnt to avoid further waste of scarce health resources.

Box 18.7 Comparative case study of physical exercise programmes (Laurant *et al.* 2003)

Physical exercise improves the health status of adults, including older adults, but many adults hardly take any physical exercise. A range of programmes in the Netherlands, focusing on walking, dancing, aerobics, etc., aim to encourage older adults to become physically active for at least 30 minutes per day on at least 5 days a week. The clinical effectiveness of many of these programmes has been proved, so the focus is on effective implementation in terms of setting up programmes and the optimal participation of older adults in these programmes.

A multiple case study project was undertaken to evaluate the implementation of ten physical exercise programmes. This study took two approaches. Firstly, structured descriptions of the programmes were produced. These showed, for instance, that a variety of methods were used to improve participation in the programmes, such as personal contact in the case of absence, obligatory indication of absence and the provision of drinks to enhance social interaction. Furthermore, project leaders were asked to describe the most important barriers and facilitators to the success of the programme. Many mentioned,

for example, problems in convincing municipalities and welfare organisations of the relevance of the programme. These data were used to provide structured descriptions of the cases.

Secondly, the study team proposed around 25 hypotheses about factors that might influence the success of implementation. For instance, it was hypothesised that the programme would be more successful if there was a local tradition of collaboration between different organisations and if the exercise sessions were three times a week rather than five. Structured questionnaires were distributed to individuals involved in organising or delivering the programmes to collect data on the variables determined by the hypotheses. Where possible, information on the success of implementation was derived from evaluations within the projects. These data were used to test the predefined hypotheses.

The results indicated that successful implementation of physical exercise programmes was associated with:

- Larger investment in the programme by organisations;
- Prevailing view that audit and evaluation were relevant;
- Local tradition of innovation in healthcare services.

is usually much lower than the number of variables, defining hypotheses *a priori* provides some protection against associations found by chance. Ideally, cases are sampled purposively so that the desired variety of cases is identified. In reality, cases are often defined by a programme or setting, so that purposive sampling is often not possible. Statistics are usually not used in the analysis of the cases, but statistics can be used in the quantitative elements that contribute to the case study.

IMPACT EVALUATIONS

If improvement strategies are targeted at a larger population in a region or country, it may be impossible to identify a relevant comparison group. In this situation,

a range of observational designs can be used to describe the impact of a strategy on the relevant outcomes. These include cross-sectional studies and studies that measure the exposure of study participants to interventions retrospectively, such as case-control studies, and retrospective and historical cohort studies (Deeks *et al.* 2003). All these studies examine variations across individual practitioners, patients, practices and hospitals (*Box 18.8*). For instance, not all practitioners may invite outreach visitors to their primary care practice to improve their prevention of cardiovascular diseases. This natural variation can be used to explore the relevance of specific determinants for change (for instance, using a case-control design) – outcomes for practitioners who received several outreach visits can be compared with those for practitioners who received only a few visits.

Box 18.8 Screening for cervical cancer (Hermens *et al.* 2000)

Different approaches are used to invite women for cervical screening– a community-based approach (invitations based on population register by local authority), an approach based on the general practice (invitations based on general practice register by general practices) and a combined approach. The impact of these three different organisational approaches was examined in a cross-sectional study. A total of 122 general practices with a computerised sex-aged register were selected; approximately 40 practices were linked with each approach. Data on attendance of women after invitations for

cervical screening were collected from the general practices. The study showed that for younger women (<45 years) the total attendance rates were highest in practices using the approach based on general practices, while for older women the rates were highest for both the general practice approach and the combined approach. The results were similar for the coverage and control rates. This resulted in a conclusion that a cervical screening approach based on general practices appeared to be necessary for the optimal impact of cervical cancer screening.

These impact evaluations usually comprise a large number of cases and, possibly, also a wide range of variables measured. Multivariate analysis techniques, such as regression analysis, are used to quantify the relationship between specific factors or differences between subgroups (*Box 18.9*). However, this evaluation design cannot assess the effectiveness of the improvement strategies reliably, as any differential uptake may be the result of a number of factors, such as self-selection by participants. Self-selection could suggest either a high apparent effectiveness of an intervention (for instance, if mainly practitioners with poor performance and therefore considerable room for improvement have high uptake) or a low apparent effectiveness (for instance, if mainly motivated practitioners with little room for improvement have high uptake). In addition, if a large number of statistical comparisons are performed it is important to recognise that some associations will be statistically significant by chance alone. Nevertheless, this type of evaluation can provide important insights into the impact of a strategy and the influence of specific factors in determining its success or failure.

COMMUNITY INTERVENTION STUDIES

If improvement programmes are targeted at larger communities, it may be possible to identify different communities and to compare relevant outcomes between these communities. This design has been called a community intervention study and has been used mainly to evaluate public health interventions (Murray 1995). A hospital or region in which a quality improvement programme is applied could be considered a community and evaluated within this design. If there are a number of communities within a population this may be regarded as a cluster trial with very large clusters. However, unless randomisation has been possible it is essentially an observational design – the researcher usually has little control over the study conditions.

If randomisation is possible, all the issues related to trials (see Chapter 17) are also relevant to this study design. However, the number of communities is usually small compared to most implementation trials and therefore power is limited – power can be enhanced by large numbers of subjects per community, but only to a certain extent (see, for an example, *Box 9.1* in Chapter 9). A consequence is that the power of the study to detect differences between groups should be based largely on the accuracy of measurements. In many studies, only a description of the changes within communities is valid. Given the sorts of interventions that are evaluated using this design, the time scale of the causal chain between intervention and health outcomes (for instance, cardiovascular mortality) is often long, so that intermediate outcomes may be more appropriate indicators for the effects of the intervention (Nutbeam 1997).

CONCLUSIONS

A range of designs for observational evaluations are available to provide insights into the processes of change and the impact of interventions and associated factors. These can be very helpful when evaluating small-scale, single-site quality improvement projects, a number of cases of quality improvement with different targets or outcome measures or large scale (national or regional) implementation programmes. In practice, these studies pose a range of methodological challenges. It is difficult to provide a standardised list of quality criteria, as has been done for trials by the CONSORT criteria, although understanding of the important dimensions of methodological quality is growing (Deeks *et al.* 2003). A danger is that observational evaluations are either all considered as 'poor quality' research or as 'everything is acceptable' research. The better evaluations use adequate sampling techniques, validated measurement instruments, rigorous analysis

---

Box 18.9 Factors associated with success of influenza vaccination (Tacken *et al.* 2002)

Most influenza vaccination programmes are targeted at citizens aged 65 years or older or at those at high-risk. A national campaign to enhance a population-based approach towards influenza vaccination was launched with a fee-for-service for family doctors and software for family practices to support the organisation of this. Practices could undertake supplementary activities, such as arranging specially designated clinics for vaccination, distributing information pamphlets or sending reminders to high-risk patients.

Data from the computerised medical record systems of 48 family practices were used to examine the influence of organisational factors. Of all patients at risk (42,426), 76% were vaccinated. A multilevel regression analysis showed that special clinics for vaccination led to significantly higher vaccination rates in older patients and in those with cardiac problems. Attendance by patients below 65 years of age was associated with the use of special information pamphlets.

methods and adequate reporting. We recommend efforts to elaborate the methodology for these types of evaluations (Deeks *et al.* 2003).

Recommended references

Deeks JJ, Dinnes J, D'Amico R, *et al.* (2003). Evaluating non-randomised intervention studies. *Health Technol Assess.* 7(27): 1–173.

Grol R, Baker R and Moss F (2003). *Quality Improvement Research. Understanding the Science of Change in Healthcare.* London: BMJ Books.

References

El Ansari W, Phillips CJ and Zwi AB (2001). Collaboration and partnerships: Developing the evidence base. *Health Social Care Community* 9:215–227.

Argyris C (1992). *On Organisational Learning.* Cambridge: Blackwell Business.

Benneyan JC, Lloyd RC and Plesk PE (2003). Statistical process control as a tool for research and health care improvement. In: Grol R, Baker R and Moss F (eds). *Quality Improvement Research. Understanding the Science of Change in Healthcare*, pp. 184–202. London: BMJ Books.

Black N (1996). Why we need observational studies to evaluate the effectiveness of health care. *BMJ* 312:1215–1218.

Campbell S, Robinson J, Steiner A, Webb D and Roland MO (2003). Improving the quality of mental health services in primary care: A longitudinal study. EQuiP Conference, Heidelberg, 13–15 November.

Deeks JJ, Dinnes J, D'Amico R, *et al.* (2003). Evaluating non-randomised intervention studies. *Health Technol Assess.* 7(27):1–173.

Eccles M, Deverill M, McColl E and Richardson H (1996). A national survey of audit activity across the primary–secondary care interface. *Qual Health Care* 5:193–200.

Harvey G and Wensing M (2003). Methods for evaluation of small-scale improvement projects. *Qual Saf Health Care* 12:210–214.

Hermens PMG, Tacken MAJB, Hulscher MEJL, Braspenning JCC and Grol RPTM (2000). Attendance to cervical cancer screening in general practices in the Netherlands. *Prev Med.* 31:35–42.

Hulscher MEJL, Van Drenth BB, Van der Wouden JC, Mokkink HGA, Van Weel C and Grol RPTM (1997).

Changing preventive practice: A controlled trial on the effects of outreach visits to organize prevention of cardio-vascular disease. *Qual Health Care* 6:19–24.

Johnston G, Crombie IK, Alder, *et al.* (2000). Reviewing audit: Barriers and facilitating factors for effective clinical audit. *Qual Health Care* 9:23–36.

Laurant M, Harmsen M and Wensing M (2003). *Implementatie van Beweegprogramma's voor Ouderen. Belemmerende en Bevorderende Factoren voor Succesvolle Implementatie [Implementation of Exercise Programmes for the Elderly. Barriers to and Incentives for Successful Implementation].* WOK: Nijmegen.

Littlejohns P, Wyatt JC and Garvican L (2003). Evaluating computerised health information systems: Hard lessons still to be learnt. *BMJ* 326:860–863.

Murray DM (1995). Design and analysis of community trials: Lessons from the Minnesota Heart Health Program. *Am J Epidemiol.* 142:569–575.

Nutbeam D (1997). *Evaluating Health Promotion: Progress, Problems and Solutions.* Geneva: World Health Organisation.

Ovretveit J and Gustafson D (2002). Evaluation of quality improvement programmes. *Qual Saf Health Care* 11:270–275.

Parr JH, Bradshaw C, Broderick W, *et al.* (1999). Improving the use of aspirin in myocardial infarction: A district strategy. *Br J Clin Gov.* 4:24–7.

Russell IT and Russell D (1990). Statistical issues in medical audit. In: Marinker M (ed). *Medical Audit and General Practice*, pp. 168–184. London: MSD Foundation.

Schon DA (1988). *Educating the Reflective Practitioner.* London: Jossey Brass.

Selim P, Bashford C and Grossman C (2001). Evidence-based practice: Tap water cleansing of leg ulcers in the community. *J Clin Nurs.* 10:372–379.

Spiegelhalter D, Grigg O, Kinsman R and Treasure T (2003). Risk-adjusted sequential probability ratio tests: Applications to Bristol, Shipman and adult cardiac surgery. *Int J Qual Health Care* 15:7–13.

Tacken M, Braspenning J, Spreeuwenberg P, *et al.* (2002). Patient characteristics determine differences in the influenza vaccination rate more so than practice features. *Prev Med.* 35:401–406.

Waterman H, Tillen D, Dickson R, *et al.* (2001). Action research: A systematic review and guidance for assessment. *Health Technol Assess.* 5:111–157.

Yin RK (1989). *Case Study Research: Design and Methods.* London: Sage.

Chapter 19

Process evaluation of change interventions

Marlies Hulscher, Miranda Laurant and Richard Grol

KEY MESSAGES

- To understand why some change interventions successfully bring about improvement while others fail to change practice, it is necessary to look into the 'black box' of interventions and study the determinants of success or failure.
- Process evaluation aims to describe the implementation of change itself, the actual exposure to the intervention and the experiences of the people involved. It is an important component in the development and understanding of potentially successful implementation interventions.
- In small-scale improvement projects, process evaluation plays a central role by providing information on the feasibility and applicability of introducing the intervention. This may result in revision of the implementation activities in the intervention.
- In experimental implementation studies or large-scale implementation programmes, process evaluation provides information that can help to explain any heterogeneity of effects.
- In the framework described in this chapter, attention is paid to the features of the target group, the features of the implementers or change agents, the frequency and intensity of intervention activities and the features of the information imparted. All of these features might influence the success of the implementation activities in question.

Box 19.1 Explaining effect, or lack of it, in implementation (Szczepura *et al.* 1994; Nattinger *et al.* 1989)

Nattinger *et al.* (1989) showed that feedback led to significant improvements in professional care, whereas Szczepura *et al.* (1994) concluded that feedback failed to change professional practice. However, careful analysis of the feedback applied in these two studies showed that the implementation activities had different characters.

In Szczepura's study, physicians in the intervention group received information about the care they had provided at three time points – at the start, after 12 months and after 24 months. This information covered cervical cancer screening, developmental screening and/or immunisation in children and the determination of risk factors in individuals aged 35–64 years, such as blood pressure, alcohol consumption, smoking and body weight. Doctors in the so-called graphic feedback group received a profile that contained, for each patient group, the minimum, maximum, median and 20th and 80th percentile values; each practice's own scores were marked clearly within each profile. The physicians in the control group received feedback in tabular form (i.e. an overview of their own values, accompanied by the minimum and maximum

scores in the total group). Neither intervention was effective. On receipt of the comparative feedback information, all practitioners were asked to rate the feedback in terms of its acceptability and intelligibility and whether or not regular feedback in this form was helpful to the practice. No differences regarding these items were reported. No information was provided by the authors on actual exposure of the target population to the intervention (e.g. how many actually read the feedback report).

Nattinger's study was performed over a period of 6 months. General internists received monthly overviews of the percentage of patients who had been treated in accordance with a mammography guideline. The first 3 months covered only the individual management of the internist in question, whereas the second 3 months covered individual management compared to the management of an anonymous group of colleagues presented as a histogram. This feedback was effective. The authors stated that they were unable to say how many physicians had actually read their feedback. Thus, no information was provided on actual exposure or the on experience of those involved.

INTRODUCTION

A wide variety of interventions can be used to change healthcare (see Section IV). Systematic reviews show that most interventions are effective in some settings, but not in others (Anonymous 1999; Bero *et al.* 1998; Grol 1997). Studies on effective intervention programmes have shown varying and often only modest improvements in healthcare performance. To understand in more detail why some interventions are successful while others fail to change practice, it is necessary to gain insight into the 'black box' of change interventions. Studying the black box of (un)successful interventions implies that we can no longer confine ourselves to describing interventions in global terms, for example as 'feedback', 'reminders' or 'a combination of a continuing medical education (CME) seminar, free office materials and one office visit by a staff member'. The examples in *Box 19.1* illustrates how two studies on apparently the same change intervention (feedback) reached different conclusions on the effectiveness of the method. The activities carried out as part of the intervention, the actual exposure of participants to these activities, and their experience of these activities may have influenced the final result (success or failure). Process evaluation illuminates the mechanisms and processes responsible for the result and their variation within target groups.

This chapter starts with a description of the different questions process evaluation can answer. It then explores the purpose and value of process evaluation and provides some examples. As in the previous chapters, we distinguish between change interventions at three stages of development – pilot studies or small-scale improvement projects, experimental studies and large-scale programmes. In addition, we address the issue of what data should be collected while performing a process evaluation.

PROCESS EVALUATION

Process evaluation is an important tool aimed at (meticulously) describing the intervention itself, the actual exposure to this intervention and the experience of the people exposed (the participants; see *Box 19.2*). This information is not only crucial to understand the success – or lack of it – of interventions, but also to provide basic data for an economic evaluation of the improvement activities. Although the latter is beyond the scope of this chapter, it enables estimates to be made of the cost in terms of time and / or money (see Chapter 20).

PURPOSE AND VALUE OF PROCESS EVALUATION

A process evaluation serves a number of different, but related, purposes:

- A description of the 'intervention as planned' acts as a blueprint to help change agents (and researchers) to apply the intervention as intended in a uniform way within the target population;
- A description of the 'intervention as performed' is important to enable others to replicate the intervention – in addition, a detailed description of the 'intervention as performed' facilitates future comparisons between studies and (meta-) analyses on crucial features of effective interventions;
- To establish the actual exposure of individuals to the intervention by checking whether the intervention worked as planned – researchers or evaluators can use the information to explain the success or lack of effect, particularly when they do not want to change the intervention during the course of a study;
- To gain detailed insight into the experiences of those involved in the intervention to revise the intervention in question – this information on influencing factors as experienced by participants can be used to improve the intervention either during its application (the developmental approach) or afterwards (the experimental approach).

Process evaluation can be applied to change interventions at any stage of their development. We dis-

---

Box 19.2 Process evaluation

Process evaluation can be used:

To describe the intervention – for example:
- What was the exact nature of the intervention?
- What material investments, time investments, etc., were required?

To check the actual exposure to the intervention – for example:
- Was the intervention implemented according to plan?
- Was the target population actually exposed to the intervention as planned?

To describe the experience of those exposed to the intervention –for example:
- How did the target group experience the intervention and the changes?
- What problems arose while implementing the changes?

tinguish between interventions at three stages of development:

■ Pilot studies or small-scale improvement projects;
■ Experimental studies;
■ Large-scale programmes.

Process evaluation plays a different role in each case.

Pilot studies and small-scale improvement projects

An evaluation of the effects of a newly developed change intervention being tested in a pilot study, or used within a small-scale improvement project, gives an estimate of the degree of change. Process evaluation can provide answers to questions on the feasibility and applicability of introducing the intervention; such answers might prompt revision of the improvement activities in the intervention. Thus, researchers and implementers of this type of change intervention can use process information to investigate whether they are on the right track or whether their approach needs adjustment (see the example in *Box 19.3*).

Experimental studies

In an experimental study on the effectiveness of a specific change intervention, the central issue is to test the effectiveness of the method in standardised circumstances. In this case, process evaluation yields information that can help to explain the effects. Process evaluation is important to check whether the planned improvement activities have, indeed, been executed in a uniform way and whether the target population has actually been exposed to these activities as planned. Researchers and implementers of these interventions can use process information to detect gaps in exposure to the intervention that might be responsible for failure or the disappointing outcome of an intervention. Another use for process evaluation in such studies is to determine how the participants experienced the activities – whether they encountered any bottlenecks while implementing the changes and whether they were satisfied with the intervention method. Together with data on the actual use of the intervention, this can explain why interventions do, or do not, work (see the examples in *Boxes 19.4* and *19.5*).

Large-scale implementation programmes

In large-scale programmes for the implementation of changes in patient care, analyses of the effects show the extent to which the goals of the intervention have been achieved, whereas process evaluation provides information about the 'intervention as performed' and about exposure to and experience with this intervention. For situations in which a control group is not available, the results of process evaluations can provide some information about the relationship between

---

Box 19.3 Intervention to improve the detection of child abuse in an emergency department (Benger and Pearce 2002)

To increase awareness of child abuse in busy emergency departments, a reminder flowchart was introduced in a suburban teaching hospital that saw about 4000 injured preschool children per year. Nurses were asked to insert a reminder flowchart sticker to assess intentional injury into the notes of all children aged 0–5 years who attended the department with any injury and to record the results of checking the child protection register. The reminder flowchart included five most commonly cited factors, like 'On examination, does the child have any unexplained injuries' or 'Is the child's behaviour and interaction appropriate?'. Doctors who assessed the patient were responsible for completing the flowchart. After an initial audit (1000 consecutive injured preschool children who attended the emergency department), the flowchart sticker was introduced for 4 weeks before the second audit was performed (1000 consecutive children).

After the introduction of the flowchart, a much greater proportion of emergency department notes recorded consideration of intentional injury than was found in the first audit (711/1000 versus 16/1000). However, the second audit showed that a flowchart sticker was included in 717 (71.7%) of eligible attendance notes. The sticker was completed in all but four cases, giving a compliance of 99.4%. Even in the 283 notes that had not had the flowchart inserted, a greater proportion of notes recorded consideration of intentional injury (17/283 versus 16/1000). The latter, the authors concluded, was probably because of heightened awareness in the department.

The authors indicated that they were disappointed that the flowchart was included in only 71.7% of the cases, but concluded that since it had to be manually added to the notes, it was inevitably forgotten at times. Automation of the process would improve inclusion rates.

Box 19.4 The effect of computerising guidelines (Rousseau *et al.* 2003; Eccles *et al.* 2002)

The study evaluated the use of a computerised decision support system (CDSS) to implement evidence-based clinical guidelines for the management of adult patients with asthma or angina seen in 60 general practices in northern England. The randomised controlled trial evaluation showed that there were no significant effects of CDSS on consultation rates, process of care measures (including prescribing) or any quality-of-life domain for either condition.

A usage log across all practices showed that levels of use of the CDSS were low. Interviews conducted with physicians in five participating practices provided insights into why. Interviewees were largely enthusiastic about the benefits of computing for general practice and were optimistic about the potential for computers to present guidelines in a manageable format. However, the CDSS was felt by most practitioners to be difficult to use and unhelpful clinically. They believed that they were already familiar with the content of the guidelines, although they did not always follow recommendations for reasons that included limitations of the guidelines, patient preferences, lack of incentives and perceived structural barriers.

The investigators concluded that even if it is possible to solve the technical hardware and software problems of producing a system that fully supports chronic disease management, there remains the challenge of integrating CDSS into clinical encounters in which busy practitioners manage patients with complex, multiple conditions.

the intervention and the changes achieved (see Chapters 17 and 18 and the example in Box 19.6).

WHAT TO MEASURE?

If a process evaluation is going to be performed, those who conduct it (researchers and change agents) are faced with the following questions, depending on the purpose of their evaluation:

■ *If the aim of the process evaluation is to describe the intervention*, what 'key features' of the intervention should be included in the description (before and/or after intervention), because they might cause or influence the effect of the intervention? This is the

Box 19.5 Improving the prevention of cardiovascular disease (Hulscher *et al.* 1998)

The study investigated the effectiveness of and experience with an, at that time, innovative method of introducing recommended best practices for the organisation of preventive activities in primary care. Over a period of 18 months, trained outreach visitors spent time solving problems in the organisation of prevention in practice. The study showed that best practices in organising prevention of cardiovascular disease in primary care could be introduced effectively (a controlled study). To evaluate the scope and limitations of the change intervention, process information was collected at the end of the project from all the participants at the intervention practices (68 doctors and 83 practice assistants at 33 practices). Information was gathered on actual exposure to the intervention, experience with the intervention in general and experience with the outreach visitors, results of the intervention regarding the number of newly detected patients at risk and the influence of the intervention on the routines of the doctors and practice assistants.

During 18 months of intervention the practices were visited between 13 and 59 times [mean 25, standard deviation (SD) nine visits]. The mean duration of a visit was 73 minutes (SD 43) with a minimum of 0 minutes (delivering materials only) and a maximum of almost 5 hours. Practices spent, on average, 45% of the visit hours on training and 52% on conferring. The number of team members with whom the outreach visitors met ranged from one to 14. In 63% of the consultations the outreach visitor met with practice assistants only, in 7% she met with the physician only and in 30% of the cases she met both practice assistants and doctors.

In 27 of the practices, change occurred for at least three of the recommended best practices, leading to a mean final adherence score of eight (minimum seven, maximum nine). These practices were visited on average 25 times for almost 31 hours. In five practices no or a very small change was shown, leading to a mean final adherence score of four. In these practices the average number of visits (20) and the total duration of the visits (19 hours) were below the group average.

The majority of physicians and practice assistants had a positive opinion of the intervention. They were satisfied about the outreach visits, but the practice assistants experienced extra workload because of the intervention. Practice assistants expressed more complaints about the paperwork involved in the project than the physicians, but they mentioned fewer patient barriers. Relationships were found between the experience of the participants and the degree to which the practice had changed – more positive experiences of the participants about the change intervention in general and more newly detected patients than expected were related to more change in recommended best practices for the organisation of preventive activities.

Box 19.6 Cervical cancer screening (Hermens *et al.* 2001)

In a national prevention programme physicians and practice assistants were exposed, over a period of 2.5 years, to a comprehensive strategy to introduce national guidelines for cervical cancer screening. The strategy comprised, on a national level, formulating and distributing guidelines, supplying educational materials and a software programme, and providing financial support. On a regional level, agreements were made between the relevant parties (general practice, municipal health services, comprehensive cancer centres and pathology laboratories) and CME meetings were organised for physicians and practice assistants. On a local level, trained outreach visitors called at practices and helped them to improve the organisation of preventive services and use the software. The evaluation (in a random, one-in-three, sample of 988 practices) showed considerable improvements at the practices – after intervention the adherence to nine out of the ten key indicators had improved.

Information on actual exposure to programme elements was collected by postal questionnaire after the intervention. Almost all practices in the study population (94%) had been informed about the national prevention programme. For practices that had received contact with an outreach visitor through a practice visit (40%), the median number of practice visits was two (range 1–13). The software programme to select eligible women was used by 474 practices (48%), either in full or in part.

Crucial elements for the successful implementation of the guidelines were:

■ Making use of the software programme [odds ratio (OR) 1.85–10.2 for nine indicators];
■ Having received two or more outreach visits (OR 1.46–2.35 for six indicators);
■ Practice assistants having attended the CME meeting (OR 1.37–1.90 for four indicators).

CME meetings for doctors were not related to change.

main question for those interested in developing a blueprint of the intervention to:

* Support uniform performance of the intervention;
* Enable replication of the intervention;
* Facilitate comparisons and meta-analysis of such change interventions.

■ *If the aim of the process evaluation is to check whether the participants were exposed as planned,* what features of the change intervention are important to measure (or monitor) while checking whether the participants were exposed as planned? This is the main question for those interested in:

* Adapting the intervention during its course;
* Explaining success or lack of success after the intervention.

■ *If the aim of the process evaluation is to describe the experience of those involved,* what are 'crucial success and fail factors' as experienced by those exposed that might cause or influence the effect of the intervention? This is the main question for people interested in revising the intervention in question.

To provide practical guidance to researchers and implementers of change interventions, we present a framework for process evaluation that can be used as a starting point to answer all three types of question.

What to measure – a framework

On the basis of several theories that underlie different approaches to changing clinical practice (Ajzen 1991;

Bandura 1986; McGuire 1985; Rogers 1983; Festinger 1954) we developed a framework that contains features of change interventions that might influence their success or failure (*Box 19.7*). We also used the checklist developed by the Cochrane Effective Practice and Organisation of Care Review Group (EPOC 1998) to guide reviewers when extracting relevant information from original studies. In addition, we used a number of reviews on the effectiveness of various interventions (Bero *et al.* 1998) and explored the literature on process and programme evaluation (Ovretveit 2000; Rossi *et al.* 1999; Swanborn 1999; Fink 1993; Rossi and Freeman 1993; Herman *et al.* 1987; King *et al.* 1987).

The resulting framework was tested on a convenience sample of 29 published studies that had used different interventions aimed at the implementation of change in practice (Laurant *et al.* 1999). Many features of the intervention were not described adequately in the publications or were not described at all, but, when approached, most authors were able to provide further information. The framework was revised based on the results of this pilot study.

In the framework (*Box 19.7*), attention is paid to features of the target group, features of the implementers or change agents, the frequency and intensity of intervention activities and the features of the information imparted. The left-hand column gives a general description of the feature of an intervention that needs to be described in more detail in the right-hand column.

Box 19.7 Framework for describing the key features of an implementation of change intervention

Background information

This framework pays attention to the features of the target group, the features of the implementers or change agents, the frequency of intervention activities and the features of the information imparted. All of these features might influence the success of the implementation of change intervention in question. The left-hand column below gives a general description of the feature of an intervention that needs to be described in more detail in the right-hand column.

Change interventions are often standardised – beforehand it is decided that each member of the target population will be exposed uniformly to the intervention (no variation is allowed across time or site). If this is not true for any of the features described below, then the 'variation is allowed' box has to be ticked for the feature in question and explanatory information must be provided. If, for example, it is decided

beforehand that each participating team or practice will receive two outreach visits, then item 4.1 below should mention 'two (planned) visits'. If, however, each team or practice may decide for itself whether or not and how many visits it will receive, then this feature of the intervention is not standardised and the item 'variation is allowed' should be ticked. After performing the intervention, the process evaluation should enable the actual number of visits per team to be described – for example, the percentage of the teams that received two practice visits or the mean (standard deviation) number of visits, respectively. Therefore, first of all, it is important to fill in whether the description of the features of the implementation of change intervention concerns a:

- ▪ Description of the intervention **as planned**;
- ▪ Description of the intervention **as performed**.

Relevant features of the intervention	How to elicit the information

1. Global typing of the intervention (see the EPOC checklist in Chapter 8 for more detail)	Describe the type of intervention concerned: *Interventions orientated towards health professionals, e.g.:*
	 a. distribution of educational materials
	 b. patient-mediated interventions
	 etc.
	
	 Organisational interventions, e.g.:
	 a. provider-orientated interventions:
	   – revision of professional roles
	   – etc.
	 b. patient-orientated interventions:
	   – mail order pharmacies
	   – etc.
	 c. structural interventions:
	   – changes to the setting/site of service delivery
	   – etc.
	
	 Financial interventions, e.g.:
	 a. care-provider financial interventions:
	   – fee for service
	   – etc.
	 b. patient financial interventions:
	   – co-payment
	 etc.
	
	 Regulatory interventions, e.g.:
	 a. management of patient complaints
	 etc.

If multiple options are mentioned above, the features of each of the options must be filled in separately	
2. Target group and/or participants *2.1. Professional status and patient categories*	*Describe the professions of the participants or the patient categories that the intervention is aimed at:* ☐ professions (e.g. nurses, internists): .... ☐ patient categories (e.g. diabetics, smokers): .... ☐ other, describe: ....
2.2. Composition of participants	*Describe whether the intervention is aimed at individuals or members of a group:* ☐ individual providers/patients ☐ group(s) of providers/patients ☐ other, describe: .... ☐ variation is allowed (e.g. in some regions the intervention is aimed at individuals, while in other regions groups are aimed at): .... *If the intervention is aimed at group members, describe whether the group is homogeneous or heterogeneous:* ☐ homogeneous group(s) for profession or patient category ☐ heterogeneous group(s) for profession or patient category ☐ other, describe: .... ☐ variation is allowed (e.g. sometimes the intervention is aimed at homogeneous groups, but then heterogeneous groups are aimed at): ....
2.3. Size of the target group	*Describe the total number of groups that the intervention is aimed at:* ☐ not applicable, the intervention is aimed at individuals (see below) ☐ it concerns a total of .... groups

	Describe the size of each group: ☐ not applicable, the intervention is aimed at individuals ☐ for each group, it concerns .... individuals ☐ other, describe: .... ☐ variation is allowed: .... *Describe per profession or per patient category the total number of* *individuals (these may be members of a number of groups) that the* *intervention is aimed at (e.g. 70 internists and 110 diabetic nurses):* ☐ in total it concerns: ....(number)........................(profession) ☐ in total it concerns: ....(number)........................(profession) ☐ in total it concerns: ....(number).................(patient category) ☐ in total it concerns: ....(number).................(patient category)
2.4. *Motivation for participation*	*Describe the motivation behind participation:* ☐ voluntary participation ☐ obligatory participation ☐ financial reward or other incentive for participation ☐ accreditation points by participation ☐ other, describe: .... ☐ variation is allowed: ....
3. 'Implementer' 3.1. *Professional status*	*Describe the professional backgrounds of the implementers, that is any* *individuals who have actual contact with the target group (the* *instructor, the feedback provider, etc.):* .... ☐ other, describe: ....

3.2. *Opinion leaders*	Describe whether the individual who implements the intervention can be considered as an opinion leader for the target group: ☐ yes ☐ no ☐ other, describe: .... ☐ variation is allowed (e.g. not all regions succeeded in engaging opinion leaders): ....
3.3. *Authority*	Describe the authority on whose basis the intervention is implemented: In the participants' eyes, the implementer: ☐ is a representative for the target group ☐ is an expert ☐ has power (to reward or punish) ☐ other, describe: .... ☐ variation is allowed (e.g. some implementers are experts while others are representatives for the target population): ....
4. Frequency 4.1. *Number*	Describe the number of identical intervention activities (e.g. sending feedback reports on four occasions, making five visits to the practice, organising one CME meeting): ☐ not applicable, it concerns a continuous activity ☐ total number of identical intervention activities: .... ☐ other, describe: .... ☐ variation is allowed (e.g. each practice or team may decide for itself whether or not and how many outreach visits it will receive): ....

4.2. *Time intervals*	*Describe the time intervals between the above-mentioned identical intervention activities:*
	☐ not applicable, it concerns only one intervention activity or a continuous activity
	☐ T_0 = starting date = ...
	$T_1 = T_0$ plus .... days/weeks/months/years
	$T_2 = T_1$ plus .... days/weeks/months/years
	$T_3 = T_2$ plus .... days/weeks/months/years
	$T_4 = T_3$ plus .... days/weeks/months/years
	$T_5 = T_4$ plus .... days/weeks/months/years
	$T_6 = T_5$ plus .... days/weeks/months/years
	$T_7 = T_6$ plus .... days/weeks/months/years
	☐ other, describe:
	....
	....
	☐ variation is allowed:
	....
	....
4.3. *Duration*	*Describe the duration of each identical intervention activity at each contact meeting:*
	☐ a specification is not possible – it concerns a continuous activity or activities with a total duration of ....minutes/hours/ days/weeks/months/years
	☐ duration T_0 = ... minutes/hours/days
	duration T_1 = ... minutes/hours/days
	duration T_2 = ... minutes/hours/ days
	duration T_3 = ... minutes/hours/days
	duration T_4 = ... minutes/hours/days
	duration T_5 = ... minutes/hours/days
	duration T_6 = ... minutes/hours/days
	duration T_7 = ... minutes/hours/days
	☐ other, describe:
	....
	....
	☐ variation is allowed:
	....
	....

5. Information about the innovation

  5.1. Type of information about the innovation

Describe the type of information that is given in the intervention about itself (e.g. the actual text of a published guideline, information on certain recommendations or indicators):

....
....
....
....
....

☐ other, describe:

....
....

☐ variation is allowed:

....
....

  5.2. *Presentation form of the information about the innovation*

Describe the presentation form of the information provided:
☐ descriptive
☐ illustrative
☐ graphic
☐ tables
☐ other, describe:

....
....

☐ variation is allowed:

....
....

  5.3. *Medium*

Describe how the information is provided:
☐ verbally
☐ written
☐ automated
☐ other, describe:

....
....

☐ variation is allowed:

....
....

6. Information about performance of target group 6.1. *Type of information about performance*	*Describe the type of information that is given in the intervention about the performance of the target group (e.g. information about individual performance regarding certain patient categories, information about the performance of the total group of participants, information about individual performance as measured with paper cases, information about national reference values, general information about practice variation, etc.):* ☐ not applicable, no information about performance is provided ☐ describe: .... ☐ other, describe: .... ☐ variation is allowed: ....
6.2. *Presentation form of the information about performance*	*Describe the presentation form of the information provided:* ☐ not applicable, no information about performance is provided ☐ descriptive ☐ illustrative ☐ graphic ☐ tables ☐ other, describe: .... ☐ variation is allowed: ....
6.3. *Medium*	*Describe how the information was provided:* ☐ not applicable, no information about performance is provided ☐ verbally ☐ written ☐ automated ☐ other, describe: .... ☐ variation is allowed: ....

| 6.4. *Feasibility of comparing information about performance* | *Describe the feasibility of comparing individual performance to that of others, or to general criteria (guidelines, recommendations, indicators, benchmarks):*
☐ not applicable, no information about performance is provided

Individual performance is compared to:
☐ performance of colleagues
☐ guidelines or recommendations
☐ indicators or benchmarks
☐ other, describe:
....
....

☐ variation is allowed:
....
.... |

HOW TO MEASURE?

Depending on the main question being addressed by the process evaluation, it is possible to take a more developmental approach (qualitative and inductive; Pope *et al*. 2002), or a more experimental approach (quantitative and deductive). Information can be gathered by on-site observation (on the spot or by audiovideo recording), self-reports (interviews and questionnaires or surveys) and from existing data sources (or secondary sources).

What methods – single or combined – should be used to gather process data?

On-site observation is feasible whenever the presence of an observer (person, camera or audiotape) is not obtrusive and will not alter the behaviour of those observed. The observational method appears attractive and simple, but can pose several problems. The method is not easily taught or quickly learnt, it is highly time consuming and sometimes produces information that is hard to summarise or analyse. As already mentioned, the method may alter the behaviour of the observed. The less structured the observation or the more complex the intervention, the more problematic the method becomes. It is therefore very important to train observers and to assess reliably.

The *self-report* technique (interviews and questionnaires) can be used either through periodic reports throughout the intervention or through retrospective reports after the intervention has ended. Periodic reports probably provide more accurate data. The number of measurements during an intervention depends on the homogeneity of the activities (the more homogeneous the activities, the less frequently data have to be gathered), the amount of time available for scoring and interpreting information, and the assessment of people's tolerance to interruptions. Reports gathered after an intervention has ended are most reliable when gathered as soon after as possible. They are also more reliable if used for interventions of relatively short duration.

Existing data sources or records can be used, that is information routinely recorded, independent of the process evaluation, in administrative and service records (e.g. the pocket diary in which the outreach visitor records appointments with practices). This is an inexpensive method, and provides data that are efficient to obtain and analyse. Records may vary from narrative reports to highly structured data forms on which personnel tick what activities have been performed. Examples of secondary sources include minutes of meetings, bills, purchase orders, invoices, certificates upon completion of activities, attendance logs, signing in and signing out sheets, checklists, referral letters, diaries, news releases, etc. Using existing records can pose some problems. They seldom cover all the information needs, so it is usually necessary to collect additional information. Providers may be concerned that a recording system will reveal negative information about themselves and so may not record data accurately or completely. Addressing such concerns and motivating people to complete records properly and in a timely fashion may, therefore, be important. In addition, if routine data are required it is important to check regularly that the information needed is actually being recorded accurately and completely.

Given the possible problems of using existing records, it is sometimes necessary to set up a project-specific recording system. To improve the likelihood of reliable and complete data, it is important to develop a system that is easy to maintain and useful for the users' purposes as well. Checklists are, for example, feasible and efficient to use – no narrative information has to be provided, as checking off various items is sufficient.

Whatever measurement method (or series of methods) is chosen, there are a number of important considerations. It is important to consider the circumstances (e.g. the amount of time available to gather and interpret data), practical issues, homogeneity of the data, privacy and confidentiality, and the estimated tolerance levels of the respondents who will be asked to provide data. In addition, the instruments should ideally be simple and user friendly so as not to be burdensome for the user. However, they must be detailed enough to answer the evaluation questions and goals. When selecting the instruments, it is necessary to consider whether the method of data gathering will have an undesirable influence on the ongoing evaluation or on the actual use of the intervention. Whether the method of data gathering has an 'undesirable' influence depends on the type of project that is being performed (small-scale improvement project, experimental study or large-scale implementation programme) and on the aim of the process evaluation. It is also important that data are gathered in a valid and reliable manner from selected population samples. Depending on the approach taken (developmental or experimental), respondent samples can be selected to reflect the diversity within a given population (purposive sampling) or to achieve statistical representativeness. Whatever method is chosen, those responsible for data gathering should have adequate training in the skills and terms associated with the use of the instruments and should be able to perform quality control checks.

Describing the intervention as 'planned' or 'performed'

To describe the features of the implementation of change intervention as planned, prior to starting the intervention, the implementers or researchers can be asked to fill in the framework. Interviews with the pro-

gramme developers and other relevant individuals can also provide information. To start or supplement the process, it may be useful to use existing documentation, such as a study plan, the programme proposal, minutes of meetings or existing records.

To describe the change intervention as performed (after finishing the intervention), interviews with the implementers of the intervention and/or the participants, or questionnaires and surveys, can be used. In this way participants provide useful information about the intervention as performed in terms of their personal participation in intervention activities. However, the reliability of data reported in retrospect decreases as the complexity and extensiveness of the intervention increases and as the interval since the start of the intervention increases, and the period since the participants were exposed to intervention activities becomes longer. Moreover, the framework involves many features and details that the respondents may not have been aware of during the intervention, which once again makes it difficult to obtain valid data after the event. Therefore, it is often preferable to gather information during the process and to use these data to describe the intervention in its final form (see below).

Checking the actual exposure to the change intervention

Participation in the intervention activities by implementers or participants can be studied prospectively (either continuously or periodically) or retrospectively (by using observation, self-reports and/or existing data sources). If possible, information should be gathered on all the features involved in 'exposure to the intervention'. However, it is no small task to verify whether the participants are performing all the intended intervention activities. Resource constraints, for example, may mean it is necessary to select a small number of key features of the intervention and pay the closest attention to these. During the performance of the intervention, it is sometimes permissible for the change process to vary across sites or time. The greater the variation permissible, the more attention must be paid to documenting exposure to the feature concerned (see the example in *Box 19.8*).

Describing the experience of those exposed to the change intervention

Participants can be asked, during and/or after the intervention, to provide information on how they experienced it. Their opinions can be explored on all the

Box 19.8 Improving the prevention of cardiovascular disease (Hulscher *et al.* 1998)

The multifaceted intervention as planned consisted of four types of intervention:

- Providing all practice members with information about the project and the recommended best practices to organise preventive services. The information was to be provided by an outreach visitor during an introductory visit (standardised with the help of a checklist).
- Providing feedback on current practice. After an analysis of the practice organisation (standardised with the help of checklists), all practice members were to receive a feedback report on current practice.
- Tailoring outreach visits from trained nurses. After receiving the feedback report, the practice members were to choose and discuss intended changes under the guidance of an outreach visitor. The outreach visitor was to help the practice to implement the changes. Outreach visits were to be arranged according to needs and wishes.
- Tailoring the provision of educational materials and practical tools. Depending on their needs and wishes, practice members were to be provided with standardised educational materials and tools.

It was decided – mainly for practical reasons such as time and money constraints – that it would be most valuable to monitor the tailoring of outreach visits and the materials received by the practice team (in which variation was allowed).

To check actual exposure to the outreach visits and materials, a simple, coded visit-registration form was developed that had to be filled in by the outreach visitor after each visit to a practice. The following features of a visit had to be recorded:

- Date and duration of the visit;
- Participants in a meeting (name and function);
- Type of activities during a meeting;
- Materials used or provided during a meeting.

The example in *Box 19.5* describes how this information was ultimately used by the researchers to describe the intervention as performed.

elements of the intervention chosen, and they can also describe features they perceived as being most related to the success or failure of the intervention. In this way, information is obtained that is closely and directly linked to the intervention *method* as experienced (see the examples in Boxes *19.9* and *19.10*).

Analysing *barriers and facilitators to change* while participating in the intervention and implementing the changes can also provide useful insights into how the intervention might be revised. This issue is discussed more extensively in Chapters 6 and 7. The framework presented in this chapter does not provide detail on this

Box 19.9 Process evaluation of a tailored multifaceted approach to changing care patterns and improving preventive care (Baskerville *et al.* 2001)

Prevention facilitators (outreach visitors) tailored the following strategies to the needs and individual circumstances of 22 practices involving 54 physicians:

- Audit and ongoing feedback;
- Consensus building;
- Opinion leaders and networking;
- Academic detailing and education materials;
- Reminder systems;
- Patient-mediated activities;
- Patient-education materials.

The interventions produced an absolute improvement over time of 11.5% in preventive care performance (13 preventive strategies, e.g. counselling for folic acid, advice to quit smoking, influenza vaccination, glucose testing, prostate-specific antigen testing).

The aim of process evaluation was to document the extent of conformity with the proposed intervention and to gain insight into why the intervention successfully improved preventive

care. Key measures in the evaluation process were the frequency of delivery of the various intervention components (i.e. the different types of intervention), the time involved, the scope of delivery, the utility of the components and physician satisfaction with the intervention.

Five data collection tools were used, as well as a combination of descriptive, quantitative and qualitative analyses. Triangulation was employed to investigate the quality of the implementation activities.

Facilitators documented their activities and progress on two structured forms known as the weekly activity sheet (hours spent on on-site and off-site activities) and the monthly narrative report (per practice – number of visits, activities and their outcomes, number of participants, plan for the following month). At 6 months and 17 months, two members of the research team conducted semi-structured telephone interviews with the participating doctors to find out whether they were happy or unhappy with the interventions, and to document their ideas about improvement and overall satisfaction (closed questions). Facilitators interviewed contact practitioners to obtain post-intervention feedback about their experience. Physicians were sent a questionnaire by mail to report any changes that had taken place over the preceding 18 months.

Facilitators visited the practices to deliver the audit and feedback, to build consensus and to introduce reminder system components. All the study practices received feedback on preventive performance, achieved consensus on a plan for improvement and implemented a reminder system:

- 90% of the practices implemented a customised flow sheet, while 10% used a computerised reminder system;
- 95% of the intervention practices wanted evidence for prevention;
- 82% participated in a workshop;
- 100% received patient-education material in a binder.

Content analysis of the data obtained during the interviews and bivariate analysis of self-reported changes compared to a non-intervention control group suggested that the audit and feedback, consensus building and development of reminder systems were the key intervention components responsible for change.

Box 19.10 Effects of a smoking cessation programme for pregnant women (Ershoff *et al.* 1989)

A prospective randomised controlled trial was performed to assess the effects of a serialised self-help smoking cessation programme in an health maintenance organisation (HMO) aimed at women during the first 18 weeks of pregnancy. Women were randomised in advance of their first visit, at which they had an individual 45 minute meeting with a health educator. At the conclusion of this meeting, the health educator conducted a 2 minute smoking-related interview with those women who smoked. Of the smokers, 165 were experimental and 158 were control (the health educator was blind to group assignment). After the smoking-related interview, in keeping with the standard practice of the medical group, all subjects were given a two-page pamphlet on the hazards of smoking during pregnancy and the importance of quitting. The health educator reinforced the written information in a 2 minute discussion and answered any questions; she also advised patients of a five-session smoking cessation class available free through the HMO.

Experimental subjects were then given the first of eight self-help booklets, together with a 3 minute overview of the programme. Women were asked to make a commitment to read *Booklet 1* within the ensuing week and to list their reasons for and against smoking. Each of the booklets had such activity assignments designed to personalise the programme. The remaining seven booklets were mailed thereafter at weekly intervals and comprised a step-by-step programme to increase motivation for quitting and to teach behavioural strategies for cessation and for relapse prevention. These 4–8 page booklets were tailored to pregnancy. All experimental group women received the programme regardless of their motivation to quit smoking or desire to receive the programme materials.

A 26th week standard telephone interview schedule was completed to collect data on health-related behaviour (including smoking and quitting) during pregnancy. The interview also assessed the degree to which the experimental group read and used the booklets, satisfaction with content and appearance, and perceived usefulness of the self-help programme.

The self-help programme yielded a 10% higher proportion of quitters than was observed among controls; more than twice the proportion of early quitters was observed (22.2% versus 8.6%).

The vast majority of women in the experimental group reported reading at least one of the eight booklets (93%), with a mean of 5.8 booklets read. Nearly half (47.7%) reported reading the entire series. The booklets were judged to be interesting, attractive, helpful and easy to understand. Half of the early quitters indicated that the booklets influenced their decision to quit, although a third rated the booklets of 'no help at all'.

---

aspect of process evaluation. Ideally, an intervention that aims to change clinical practice is designed on the basis of a systematic scientific approach that (a) analyses barriers and incentives to change, and (b) links the intervention to these influencing factors. A complete analysis of the experience of participants with the aim of gaining insight into how the change intervention might be revised should therefore also check whether barriers and facilitators were handled successfully in the implementation plan.

CONCLUSIONS

Process evaluation can illuminate the mechanisms and processes responsible for the (lack of) change in the target group. In so doing, process evaluation makes a very relevant and important contribution to the development of potentially successful interventions to implement changes in patient care.

The framework presented in this chapter gives the key features necessary to describe an implementation of change intervention in detail, to check whether the intervention was performed as planned and to assess the experience of participants.

Recommended literature

Fink A (1993). *Evaluation Fundamentals Guiding Health Programs, Research, and Policy.* Newbury Park: Sage.

Grol R, Baker R and Moss F (2003). *Quality Improvement Research. Understanding the Science of Change in Health Care.* London: BMJ Books.

Ovretveit J (2000). *Evaluating Health Interventions: An Introduction to Evaluation of Health Treatments, Services, Policies and Organizational Interventions.* Buckingham: Open University Press.

Rossi PH, Freeman HE and Lipsey MW (1999). *Evaluation. A Systematic Approach.* Thousand Oaks: Sage.

References

Ajzen I (1991). The theory of planned behaviour. *Organ Behav Hum Decis Process* 50:179–211.

Anonymous (1999). Getting evidence into practice. *Effective Health Care*, Vol. 5, pp. 1–15. Leeds: University of Leeds.

Bandura A (1986). *Social Foundations of Thought and Action: A Social Cognitive Theory.* New York: Prentice-Hall.

Baskerville NB, Hogg W and Lemelin J (2001). Process evaluation of a tailored multifaceted approach to changing family physician practice patterns and improving preventive care. *J Fam Pract.* 50:W242–W249.

Benger JR and Pearce AV (2002). Simple intervention to improve detection of child abuse in emergency departments. *BMJ* 324:780–782.

Bero L, Grilli R, Grimshaw JM, *et al.* (1998). Closing the gap between research and practice: An overview of systematic reviews of interventions to promote implementation of research findings by health care professionals. *BMJ* 317:465–468.

EPOC (1998). *The Data Collection Checklist.* Cochrane Effective Practice and Organisation of Care Review Group. Oxford: Update Software.

Eccles M, McColl E, Steen N, *et al.* (2002). A cluster randomised controlled trial of computerised evidence based guidelines for angina and asthma in primary care. *BMJ* 325:941–947.

Ershoff DH, Dolan Mullen P and Quinn VP (1989). A randomized trial of a serialized self-help smoking cessation program for pregnant women in an HMO. *Am J Public Health* 79:182–187.

Festinger L (1954). A theory of social comparison processes. *Human Relations* 7:117–140.

Fink A (1993). *Evaluation Fundamentals Guiding Health Programs, Research, and Policy.* Newbury Park: Sage.

Grol R (1997). Beliefs and evidence in changing clinical practice. *BMJ* 315:418–421.

Herman JL, Morris LL and Fitz-Gabbon CT (1987). *Evaluator's Handbook*, Vol. 1 in *Program Evaluation Kit*, Herman Jl (ed). Newbury Park: Sage Publications.

Hermens RPMG, Hak E, Hulscher MEJL, *et al.* (2001). Adherence to guidelines on cervical cancer screening in general practice: Programme elements of successful implementation. *Br J Gen Pract.* 51:897–903.

Hulscher MEJL, Drenth BB van, Mokkink HGA, *et al.* (1998). Tailored outreach visits as a method for implementing guidelines and improving preventive care. *Intern J Quality Health Care* 10:105–112.

King JA, Morris LL and Fitz-Gabbon CT (1987). *How to Assess Program Implementation.* Vol. 5 in *Program Evaluation Kit*, Herman Jl (ed). Newbury Park: Sage.

Laurant M, Hulscher M, Wensing M and Grol R (1999). *Analysing and Monitoring Implementation Strategies for Changing Professional Practice.* Nijmegen: WOK.

McGuire WJ (1985). Attitudes and attitude change. In: Lindsay G and Aronson E (eds). *The Handbook of Social Psychology*, Third Edition, pp. 233–346. New York: Random House.

Nattinger AB, Panzer RJ and Janus J (1989). Improving the utilization of screening mammography in primary care practices. *Arch Intern Med.* 149:2087–2092.

Ovretveit J (2000). *Evaluating Health Interventions: An Introduction to Evaluation of Health Treatments, Services, Policies and Organizational Interventions.* Buckingham: Open University Press.

Pope C, van Royen P and R Baker (2002). Qualitative methods in research on healthcare quality. *Qual Saf Health Care* 11:148–152.

Rogers EM (1983). *Diffusion of Innovations.* New York: The Free Press.

Rossi PH and Freeman HE (1993). *Evaluation: A Systematic Approach.* Newbury Park: Sage.

Rossi PH, Freeman HE and Lipsey MW (1999). *Evaluation. A Systematic Approach.* Thousand Oaks: Sage.

Rousseau N, McColl E, Newton J, Grimshaw J and Eccles M (2003). Practice based, longitudinal, qualitative interview study of computerised evidence based guidelines in primary care. *BMJ* 326:314–322.

Swanborn PG (1999). *Evalueren. Het Ontwerpen, Begeleiden en Evalueren van Interventies: Een Methodische Basis voor Evaluatie-Onderzoek.* [*Evaluation. The Design, Support and Evaluation of Interventions: A Methodological Basis for Evaluation Research.*] Amsterdam: Uitgeverij Boom.

Szczepura A, Wilmot J, Davies C, *et al.* (1994). Effectiveness and cost of different strategies for information feedback in general practice. *Br J Gen Pract.* 43:19–24.

Chapter 20

Economic evaluations of implementation strategies

Johan L Severens, Jody D Martens and Michel Wensing

KEY MESSAGES

- Economic evaluations of implementation strategies are based on an explicit comparison of alternative methods of introducing desirable changes into healthcare. When performing a complete economic evaluation, the costs incurred by the efforts of people and any use of resources are related to the (health) outcomes obtained.
- In implementation studies, economic evaluations can be very informative, but have only been performed on a limited scale so far.
- In improvement projects and large-scale implementation projects, an integrated economic evaluation is usually not performed. Instead, the costs and changes in healthcare processes or patient health outcome are described separately.
- Economic evaluation research of implementation strategies is most beneficial if the cost effectiveness of the desired professional behaviour or healthcare process in optimal conditions is known and found to be acceptable, because active implementation can only be cost effective given this prerequisite.
- Unlike economic evaluations of medical interventions, in economic evaluations of implementation strategies both care process and patient outcomes can be incorporated into cost-effectiveness measures.

Box 20.1 Randomised controlled economic evaluation of asthma self-management in primary healthcare (Schermer *et al.* 2002)

In this randomised controlled economic evaluation, guided asthma self-management was compared with usual asthma care according to guidelines for Dutch family physicians. 19 family practices were randomised, and 193 adults with stable asthma (98 self-management, 95 usual care) were included and monitored for 2 years. Patient-specific cost data were collected, preference-based utilities were assessed and incremental cost per quality-adjusted life year (QALY) and incremental cost per successfully treated week gained was calculated. Self-management patients gained 0.039 QALY and experienced 81 successfully treated weeks in the 2 years; the corresponding figures for usual care were 0.024 and 75, respectively. Total costs were 1084 euros for self-management and 1097 euros for usual care. Self-management patients consumed 1680 puffs of budesonide, and usual care patients 1897. When all the costs were included, self-management was cost-effective on all outcomes. It was concluded that guided self-management is a safe and efficient alternative approach compared with the asthma treatment usually provided in Dutch primary care.

INTRODUCTION

In the previous chapters, the effects and process evaluation of implementation projects, implementation studies and large-scale implementation studies are discussed. In this chapter, a further element is added to the evaluation by including the costs of the implementation strategy and its consequences, as well as the explicit relationship between these costs and the results obtained.

So far, there are few examples of good economic evaluations of implementation strategies. In a recent review of 235 studies reporting 309 comparisons of strategies to implement clinical guidelines only 29% of the comparisons reported any economic data (Grimshaw *et al.* 2004). Overall, the methods of the economic evaluations and cost analyses were poor. Eleven comparisons reported cost-effectiveness analyses, 38 reported cost-consequence analyses (in which differences in cost were set against differences in several measures of effectiveness) and 14 reported cost analyses (in which some aspect of cost was reported, but not related to benefits). The majority of studies only reported costs of treatment; only 25 studies reported data on the costs of guideline development or guideline dissemination and implementation. The majority of studies used process measures for their primary endpoint despite the fact that only three guidelines were explicitly evidence based (and therefore may not have been efficient). The viewpoint adopted in economic evaluations was only stated in ten studies. The methods used to estimate costs were comprehensive in about half of the studies, and few studies reported details of resources use. The poor quality of reporting of economic evaluations means data on resource use and cost of guideline development, dissemination and implementation were not available for most of them.

However, healthcare managers and policy makers often make an implicit calculation about the costs and results of a particular implementation strategy, or the competing costs of different strategies to introduce a guideline or change in physician's practice. In an economic evaluation this calculation is made explicitly. In this chapter, the principles of economic evaluations are described and applied to implementation research, and many of the shortcomings identified in the review above are discussed. We discuss the core, methods and starting points of economic evaluations, and the principles of cost-effectiveness analysis. We end the chapter with a brief evaluation of the usefulness of economic evaluations during implementation research.

THE BASIS OF ECONOMIC EVALUATIONS

As discussed earlier in this book, there is a range of implementation strategies designed to change healthcare processes and encourage particular behaviours by healthcare professionals, such as doctors, paramedical staff and nurses. These strategies differ not only in their form, but also in their effects – in their impact on the behaviour of healthcare professionals and on the health, quality of life or satisfaction with care of patients (Wensing *et al*. 1998; Grimshaw and Russell 1993). They also vary greatly in terms of the amount of time and effort they require from healthcare professionals.

Implementation research determines both the positive and negative consequences of the application of implementation strategies. Therefore, it is important to consider not just the overall results, but also the efforts required to achieve them. If an implementation strategy is very expensive, the costs (use of people, time and other resources) incurred come at the expense of other healthcare activities. It is possible that a clinical intervention that is cost effective in the context of a clinical trial requires so much resource to implement in a routine care setting that its cost effectiveness deteriorates. The application of an implementation strategy can, therefore, be considered an investment that can be judged according to its cost effectiveness.

Economic evaluations are a specific form of evaluation that focusses on the relationship between the benefits achieved and the resources required to achieve those benefits. Therefore two criteria must be met (*Figure 20.1*). First, there needs to be a choice between interventions. In implementation research, the choice consists of a comparison of two or more different implementation strategies or the comparison of an implementation strategy with 'doing nothing' or 'usual healthcare'. Second, in economic evaluations an explicit relationship is made between the inputs (use of people and resources) and the related consequences or actual outcomes. The use of people and resources is usually expressed in monetary units (euros or dollars), so that they can be considered expenses. The effects and costs of an implementation strategy can then be considered in comparison with an alternative option that

Figure 20.1 Criteria for a complete economic evaluation (based on Drummond *et al*. 1997)				
		Are both outcomes and costs taken into consideration?		
		Description of outcomes	**Description of costs**	**Description of cost–effects**
Are alternatives being compared?	**No**	Outcomes only	Costs only	Both outcomes and costs
	Yes	Evaluation of outcomes	Evaluation of costs	Economic evaluation

is relevant to the sector; this is known as the incremental cost effectiveness or relative cost effectiveness of an implementation strategy.

In this book, a distinction is made between implementation projects, implementation studies and large-scale implementation projects. Since both implementation projects and large-scale implementation projects usually include the application of an implementation strategy without the involvement of a control or comparison intervention, the comparison criteria mentioned above are not met. However, in projects such as these it can be useful, for healthcare professionals, institutions and policy makers, to describe the costs of an implementation strategy. In this case, separate descriptions of costs and changes are reported in a table.

Definition of cost effectiveness

The term cost effectiveness can be misunderstood (Doubilet *et al.* 1986). *Figure 20.2* shows the definition of cost effectiveness in clinical research. In the case of patients given experimental treatment A experiencing less therapeutic effect and incurring higher costs than those given experimental treatment B, there is an inferior treatment (A) and the introduction of that therapy into routine healthcare should not occur. The opposite occurs when an experimental therapy has a greater effect than the comparison and also incurs lower costs; this is known as dominance. The other two cases (higher costs and better outcomes, or lower costs and worse outcomes) are known as consideration problems and there is then a need to decide on an acceptable ratio between costs and effects.

METHODS OF ECONOMIC EVALUATIONS

There are four basic types of economic evaluations: cost-minimisation analysis, cost-effectiveness analysis,

cost–utility analysis and cost–benefit analysis. Cost-consequence analyses are often considered a type of economic evaluation. However, this method does not explicitly relate costs to a measure of effectiveness, the prerequisite for a full economic evaluation.

A *cost-minimisation analysis* is characterised by the assumption or knowledge that the outcome (consequences, benefits) of the studied strategies is identical. This can occur within a study or be known from previous research in the scientific literature. In the face of such equivalence of effect only the costs of the alternatives are determined, and the least-expensive alternative is usually preferred (*Box 20.2*).

Unlike cost-minimisation analysis, the other types of economic evaluations integrate the outcomes of interventions and the evaluation, usually aiming to produce a single summarising unit. *Cost-effectiveness analyses* express outcomes in natural measurable outcome parameters. In implementation research, this could be measures such as:

- Number of physicians' practices reached by the implementation strategy (e.g. mailing of guidelines);
- Number of practices, departments or professionals that work in accordance with a specific guideline;
- Number of patients who received treatment in accordance with a protocol;
- Health condition of the patients concerned or their satisfaction with the healthcare provided.

Process parameters, such as the number of physicians who work in accordance with a protocol or the number of patients who have received treatment in accordance with that protocol, can be considered intermediary parameters that (should) have a relationship with patient outcomes. In doing so, the analysis is limited to the level of healthcare provider or institution (Wood and Freemantle 1999).

Figure 20.2 Classification of the outcomes of economic evaluations that compares two alternative treatments (A and B) with each other (based on Sculpher 2000)

		Consequences of treatment A compared to treatment B	
		A is worse than B	A is better than B
Costs of A compared to B	Higher	A is inferior compared to B	Is a better outcome worth the higher costs?
	Lower	Is a worse outcome acceptable, considering the lower costs?	A is dominant compared to B

Box 20.2 Individual feedback to care physicians about diagnostic test requests (Winkens *et al.* 1996)

In this study, the influence of individual feedback on physicians' requests for diagnostic tests was examined. Based on an extensive retrospective study, it was shown that individual feedback led to a significant reduction in costs. To estimate the relative impact of the implementation strategy, comparator data were used from a laboratory in another part of The Netherlands. In the feedback laboratory group fewer tests were ordered and costs were lower. Although data about patient outcomes were not available, possible unwanted effects of the decline in diagnostic test requests were sought and none could be demonstrated. Therefore, it was assumed that the provision of care was equivalent between the two sites. Since no explicit analytical connection was made between costs and outcomes, this study can be defined as a cost-minimisation analysis.

In *cost–utility analyses*, patient health is the focus and these analyses always refer to patient outcomes. It is a characteristic of cost–utility analyses that patients' eventual physical health is rated through the use of a utility measure. This health rating is indicated by a number between 0 and 1, where 1 equals perfect health and 0 the worst imaginable condition. For this rating, either a societal or individual rating for the health condition can be used. Utilities can be used as the basis for the calculation of metrics, such as the QALYs, a measure that uses societal ratings of a patients' health condition and relates these to life span. Self-evidently, cost–utility analyses require patients to participate in a study and complete questionnaires. Within clinical evaluation studies this method of analysis is frequently used, but within implementation research they are used only sporadically. For situations in which they are used it is important to realise that the effects on patient outcomes are determined not only by the implementation strategy used, but also by the cost effectiveness of the clinical interventions implemented.

Cost–benefit analyses are distinguished from other types of economic evaluations by the fact that they measure both costs and consequences in financial terms – patient survival or quality of life would be expressed in euros or dollars. There are many issues involved in such analyses and they are not often used in healthcare evaluations. However, the term cost–benefit is often used incorrectly in situations where there are financial savings. The use of the term cost–benefit suggests that such savings are benefits, whereas they are merely lower costs.

It is often the case that the relationship between costs and effects is expressed in a single unit, such as a cost-effectiveness ratio. This requires a single effect, an unusual situation for implementation strategies. An alternative is a *cost–consequence analysis*. This method presents an overview of the costs and consequences without attempting to amalgamate these into one single unit. It simply displays the costs and consequences without indicating a value or preference. These are then presented to those clinicians or policy makers who have to make a decision about the use of the intervention (Mauskopf *et al.* 1998). McIntosh *et al.* (1999) introduced the so-called balance sheet approach, which can be considered a specific type of cost–consequence analysis in which positive and negative consequences are simply stated in a table.

An overview of the methods of economical evaluations is shown in *Table 20.1*.

Table 20.1 Methods of economic evaluations

Method	Measurement level	Measurement unit
Cost-minimisation analysis	Not relevant, because consequences of the implementation strategies are identical	Not applicable
Cost-effectiveness analysis	Multiple – healthcare agencies, healthcare professional or patient	Statement of effect in several measuring units
Cost–utility analysis	The patient	Health status
Cost–benefit analysis	The patient	Monetary units
Cost–consequence analysis	Multiple – healthcare agency, healthcare professional or patient	Statement of consequences in several measuring units

POLICY COST-EFFECTIVENESS

The cost-effectiveness ratio of an implementation strategy expresses how the costs relate to the results obtained. These can be formulated in terms of process parameters (e.g. adherence to guidelines) or patient outcomes – the implementation costs per guideline-treated patient (with process parameters as the outcome unit) or the implementation costs plus treatment costs per successfully treated patient (with outcome parameter as the outcome unit), for example. By comparing the effects and costs of alternative implementation strategies with each other, the incremental cost-effectiveness ratio can be determined. Whether or not this ratio is acceptable cannot be determined through an economic evaluation, since it is a choice of policy.

The ultimate goal in health economists' research is to express efficiency of an implementation project in terms of patient outcome to help decision makers explore whether investing in change is worthwhile (see *Box 20.1*). Mason *et al.* (2001) made an important step forward by developing a more advanced approach in which implementation cost-effectiveness was combined with treatment cost-effectiveness. This model shows that multiple influences determine whether investing to achieve behavioural change is worthwhile. The preconditions are that there is an evidence-based message of clinical and cost-effective care, and existing care is suboptimal (*Box 20.3*).

Worthwhile improvement of healthcare from a policy viewpoint demands an implementation method that does not load treatment cost-effectiveness too much (Mason *et al.* 2001). An example of the estimation of overall policy costs and benefits can be expressed in Equation (20.1), which gives the policy cost-effectiveness ΔCE_p in terms of (Mason *et al.* 2001):

- Net health gain Δb_t, cost of care Δc_t and treatment cost-effectiveness per patient ΔCE_t ($=\Delta c_t / \Delta b_t$);
- Net cost Δc_i, proportion of patient care changed Δb_i and implementation cost-effectiveness per practice ΔCE_i ($= \Delta c_i / \Delta b_i$);
- Duration of effect of the implementation method d;
- Average practice size n_p and population prevalence p_d of the condition targeted;
- Loading factor on treatment cost effectiveness L_{CE}.

$$\Delta CE_p = \frac{1}{d \cdot n_p \cdot p_d \cdot \Delta b_t} \cdot \Delta CE_i + \Delta CE_t = L_{CE} + \Delta CE_t$$

(20.1)

KEY DECISIONS IN ECONOMIC EVALUATIONS

Choice of comparator

The choice of the comparator is a fundamental aspect of any evaluation. It is important to decide what the costs and effects of an implementation strategy are to be compared with:

- An alternative workable implementation strategy (perhaps a combination of interventions);
- A routinely used implementation strategy (such as the publication of guidelines);
- No specific implementation strategy (usual healthcare).

Clearly, the implications of such differing comparisons could vary widely.

Box 20.3 A randomised controlled trial examining three training and support strategies to promote the use of a brief intervention to decrease risky drinking (Kaner *et al.* 1999)

This study reports the evaluation of three training and/or support strategies that were intended to motivate primary care physicians to use a screening and brief intervention (SBI) package targeted towards risky drinking of alcohol. The strategies were:
(1) Distribution of guidelines;
(2) Distribution of guidelines plus training;
(3) Distribution of guidelines plus training and telephone support.
The 'guideline plus training and telephone support' strategy turned out to be the most cost effective, in terms of costs per patient screened and the costs per patient on whom an intervention was performed. In this study, the cost-effectiveness for each strategy was determined separately. Therefore, the cost-effectiveness that was reported was the relative cost-effectiveness compared with doing nothing, an alternative not included in the study. Further analysis showed that the relative cost-effectiveness of intervention (2) compared to (1) was more positive than that for intervention (3) compared to (1) and the relative cost-effectiveness of (3) compared to (2) was less positive than either.

Time horizon of a study

The time horizon of a study is the time period about which a study aims to make a statement, for instance 1 year or 10 years. A time horizon should be chosen to allow all the anticipated costs and consequences of the implementation strategies to be included in the study. If a study was to evaluate the impact of a strategy to modify the management of cardiovascular disease and the chosen endpoint was patient mortality, the time horizon could be a period of several years. However, such extended time periods are often not acceptable – decision makers do not want to wait that long, and long-term research is very costly (Black 1996).

However, implementation research is frequently not about the question of whether or not there have been effects on patients and at what cost, but rather about questions of how professional behaviour or healthcare processes can be improved and at what cost. So patient outcomes may not be measured. If the relationship between a health action and patient outcomes is well understood from clinical research studies, a short time horizon may be sufficient as, under these circumstances, it is only necessary to demonstrate change in process – whether the acting physicians treat their patients in accordance with the guidelines (*Box 20.4*). Such intermediary results could potentially be used as a basis for the prediction of outcomes over longer time horizons using modelling studies, such as decision analytic models, Markov models and Monte Carlo simulations (Brennan and Akehurst 1999; Buxton *et al.* 1997). For situations in which the clinical effectiveness of one or more interventions is not known, researchers may have to conduct longer studies and ensure that they capture the relevant clinical outcomes within an implementation evaluation.

Study perspective

Economic evaluations can be conducted from a number of perspectives, such as financial, healthcare or societal. The perspective that is chosen determines the range and nature of the costs considered.

From a *financial perspective* (an insurer's or third-party payer perspective), the focus is on tariffs for efforts in healthcare (cost of annual cover, actual handling, nursing days, resting days, etc.). From a *healthcare perspective*, the costs are rated in terms of actual costs incurred by the healthcare system. An example to make the difference between these perspectives clear is the payment of physician's services. Based on a system of annual cover (as is the case for patients insured by a sick fund in the Netherlands) the medical specialist receives a standard compensation for consultations, regardless of the actual number of contacts with the patient during a full year; within a financial perspective this standard cost is an appropriate figure, while within a healthcare perspective the number and cost of every consultation would be considered. A societal perspective includes the total costs as nearly as possible. This includes both costs within the healthcare sector and costs outside the healthcare sector that affect patients or third parties (such as costs related to sick leave).

While the *societal perspective* is the most inclusive, the choice of perspective will be influenced by the relative contribution of health and non-health costs and pragmatic considerations around the logistics of collecting data.

A study perspective that is not part of the common perspectives of economic evaluations of medical technologies, yet very important for implementation, is the *perspective of the healthcare provider and healthcare institution*. This perspective is relevant, since it concerns the costs and consequences that are experienced directly

---

Box 20.4 Cost–effectiveness of audit in case of thrombolysis (Robinson *et al.* 1998)

An example of the problems concerning process parameters versus patient outcomes as cost-effectiveness parameters is a study that examined the cost-effectiveness of audits of thrombolysis in patients who were suspected of having an acute myocardial infarction.

This study examined the costs for each extra patient who was treated for thrombosis. Thus, instead of patient outcomes,

a process parameter was used, which resulted in an estimated £101–£395 per extra patient treated.

The authors based their choice for such an outcome measure on the overwhelming evidence that the clinical actions being encouraged were effective. This legitimises the assumption that the increase in thrombolysis treatment leads to better patient outcomes.

by healthcare providers or healthcare institutions trying to implement an innovation and participate in a change strategy. In contrast to the above-mentioned healthcare perspective, this approach indicates in the implementation strategy which party is responsible for the costs or consequences. This approach maps well onto the cost–consequence analysis. For example, *Table 20.2* shows a cost–consequence table that is related to an implementation strategy intended to reduce the waiting lists for treatment (McIntosh *et al.* 1999). This method indicates which party is really responsible for the costs or consequences.

COST ANALYSIS

The execution of cost analyses is a main part of each economic evaluation of implementation strategies. There are several types of costs, the relevance of which depends on the perspective chosen.

Directly attributable, indirectly attributable, fixed and variable costs

When considering healthcare provision for an individual patient, a distinction is made between those costs directly attributable to the healthcare process and other, indirectly attributable costs. Directly attributable costs include the time a physician spends with a patient and the materials used during that time. Indirectly attributable costs (also known as overhead costs) include the time a physician spends on extra education, any activities of the practice assistant that cannot be attributed to a specific patient, the time a consultant spends providing individual feedback to healthcare providers and the costs of developing a change proposal or new procedure.

Within a cost analysis, further distinctions are made between fixed and variable costs. Fixed costs are costs that have no link to the scale of use of the specific (healthcare) provision in the short term. For example, if consensus meetings are used to develop a protocol or pathway, the costs remain the same, whether one or 100 physicians later use the guideline. Attribution of the fixed costs to patients or healthcare providers occurs on the basis of a simple division. A fixed cost of 10,000 euros for consensus meetings and ten physicians subsequently using the pathway with ten patients each gives fixed costs for that pathway of 1000 euros per physician and 100 euros per patient. If 20 physicians and nurses follow a protocol with ten patients each, these costs become 500 euros per professional and 50 euros per patient.

The variable costs of an implementation strategy are dependent on both intensity and the degree to which a protocol, guideline or procedure is followed. Thus, education that lasts 2 days is more expensive than education that lasts 2 hours. The variable costs related to the degree to which a protocol or guideline is followed are illustrated with a guideline recommendation that advises that patients at increased risk of cardiovascular disease be called on a regular basis for check-ups to measure blood pressure. Here, the number of patients affected by the recommendation determines the amount of the costs. If the number of patients is zero, the number of consultations based on the guideline is zero, incurring zero (variable) costs; equally, 130 patients invited and consulting incur 130 unit costs. Therefore, unlike fixed costs, variable costs always have to be measured empirically because they cannot be calculated through a simple division per measuring unit (practice, physician or patient).

Table 20.2 Hypothetical example of a cost–consequence analysis of waiting lists for treatment from a healthcare provider's perspective (based on McIntosh *et al.* 1999)

Costs	Responsible party	Consequences	Responsible party
Appointment of consultant	Institution	Reduced waiting list	Patient
Investment of 20-hour preparation and administration by physician	Physician	One polyclinic visit less per patient	Physician and/or patient
Patient's saving time and travelling expenses	Patient	Time for other activities, such as paid work	Patient
Reduction of emergency operations	Institution and/or physician	Extra free rooms in polyclinic	Institution and/or physician

Types of costs

Within economic evaluations in the healthcare sector, distinction is made between several types of costs whose inclusion are dependent on the choice of study perspective. Medical, nursing or paramedical costs are costs linked directly to a patient's healthcare process, such as the costs for diagnostics or therapy. The directly attributable costs of implementation strategies are also part of this cost category. The costs of implementation strategies focused on innovations for healthcare professionals can be subdivided into different phases of the implementation process (Severens 2003). Firstly, there are costs related to the *development of the innovation* itself. Ideally, these (fixed) developmental costs should be part of a cost analysis. In reality, however, the availability of an innovation (a new procedure, a protocol or a guideline) is usually taken as a given and not included in an economic evaluation. Next, there are costs associated with the *development of a specific implementation strategy*. For example, if implementing a guideline includes using outreach visitors who need to visit practices, teams or physicians, training of the visitors would be desirable. Such costs are usually one-off costs and therefore can also be considered fixed costs. In contrast, the costs of the *execution of the implementation strategy* (e.g. visitors spending time visiting physicians or practices) are not relevant until the moment the strategy is executed. These are usually considered as variable costs. Variable costs are also those costs associated with a *change in healthcare provision* as a result of the application of an implementation strategy, for instance a decrease of test ordering.

Non-medical costs are costs incurred outside the healthcare sector. These include the patients' costs, such as costs for time and travelling (direct non-medical costs) and other societal costs, also known as indirect non-medical costs, such as costs that result from absence from work through health problems, costs of special education and legal costs. *Table 20.3* shows the relevance of the costs in the different stages of implementation strategies and *Box 20.5* illustrates a cost analysis of an implementation strategy.

Volumes and cost prices

An important part of a cost analysis is to determine volumes, such as number of consultations, tests, treatments, etc. Volumes are all the units of 'expenditure', measured in some way, that form the basis for the cost analysis. When looking at the number of professionals, physicians that work in accordance with a protocol or shared care pathway, for example, the number and duration of the contacts between a general practitioner (GP) and a consultant can be used as a volume parameter. If, however, the health condition of the individual patient is used as the cost-effectiveness measure, the number of contacts between the physician and patient is relevant as well.

Once the volumes to be measured have been defined, the next step is to attribute cost prices to each unit of volume. In reality, it is almost impossible to collect specific cost-price data empirically for all volumes. Therefore, it is customary to use pre-existing data of cost prices, for which several sources can be used. Firstly, volumes and corresponding cost prices may have been reported in the *scientific literature*. When using these data, researchers need to ask themselves whether or not the definition of the volume unit agrees with that in their own study and whether or not the sit-

Table 20.3 Costs in the different stages of implementation strategies	
Stages	Relevance
Development of a guideline, protocol or procedure	Ideally, these fixed costs are passed on to the cost-effectiveness measure through a division calculation
Development of the implementation strategy	See above
Execution of the implementation strategy	These costs are always taken into consideration
Change in healthcare provision and patients' use of healthcare	These costs are taken into consideration when measurement at patient level is conducted
Non-medical costs	These costs are taken into consideration when measurement at patient level is conducted

Box 20.5 Cost analysis of an implementation strategy

The explanation of cost analyses of implementation strategies can be illustrated using the Dutch Cardiovascular Risk Prevention (CARPE) study to reduce cardiovascular risk in primary care . The focus of this randomised, controlled before-and-after study (Frijling et al. 2001) was to evaluate the use of trained outreach visitors or facilitators to adherence to the use of the recommendations of seven national primary care guidelines (hypertension, cholesterol, diabetes mellitus II, peripheral arteriosclerosis, angina pectoris, heart failure and cerebrovascular accident or transient ischaemic attack) with those patients in the primary care physician's practice with cardiovascular risk indicators or diseases. The cost analysis addressed the question "what are the costs of the intervention compared to no active implementation strategy (zero costs)?". The analysis used a healthcare perspective and the time horizon was limited to the 18 months during which the visitors were active. The cost analysis of the several stages of implementation was limited to the execution of the implementation strategy. During the study the facilitators prospectively recorded cost volumes for each visit to the primary care physicians' practices. This involved the number of visits by the visitor to each practice as well as the preparation, travel and consultation time per visit, the preparation and execution time that primary care physician(s) and practice assistant(s) spent during each visit and the number of miles the visitor had to travel. The recorded volumes were rated against the actual cost prices (1999 prices) in accordance with Dutch guidelines (Oostenbrink et al. 2002). Data were collected on 934 consultation visits at 62 primary care physicians' practices. Results are shown in the table below. The number of visits to each practice ranged from three to 17 (mean 14.8 visits). Partly because of this, the costs per practice varied. It was also the case that the number of primary care physicians and assistants who actively participated in the implementation strategy (by preparing and attending consultation visits) varied for each practice – one to four primary care physicians and zero to five assistants per practice, respectively. In particular, it turned out that the costs of the time investment of the primary care physicians largely determined the variation in costs of the implementation strategy.

Costs of the outreach visitor intervention (in Euros) per practice

	Mean costs	Minimum	Maximum
Travelling expenses outreach visitor	339	0	1522
Time costs outreach visitor:			
costs for preparation time and/or travelling	935	184	1609
costs for presence at a practice visit	276	53	419
Time costs practice assistant:			
costs for preparation time	271	0	1395
costs for presence at a visit	296	0	728
Time costs general practitioner:			
costs for preparation time	1245	53	4493
costs for presence at a visit	955	239	3084
Total time costs per practice	3978	574	8673

uation on which the cost price is based is comparable. All cost prices must be based on the same year of analysis or indexed to one specific year. Secondly, *guideline prices* may be available. These are (usually) national data on the costs and production volume of healthcare institutions that give estimates of the average integral cost prices. Using such national guideline prices is therefore recommended only if the general approach suffices. Thirdly, *current tariffs* can be used. As men-tioned before, current tariffs are used for evaluations from a financial perspective. Tariffs can also be used in situations in which it can be assumed that the tariff does not deviate much from the actual cost price. However, for those volumes for which it is decided that an exact cost price needs to be determined, a *cost-price study* has to be performed. Obviously, this also has to be done for those volumes for which no approximate cost price is available at all, such as for new methods of treatment or for a new implementation strategy, for example. A cost-price study is also recommended for those volumes that make a large contribution to the cost differences between several implementation alternatives. In general, cost price research is a specialist and time-consuming job.

SENSITIVITY ANALYSIS, MODELLING AND BUDGET IMPACT

Sensitivity analysis

Cost and cost-effectiveness outcomes are composed of stochastic and deterministic variables. Stochastic variables are those that have been measured per analysis unit (patient, physician, hospital, practice) of the study. Therefore, it is possible to calculate a mean value with a corresponding standard deviation and the uncertainty can be expressed as a confidence interval. Deterministic variables are those that have been determined once in a 'point estimate'. For example, the *number* of physician–patient consultations per patient is a stochastic variable and the *cost price* for a consultation (which can be an estimate, a derivation or a measurement) is a deterministic variable one. Even if the cost price is based on cost-price research with more than one work place measurement, only one single (deterministic) average cost price for the volume unit can be used.

However, a policy maker or researcher may want to know how much the results of the study have been influenced by the deterministic variables. To determine how changes in deterministic variables influence the results, a sensitivity analysis can be performed (Briggs *et al.* 1994). In such an analysis, the effect of changes on the most important factors on overall cost and cost effectiveness is examined. There are several techniques for sensitivity analysis. For instance, the estimate of a deterministic variable (e.g. 20 euros for a consultation with a primary care physician) is either slightly decreased (to 15 euros) or increased (to 25 euros) to judge the influence of these changes on the outcomes of the analysis. This is called a one-way sensitivity analysis. When several deterministic variables are varied at the same time, it is called a multiple sensitivity analysis.

Sometimes, stochastic variables are also considered in a sensitivity analysis. As each variable has a confidence interval it is possible to examine the impact of using the value of the upper or lower confidence interval instead of the mean. It can also be used to compensate for research design problems. For example, in a clinical trial patients may visit their physicians more frequently, not only for their routine healthcare, but also for pre-specified contacts for trial-related measurements. The latter contacts and their costs are driven by research protocol (Drummond *et al.* 1997), and should not be part of a cost analysis. However, if these two types of contact cannot be distinguished reliably, the stochastic parameters of the total number of contacts with primary care physicians can be decreased arbitrarily in a sensitivity analysis.

Modelling in economic evaluation

Empirical evaluation of health effectiveness is not always possible. When this is the case, or policy makers need information before empirical data are available, modelling can be used. Modelling combines data and assumptions to predict costs and outcomes of health interventions (*Box 20.6*).

Health economic models are used to generalise from the data observed in one situation to others, such as from trials to routine healthcare practice. Health economic models are generally used in two situations. Firstly, decision-analytic models are used to adjust or extrapolate data when the relevant clinical trials have not been conducted or did not include economic data. Secondly, statistical models, like extrapolation models, epidemiological models and Markov models, can be used where intermediate outcomes need to be con-

---

Box 20.6 CARPE project (Lobo *et al.* 2003)

In the CARPE study, as described in *Box 20.5*, the costs of the implementation strategy were calculated for each practice. The costs seemed unacceptably high. However, from a societal point of view, costs might be counterbalanced by long-term (financial or non-financial) revenues, such as lower medical costs through declining medical consumption by patients, or life years gained and QALYs gained. The limited duration of the CARPE project meant only intermediate endpoints were expressed. Extrapolation of these intermediate outcomes to final patient outcomes by modelling could offer decision makers important information about the long-term health outcomes.

nected with final outcomes or to extrapolate beyond short-term follow-up (Buxton *et al.* 1997; Gold *et al.* 1996).

It is important to regard models and their results as aids to decision making and not as scientific truths, because they are partly based on assumptions rather than on data. Although modelling is commonly used in economic evaluations, a number of concerns are regularly raised. The main disadvantage of decision-analytic modelling is that pieces of information from different studies and populations are combined into the same model; this has been termed a 'Frankenstein's monster' form of economic evaluation because the analyst brings different parts together to form a model (or monster) that hopefully will behave in a predictable way (O'Brien 1996).

A number of criteria can be given to assess the quality of models. Most of them fall into three areas – model structure, data used as inputs and model validation. Model assumptions about causal structure and parameter estimates should be assessed continually against data, and models should be revised accordingly. Structural assumptions and parameter estimates should be reported clearly and explicitly, and opportunities for users to appreciate the conditional relationship between inputs and outputs should be provided through sensitivity analyses.

Model-based evaluations can be an important resource for healthcare decision makers. Therefore, it is an important responsibility of model developers to conduct modelling studies to the highest standards and to complement the model results with a faithful disclosure of the underlying assumptions and with the caution that conclusions are conditional upon the assumptions and data on which the model is build (Weinstein *et al.* 2003).

Budget impact analysis

An economic evaluation leads to insights into the additional costs per analysis unit (patient, physician, hospital, practice) and the additional cost effectiveness of the implementation strategy compared to a different strategy. However, this does not provide information about the influence of a large-scale application of an implementation strategy in the healthcare sector. A budget impact analysis makes clear the effects of the broad introduction of an implementation strategy within a healthcare system. In other words, it makes clear what the costs and impacts are if a health intervention is implemented on a national scale. For this analysis it is necessary to know – in addition to investments and possible savings at the level of patients, healthcare providers or practices – how many patients, healthcare providers and practices are eligible for the implementation strategy. From the appropriate multiplication of these two sets of figures, researchers can offer policy makers the likely total costs and savings generated by a wide distribution of the implementation strategy.

CONCLUSIONS

The cost effectiveness of an implementation strategy is an amalgamation of four things (Sculpher 2000):
- Cost effectiveness of the desired medical actions;
- Degree to which these desired actions already take place;
- Costs of an implementation strategy;
- Effectiveness of an implementation strategy.

Economic evaluations of implementation projects, implementation studies and large-scale implementation projects have, as yet, been performed on a limited scale only compared to economic evaluations of medical interventions. In implementation projects and large-scale implementation studies there is usually no comparator, which makes a complete and reliable economic evaluation impossible. Implementation trials, however, generally contain an explicit (empirical) comparison of at least two alternative strategies to encourage the desired clinical behaviour. It is characteristic of a complete economic evaluation that both costs and outcomes are examined and that these are related to each other or at least listed next to each other in a cost–consequence chart. As opposed to economic evaluations of medical interventions, economic evaluations of implementation strategies can use both process and patient outcomes in cost-effectiveness measurements. However, economic evaluation research of implementation strategies is only useful if the cost-effectiveness ratio of the desired medical behaviour is known and found acceptable or if it can, at least, be assumed to be favourable.

Recommended literature

Mason J, Freemantle N, Nazareth I, Eccles M, Haines A and Drummond MF (2001). When is it cost-effective to change the behaviour of health professionals? *JAMA* **286**:2988–2992.

McIntosh E, Donaldson C and Ryan M (1999). Recent advances in the methods of cost–benefit analysis in health-care. Matching the art to the science. *PharmacoEconomics* **15**:357–367.

Sculpher M (2000). Evaluating the cost-effectiveness of interventions designed to increase the utilization of evidence-based guidelines. *Fam Pract.* **17**(Suppl. 1):S26–S31.

Severens JL (2003). Value for money of changing healthcare services? Economic evaluation of quality improvement. *Qual Saf Health Care* **12**:366–371.

References

Black NA (1996). Why we need observational studies to evaluate the effectiveness of health care. *BMJ* **312**:1215–1218.

Brennan A and Akehurst R (1999). Modelling in economic evaluation: What is it place?; What is its value? *PharmacoEconomics* **17**(5):445–459.

Briggs AH, Sculpher M and Buxton MJ (1994). Uncertainty in the economic evaluation of health care technologies: The role of sensitivity analysis. *Health Econ.* **3**:95–104.

Buxton MJ, Drummond MF, Van Hout BA, *et al.* (1997). Modelling in economic evaluation: An unavoidable fact of life. *Health Econ.* **6**:217–227.

Doubilet PM, Weinstein MC and McNeil BJ (1986). Use and misuse of the term 'cost effective' in medicine. *N Engl J Med.* **314**(4):253–255.

Drummond MF, O'Brien BJ, Stoddart GL and Torrance GW (1997). *Methods for the Economic Evaluation of Health Care Programmes*, Second Edition. Oxford: Oxford Medical Publications.

Frijling BD, Spies TH, Lobo CM, Hulscher MEJL, van Drenth BB and Braspenning JCC (2001). Blood pressure control in treated hypertensive patients: Clinical performance of general practitioners. *Br J Gen Pract.* **51**:9–14.

Gold MR, Siegel JE, Russell LB and Weinstein MC (1996). *Cost-Effectiveness in Health and Medicine.* New York: Oxford University Press.

Grimshaw GM and Russell IT (1993). Effect of clinical guidelines on medical practice: A systematic review of rigorous evaluations. *Lancet* **342**:1317–1322.

Grimshaw GM, Thomas RE, MacLennan G, *et al.* (2004). Effectiveness and efficiency of guideline dissemination and implementation strategies. *Health Technol Assess.* **8**(6):1–84.

Kaner EFS, Lock CA, McAvoy BR, Heather N and Gilvarry E (1999). A RCT of three training and support strategies to encourage implementation of screening and brief alcohol intervention by general practitioners. *Br J Gen Pract.* **49**:699–703.

Lobo CM, Euser L, Kamp J, *et al.* (2003). Process evaluation of a multifaceted intervention to improve cardiovascular disease prevention in general practice. *Eur J Gen Pract.* **9**:77–83.

Mason J, Freemantle N, Nazareth I, Eccles M, Haines A and Drummond MF (2001). When is it cost-effective to change the behaviour of health professionals? *JAMA* **286**:2988–2992.

Mauskopf JA, Paul JE, Grant DM and Stergachis A (1998). The role of cost–consequence analysis in health care decision making. *PharmacoEconomics* **13**:277–288.

McIntosh E, Donaldson C and Ryan M (1999). Recent advances in the methods of cost–benefit analysis in health-care. Matching the art to the science. *PharmacoEconomics* **15**:357–367.

O'Brien BJ (1996). Economic evaluation of pharmaceuticals: Frankenstein's monster or vampire of trails? *Med Care* **34**(Suppl.):DS99–DS108.

Oostenbrink JB, Koopmanschap MA and Rutten FFH (2002). Standardisation of costs; the Dutch manual for costing in economic evaluations. *PharmacoEconomics* **20**:443–454.

Robinson MB, Thompson E and Black NA (1998). Why is the evaluation of the cost-effectiveness of audit so difficult? The example of thrombolysis for suspected acute myocardial infarction. *Qual Health Care* **7**:19–26.

Schermer TR, Thoonen BP, Boom Gvd, *et al.* (2002). Randomized controlled economic evaluation of asthma self-management in primary health care. *Am J Resp Crit Care Med.* **166**:1062–1072.

Sculpher M (2000). Evaluating the cost-effectiveness of interventions designed to increase the utilization of evidence-based guidelines. *Fam Pract.* **17**(Suppl. 1):S26–S31.

Severens JL (2003). Value for money of changing healthcare services? Economic evaluation of quality improvement. *Qual Saf Health Care* **12**:366–371.

Weinstein MC, O'Brien BJ, Hornberger J, *et al.* (2003). Principles of good practice of decision analytic modelling in health care evaluation: Report of the ISPOR Task Force in Good Research Practices.Modelling Studies. *Value Health* **6**:9–17.

Wensing M, van der Weijden T and Grol R (1998). Implementing guidelines and innovations in general practice: Which interventions are effective? *Br J Gen Pract.* **48**:991–997.

Winkens RAG, Ament A and Pop P (1996). Routine individual feedback on requests for diagnostic tests: An economic evaluation. *Med Decis Making* **16**(4):309–314.

Wood J and Freemantle N (1999). Choosing an appropriate unit of analysis in trials of interventions that attempt to influence practice. *J Health Serv Res Policy* **4**(1):44–48.

Epilogue

Richard Grol

Box 1 Experiences in 16 local implementation projects (Dunning *et al.* 1999)

In 16 districts in the UK projects were prepared to achieve changes in patient care, the PACE (promoting action on clinical effectiveness) project. These concerned a variety of topics such as the care for patients with cardiovascular diseases, prevention and management of stroke, management of mentally ill patients and the management of low back pain and pressure ulcers. The evaluation showed that a multifaceted approach with different implementation strategies linked to the topic, the target group and the setting could be effective. However, it also became clear that effective implementation includes hard work, good planning, flexibility, and time and money.

This book presents a large number of theories, ideas, scientific findings, best practices, methods and experiences in the field of changes in the practice of in patient care. We have tried to present these in an accessible, understandable way and guide you step-by-step through this complex area. We suppose that, from time-to-time, you have felt rehearsal and overlap of the information provided. This was a deliberate decision to ensure the main argument and messages in the book remain clear.

You must also have noticed that much in the field of the implementation of change is yet unclear. Sometimes theories and research results contradict each other. This should not result in a delay in starting with the implementation of change in practice. Good planning and preparation, a systematic approach as presented in this book, and the use of experiences and best practices from elsewhere will help a successful implementation of change in practice.

We frequently stress the time and resources required for effective implementation. This is often forgotten or underestimated. However, this should not be an obstacle to an effective improvement action. Start small in a safe environment and don't be too ambitious.

As Don Berwick, one of leaders of quality improvement, once said: "You win the Tour de France not by planning for years for the first perfect bicycle ride, but by constantly making small improvements."

References

Dunning M, Abi-Aad G, Gilbert D, *et al.* (1999). *Experience, Evidence and Everyday Practice*. London: King's Fund.

Index